GIS and Public Health

GIS and Public Health

Ellen K. Cromley
Sara L. McLafferty

THE GUILFORD PRESS
New York   London

© 2002 The Guilford Press
A Division of Guilford Publications, Inc.
72 Spring Street, New York, NY 10012
www.guilford.com

Printed in the United States of America

This book is printed on acid-free paper.

Last digit is print number: 9 8 7 6 5 4 3 2 1

Library of Congress Cataloging-in-Publication Data

Cromley, Ellen K.
   GIS and public health / Ellen K. Cromley, Sara L. McLafferty.
      p. cm.
   Includes bibliographical references (p.).
   ISBN 1-57230-707-2
   1. Geographic information systems. 2. Public health—Data
processing. I. McLafferty, Sara, 1951– II. Title.
RA566 .C764 2002
614.4′2′0285–dc21   2001054821

To Robert, Gordon, and Eddie
and
Avijit, Smita, and Priya

Contents

Acknowledgments

In the mid-1990s we found ourselves "doing" GIS and public health. We were working with public health analysts on health issues ranging from Lyme disease to breast cancer. We were supervising student research, teaching courses, and educating public health workers about GIS and public health. A community of scholars and practitioners was emerging, but there was no book to serve as a guide. We set out to fill this gap and embarked on the long journey that produced this book. From the very beginning, Peter Wissoker, former editor for geography at The Guilford Press, provided strong support and encouragement. His patience and gentle prodding were crucial for getting this work done. We also thank the reviewers, Gerard Rushton and Stephen Matthews, for their careful reading of the first draft of the manuscript and their constructive and insightful comments, and all of those at Guilford who helped us see this project to completion.

Like most good GIS applications, this book has been a collaborative effort in the best sense of the word. It also reflects what we have learned in our work over the past decade with state, local, and federal public health agencies, community groups, colleagues, and students around a wide set of issues related to GIS and public health. We are grateful to all the people we have worked with for providing opportunities "in the field" to learn from them and to use emerging geographic technologies to improve public health.

We acknowledge Andrea Boissevain of Health Risk Consultants, Inc., the Connecticut Hospital Research and Education Foundation, Garry Lapidus of the Injury Prevention Center at the Connecticut Children's Medical Center, and staff of the Connecticut Department of Public Health including Gary Archambault, Diane Aye, Matthew Cartter, MD, Marcie Cavacas, Gerald Iwan and the GIS team in the Water Supplies Section, Mary Kapp, and Richard Melchreit, and graduate students in the Department of Geography at the University of Connecticut who also participated in various research projects, including Marc Bailey, Kevin Joy, Steve McGee, Dave Merwin, Ted Milligan, Kristine Noviello, Paul O'Packi, Brian Pope, Jennifer Roberts, Christine Seidel, Xiaojing Wei, and Adam Winters. We also express our appreciation to Richard Gaulin, Planning Department, and Gene Interlandi and Roseann McCorkle, Accident Records Section, of the Connecticut Department of Transportation. Robert Cromley, Professor, and Richard Mrozinski, GIS Lab Manager, in the Department of Geography at the University of Connecticut and T. Patrick McGlamery, Map Librarian, Homer Babbidge Library, University of Connecticut, also deserve thanks.

In addition, we thank Howie Sternberg, Deborah Dumin, Diana Danenberg, Jon Scull, and Steven Fish of the Connecticut Department of Environmental Protection for their efforts to make spatial databases publicly available and for their willingness to share their considerable GIS expertise.

During the preparation of this volume, Sara McLafferty was on the faculty at Hunter College in New York City. There she was fortunate to be able to work with many colleagues in exploring health issues in the New York metropolitan region. Special thanks to Keith Clarke, Victor Goldsmith, Nick Freudenberg, and Jack Caravanos, who are or were on the faculty at Hunter College; Professor Roger Grimson of SUNY Stony Brook; the members of the West Islip Breast Cancer Coalition; Dr. Christina Hoven of Columbia University; Dr. James Childs of the Centers for Disease Control and Prevention; and Dr. Camillo Vargas and James Gibson of the New York City Department of Health. The New York City Department of Health generously gave permission to use individual-level rat bite data to prepare several figures in this book. The graduate program in geography at Hunter provided a rich environment for pushing the boundaries of GIS and public health and developing real-world applications. This book benefited greatly from the expertise and insights of a talented group of Hunter graduate students whose interests encompass GIS and health: Henry Sirotin, Barbara Tempalski, Cheryl Weisner Itkin, Linda Timander, Brett Gilman, Delene Pratt, Steve Evans, Katy McSorley, Julie Kranick, Sonia Tatlock, Colin Reilly, Chris Hanson-Sanchez, Doug Williamson, and Sue Grady.

The highways—real and virtual—that connect Storrs and New York City became a conduit for ideas about what public health practitioners need to know about GIS and how GIS can contribute to improving public health. This book is dedicated to our families for their continued love and support. They were the ones who kept everything in perspective.

List of Figures

xvi / List of Figures

List of Tables

Introduction

Geographic information systems (GIS) are transforming the way we describe and study the earth. Throughout history, geographers have attempted to understand the surface of the earth as the living environment of human populations and the forces of change that alter the earth's environments. The environment affects our health and well-being and we, through our activities, reshape the environment. GIS provide a digital lens for exploring the dynamic connections between people, their health and well-being, and changing physical and social environments.

This book is an introduction to the use of GIS in analyzing and addressing public health problems in the United States. GIS are computer-based systems for integrating and analyzing spatial data. Our book considers how GIS can be used to map and analyze the geographical distributions of populations at risk, health outcomes, and risk factors; to explore associations between risk factors and health outcomes; and to address health problems.

The book is written for geographers, public health practitioners, epidemiologists, and community members interested in applying GIS to the study of human health problems. The main question we seek to answer for the reader is "What do I need to know about GIS for public health?" Our answer is that to use GIS to establish a geographic foundation for public health, we need to know about GIS data and systems, the methods for analyzing GIS data, and how and for whom GIS are used.

GEOGRAPHIC FOUNDATIONS FOR PUBLIC HEALTH

At its most basic level, a geographic foundation for public health looks at the question "Where?" Where do people live? Where are the agents of dis-

1

ease? Where can we intervene to eliminate risks or to improve health services delivery? People and the factors that cause disease are dispersed, often unevenly, across communities and regions. The processes that bring people into contact with disease agents are also geographically variable.

Health is not just the absence of disease, it is a state of physical, social, and emotional well-being. Because people are affected by their environments, health has the environment of the person as its geographical context. This environment is connected to natural, social, and economic processes that operate on the local, regional, and global scales. How people behave contributes to their health status, but we cannot divorce behavior from the environmental and social contexts in which it occurs. Not all of the factors that affect our well-being are under the immediate direct control of the individual. The environment of the person is one starting point for public health GIS.

Populations at Risk

GIS are being used in public health studies to model where people live and the environments they experience throughout their lives. GIS make it possible to view residential distributions in great detail (Figure I.1). Because of the economic and social processes that structure residential development, age, sex, and race–ethnicity of the population are usually not uniform throughout the region of settlement. Instead, different neighborhoods or communities often have different demographic characteristics. GIS make it possible to view these differences in detail also.

The distribution of population by residence is perhaps the most frequently considered geographical distribution in public health and epidemiology. The residence, however, is only one activity site in the environment of the person, albeit an important one. The *activity space* is the area where a person spends time (Golledge & Stimson, 1997). It is comprised of a home base or residence; other activity sites like workplaces, schools, stores, restaurants, and recreational areas that are regularly visited; and the pathways traveled to and from the home and other activity sites. The size and shape of an individual's activity space will vary depending on the activities the person is obligated or chooses to perform, the modes of transportation available, and the geographical locations where activities may take place. Individuals sharing the same home base may have very different travel and activity patterns, and as a result different activity spaces. The activity space is important because it represents the zone where the individual can be exposed to risks or resources. In addition to modeling population distribution by residence, GIS are being used to analyze travel diaries (McCormack, 1999) and represent activity spaces (Figure I.2).

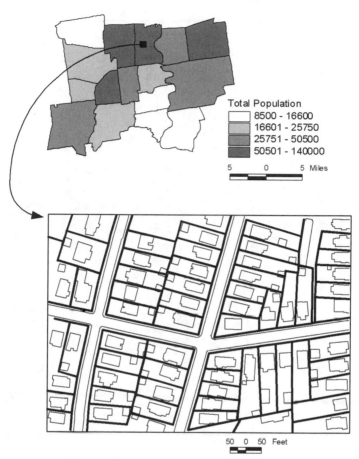

FIGURE I.1. GIS can be used to make conventional maps of population distribution but they can also display maps showing the locations of buildings where people live.

Migration is a process that results in the permanent or semipermanent relocation of the home (Golledge & Stimson, 1997). Although most people who move stay within the same community and relocate only a short distance from their previous homes, some make longer distance moves. These moves result in a complete displacement of the individual's activity space, exposing the person to a new set of risks. Furthermore, migration rates are rarely similar across all social and demographic groups. Migration complicates the study of disease when the time between exposure and onset is long.

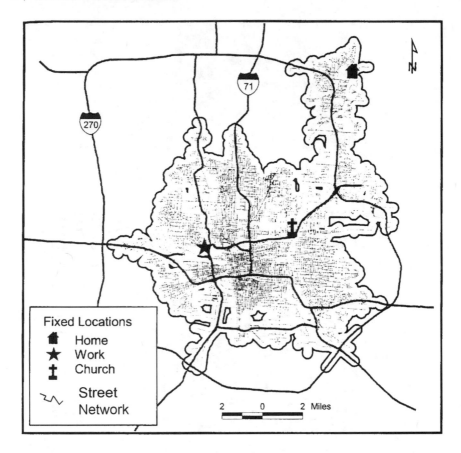

FIGURE I.2. The potential area where an individual could travel based on the person's home location, workplace, and church. From Kwan (1999). Copyright 1999 by Association of American Geographers. Reprinted by permission.

The distributions of population and changes in population due to natural increase and aging are relatively easy to model because of the availability of census and vital statistics data. Migration flows and changes in population due to migration are more difficult to study in the United States because we do not normally maintain detailed residential histories for individuals. Nevertheless, some health records contain information on place of birth and place of residence at the time the health event is registered. Detailed surveys are also conducted to re-create residential histories. These data can be used to explore differences in health outcomes in the context of migration (Greenberg & Schneider, 1992) and migration for medical care (Davis & Stapleton, 1991). In places where detailed migration data exist, the use of GIS has been proposed to improve estimation of populations at risk (Kohli et al., 1997). The use of GIS in public health enables us to describe more accurately the environment of the person and its temporal and spatial complexity.

Health Outcomes

Although the health event is the outcome of a complex process exposing human populations at risk to risk factors, many public health investigations and epidemiological studies start with outcomes. In many of the sources of data on mortality (death) and morbidity (illness), residential location at the time of death or diagnosis is reported. This makes it possible to map cases and rates and to search for clusters of health events.

Incidence and prevalence of disease vary geographically. *Incidence* is the number of new cases of the disease or health event observed within a specified period of time. *Prevalence* is the number of existing cases of disease at a particular point in time. Prevalence is related to incidence but is also influenced by the duration of the disease. A disease process that results in death shortly after onset would probably have a higher incidence than prevalence in a community. A chronic illness that was rarely fatal might have higher prevalence than incidence.

Disease mapping has made contributions to public health and epidemiology for centuries (Gilbert, 1958; Shannon, 1981). As many of the examples in this book illustrate, GIS make it easier to map large databases of health events at a high level of spatial disaggregation and to link data from surveillance systems to other information about the environment, including information on the distribution of risk factors (Figure I.3).

A common practice in mapping incidence and prevalence has been to calculate disease rates for political or administrative units like towns or census tracts, primarily because population and health outcome data are often reported for these areas. A problem with this approach is that the boundaries of these units often arbitrarily partition the underlying distribution of population or cases or both. GIS make is possible to overlay the distributions of cases and populations at risk and to display multiple views of the distribution of health outcomes.

GIS are also supporting analyses to search for disease clusters using methods that do not rely on aggregated data. Areas of high and low incidence can be identified by searching around individual cases to find areas that have high numbers of cases relative to the local population.

Risk Factors

Like populations at risk, the risk factors for disease are also not usually concentrated at a single point. Contaminants and biological agents of disease are present in our ecosystem. GIS have proven to be powerful tools for

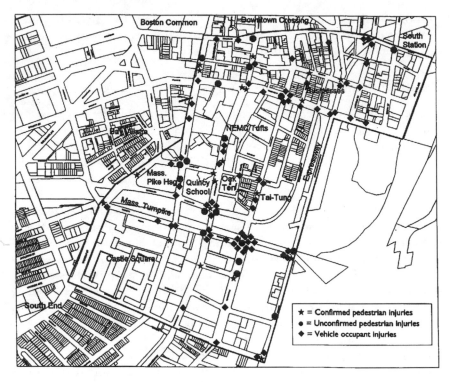

FIGURE I.3. Locations of confirmed pedestrian injuries in the context of reported total traffic injuries in a neighborhood in Boston. From Brugge, Leong, and Lai (1999). Copyright 1999 by Oxford University Press. Reprinted by permission.

modeling environmental conditions across the full ranges of geographical scales, from local to global.

Many GIS applications model temporal and spatial patterns of hazards for environmental health problems and infectious diseases (Figure I.4). These models are increasingly sophisticated and the scale and quality of the spatially referenced data they incorporate continue to improve. Public health GIS applications may model the spread of contaminants and vector and host habitats.

The ability to model the distribution of known or potential risk factors for health problems is important for public health intervention activities. GIS are being used at the community level to notify people living in neighborhoods where hazards have been identified so that they can take appropriate action to prevent health problems from occurring. While these analyses can be performed without reference to health outcomes,

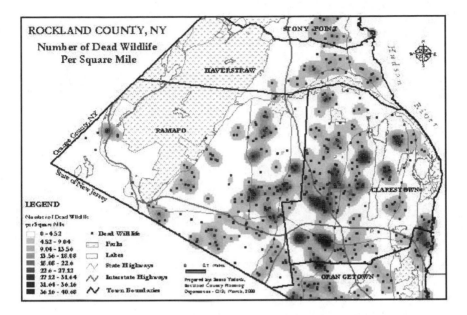

FIGURE I.4. Number of dead wildlife per square mile in Rockland County, New York, mapped as part of the surveillance effort for West Nile virus. From Rockland County Planning Department GIS (2000). Reproduced by permission of Rockland County, New York. We hold Rockland County harmless regarding the accuracy of the map.

studies of the geographical patterns of risk factors can also be used to investigate the causes of disease.

Associations between Risk Factors and Outcomes

Epidemiological studies involve comparing the incidence rate of disease observed in a study group at risk against the incidence rate of disease in a comparison group. A number of measures are used to compare the rate of disease observed in the exposed group to the rate of disease observed in the comparison group (Woodward, 1999). The *relative risk*, or *risk ratio*, is the ratio of the risk of disease among those who have the risk factor to the risk of disease for those without the risk factor (Table I.1). A second measure, the *odds ratio* is also used by epidemiologists. *Risk* measures the number of times the health event occurs relative to the total number of people in the study group. The *odds* measures the number of times the health event occurs relative to the total number of times it does not occur. The numerator of the *odds ratio* is the ratio of health events to no health events in the exposed pop-

TABLE 1.1. Associations between Risk Factors and Outcomes for Disease Incidence in a Population

| Risk factor | Disease status | | Total |
	Disease	No disease	
Exposed	a	b	$a + b$
Not exposed	c	d	$c + d$
Total	$a + c$	$b + d$	$n = a + b + c + d$

Risk = $(a + c)/(a + b + c + d)$

Exposure-specific risk for those with risk factor = $a/(a + b)$

Exposure-specific risk for those without risk factor = $c/(c + d)$

Relative risk = $\dfrac{a/(a+b)}{c/(c+d)} = \dfrac{a(c+d)}{c(a+b)}$

Odds ratio for those with risk factor compared to those without = $\dfrac{a/b}{c/d} = \dfrac{ad}{bc}$

Note. Adapted from M. Woodward. (1999). *Epidemiology: Study design and data analysis.* Boca Raton, FL: Chapman & Hall/CRC. Reproduced with permission of the publisher.

ulation. The denominator of the odds ratio is the ratio of health events to no events in the unexposed population. Standardized event ratios like the *standardized mortality ratio* and the *standardized incidence ratio* are statistics frequently used for comparing mortality or incidence observed in exposed persons to mortality or incidence previously observed in a standard population (Fleiss, 1981; Selvin, 1991; Kelsey, Whittemore, Evans, & Thompson, 1996).

Although these measures are well established in epidemiological research, it is not always easy to determine meaningful numerators and denominators to calculate them. GIS are making it possible to explore some of the most important methodological issues in applying these measures to identify significant patterns of disease. Epidemiological surveys and case–control studies involve drawing samples from the population. Assumptions are made about the probabilities of inclusion in the sample. Because populations or population subgroups are not distributed evenly across communities, a random sample of all people with the demographic and health characteristics of interest will not be a random sample of all places (Goodchild, 1984). GIS can provide the means for exploring distributions of populations and health events to develop spatially stratified sampling techniques.

In order to obtain enough cases to ensure statistical power, analysts sometimes increase the size of the study population, usually by increasing the geographical area of analysis. This approach can be misleading when the underlying geography of risk factors, exposure, and health outcomes are ignored. Enlarging the study area introduces other geographical differences besides the health outcome in question, such that it becomes difficult to tell whether there is an inherent difference between groups or between areas.

These problems are exacerbated by controlling for confounding factors through techniques like age standardization. A *confounding factor* is a variable that is causally related to the health problem under study or is a proxy for an unknown causal variable but is not a consequence of the exposure of interest. Age is a confounding factor commonly controlled for in epidemiological studies because "age almost always strongly influences disease risk" (Selvin, 1991, p. 29). To compare disease incidence rates for two groups—for example, white women and African American women living in a region—age-standardized rates would be calculated to adjust for differences in age between the two groups. As noted, the argument for this is that, since disease risk is higher in particular age groups, we would expect more cases of disease in a population that contains more people in those age groups.

However, if the cause of the disease is believed to be environmental, then we would expect disease risk to be higher in those geographical areas where environmental risk is higher. This would be particularly important in comparing rates for white and African American women if white and African American women of the same age were residentially concentrated in different areas within the larger community. Such areas would likely be associated with different levels of exposure to disease risk factors that are unevenly distributed in the environment.

An important criticism of adjustment of rates is "that if the specific rates vary in different ways across the various strata, then no single method of standardization will indicate that these differences exist. Standardization will, on the contrary, tend to mask these differences" (Fleiss, 1981, p. 239). An empirical study of age-specific death rates for males in the United States revealed that, up to age 40, rates in metropolitan counties were lower than rates in nonmetropolitan counties (Kitagawa, 1966). After age 40, the reverse was true. A single, summary comparison would fail to reveal this geographical pattern.

The spatial data-handling capabilities of GIS make it possible to identify exposed and unexposed groups and to explore geographic variations in health outcomes between those groups. Better identification of the numerators and denominators in these epidemiological measures supports the development of more meaningful comparisons of health outcomes across groups *and* areas.

Health Interventions

The geography of health services has been called "the *sine qua non* of medical geography" (Hunter, 1974, p. 16). Setting aside the fact that health services utilization is one of the main, if biased, sources of information we have about health and morbidity in the population, what is the point of studying patterns of environmental contamination or uncovering the causes of disease if we are not willing to go the next step to intervene or to support the education, enforcement, environmental modification, and medical care intervention efforts of those committed to advancing human health? As long as our activities occur in time and space, knowing how patterns of health, disease, and health services characterize regions will be essential to this effort.

GIS are reviving interest in the location of medical care services and are used by many medical care providers to evaluate spatial patterns in service utilization and the geographic structure of delivery systems (Villalon, 1999). The role of GIS in health services delivery and planning, however, is potentially much broader. A geographic foundation for public health also means considering the locational impacts of health policy. During the debate over health care reform at the national level in the 1990s, managed competition was offered as a policy for reorganizing medical care delivery. In "The Demographic Limitations of Managed Competition" (Kronick, Goodman, Wennberg, & Wagner, 1993), some very straightforward concepts of economic geography were used to answer a simple question: Where are the places in the United States where managed competition as a market-driven approach to health care reform can work? Estimates of the minimum population required to support several independent competing provider groups were based on the extent to which the competing groups were independent, the number of organizations needed to provide competition, the threshold populations for services, and the geographic boundaries of health service markets. The results indicated that reform of the U.S. health care system by managed competition would be feasible only in major metropolitan areas (Figure I.5). More than one-third of the population lived in places where managed competition could not be supported.

This illustrates the tensions between top-down versus bottom-up approaches to public health. In a top-down approach, priorities are identified at the national or state level based on aggregated data. Because of geographical variations in health problems or access to care, problems that are important at the state level may not be equally present in every community, and health care interventions that might work in some places may not work equally well in others. GIS are providing citizens at the local level with information to identify health problems of local concern, even if these are not the highest priority on a state or national level, and to advocate for public health policies. And they are creating an opportunity for policymakers at the national level to view and analyze health problems and policies in their full complexity.

When we use GIS to understand patterns of ill health and to plan public health interventions, our efforts are rooted in place and space. Ge-

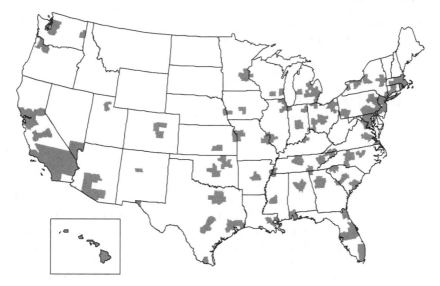

FIGURE I.5. Health markets with populations greater than or equal to the threshold needed to support managed competition. From Kronick, Goodman, Wennberg, and Wagner (1993). Copyright 1993 Massachusetts Medical Society. All rights reserved.

ographers have written about the concepts of space and place as overarching themes in the geography of health (Kearns, 1993). *Space* refers to position or location. It describes the geographical distributions of constraints and opportunities that influence and result from human activities and interactions. In contrast, *place* is a relational concept that addresses the human meanings and experiences associated with particular locations. Social relations and the physical sites of everyday life are intertwined in the concept of place.

By definition, GIS are concerned with space. The geographical coordinates that link diverse data layers together in a GIS identify location in space. However, GIS are also rooted in place. Each is used in a particular context that is a composite of social, political, and historical conditions and trends. When people use a GIS, their "sense of place" defines what questions to ask and molds their interpretation of results. While our book emphasizes the spatial dimensions of GIS in public health, these cannot be divorced from the place contexts in which GIS are used.

The geographic foundations for public health we have briefly summarized here are receiving more attention through the application of GIS technology in public health. People adopting GIS technology for public health need to understand GIS materials, GIS methods, and the institutional context of GIS in public health practice, which affects the kind and quality of GIS data available. Our book is organized to foster this understanding.

ORGANIZATION AND SCOPE

The first section of the book focuses on GIS materials, including spatial databases and the generic hardware and software needed to manage them. It also introduces PUBLIC HEALTH GIS, a geographic information system designed especially for this book. Many of the figures illustrating key points in the book were prepared from analyses of data from the PUBLIC HEALTH GIS. Chapter 1 provides an overview of geographic information systems, their development, and their main functions. Chapters 2 and 3 describe important attributes of geographic databases and the foundation and other databases most commonly used in public health GIS.

The emphasis on geographic data is necessary. Many public health analysts maintain or use large databases of health events or health services. Most of these databases have some geographical information like a street address, a town name, or a county. Often, however, these databases are not structured in a way that makes it possible to map and analyze geographical relationships. GIS incorporate the foundation databases that make the mapping of health events and health services possible.

GIS implementation requires data. Adopting GIS for public health analysis therefore requires a commitment to acquiring, managing, and maintaining large *spatial* databases in digital form. Technological advances in computing and the growth of the Internet have made foundation databases more accessible to public health organizations, provided they are willing to acquire the hardware and software necessary to develop applications or to access them over the Internet.

The second section of the book considers GIS methods for mapping and analyzing spatial data on population, health events, risk factors, and health services. Chapter 4 provides an overview of the mapping process, the different approaches available for mapping and querying health data, and the impact of developments in computer-assisted and web-based cartography on the kinds of maps that are being developed and published. Chapter 5 reviews the range of methods available for identifying areas of high and low incidence of disease, including spatial clustering methods. The uses of GIS in analyzing risk factors and health outcomes for environmental health problems, communicable disease, and vector-borne disease are discussed in Chapters 6 through 8.

GIS implementation implies a commitment to spatial analysis methods as part of the research approach. Such methods may not always be emphasized in traditional public health curricula or research. Our book provides an introduction to a range of techniques used in spatial data analysis and points the reader to more detailed discussions of these techniques. Some of the studies we cite as examples use GIS in ways that can be criticized, often as a result of data limitations, but they have been included because they contribute to our understanding of GIS and public health in other ways.

The final section of the book deals with the institutional context of public health GIS, particularly as it affects public health policy and intervention efforts. Chapters 9 and 10 discuss how GIS are used to evaluate accessibility to health services and the geographical aspects of health care delivery. Chapter 11 looks at the main settings where public health GIS applications are being developed, including community-based GIS, and considers how these institutional contexts affect the availability and use of data for public health GIS and where public health GIS may be headed.

Although GIS are being used to study public health issues around the world, our book focuses on the United States. In part, this is because the United States is the place we know best from life experience and from our own research. There are other reasons why the United States is an appropriate geographical focus for this book. For place-based studies of health, the United States offers a wide range of natural and built environments. The population is also diverse and experiences the full range of health conditions. The widespread public availability in the United States of digital spatial databases creates a foundation for GIS-based analyses of health problems that does not exist in many other countries.

Although the federal government has played a major role in developing these foundation databases and others of relevance to public health GIS, state and local governments have the main responsibility for health surveillance, public health intervention, and licensing and regulation of health providers and health services. As a result, public health GIS applications based in any region of the country are highly dependent for their success on the level of development of health and other GIS databases and systems in that region and on state and local policies governing use and distribution of data. This is an important reason why our book does not attempt to tell readers how to use a particular GIS software package with their own data.

GIS AND PUBLIC HEALTH

Everything that occurs on the earth that can be spatially referenced can be represented in a GIS. That is, we can use GIS to make maps of almost anything. Because of their visual power, GIS maps can become metaphors for the social and environmental conditions that are "contained" in geographic space. We are often tempted to look for spatial solutions to problems that arise from these conditions. Although health problems have a spatial dimension and many can be addressed by changing locational relationships, by closing down a polluting manufacturing plant or opening a clinic, GIS may not be an aid to analysis for other problems.

The role of GIS in public health is potentially great. As computer technology continues to transform our ability to gather, analyze, and map health data, new roles for GIS in public health may emerge. GIS, as a means for exploring health problems and finding ways to address them, will take its place in the conceptual and methodological foundations of public health.

CHAPTER 1

Geographic Information Systems

Geographic information systems (GIS) are computer-based systems for the integration and analysis of geographic data. *Geographic data* are spatial data that "result from observation and measurement of earth phenomena" referenced to their locations on the earth's surface (Tomlinson, 1987, p. 203). Whenever public health professionals or epidemiologists use disease registries with address information, consider the locations of toxic waste disposal sites, or look at air quality and water quality reports from monitoring stations, they are working with geographic data.

This chapter considers GIS as an "enabling" technology, applicable to the integration and analysis of many different types of spatial data—not just health data—by people in different organizational settings asking very different questions. One of the most striking features of GIS is their broad applicability. The first two sections of this chapter offer a definition of GIS and describe the major functions of GIS software: spatial database management, visualization and mapping, and spatial analysis, including the emerging role of GIS in distributing spatial data and GIS applications over the Internet. The last sections of the chapter trace the development of GIS applications in public health.

DEFINITIONS OF GIS

In part because GIS is an enabling technology, a consensus definition of GIS has been difficult to achieve. The acronym has several usages: "as a technology, as a research field, and as a community" (Goodchild, 1995b, p. 35). As a technology, GIS rely heavily on computer hardware and peripheral equipment like scanners, digitizing tablets, plotters, and printers that may not be part of the hardware configurations available to a public health analyst. The definition of GIS as "computer-assisted systems for the capture, storage, retrieval, analysis, and display of spatial data" (Clarke, 1986, p. 175) might lead one to assume that the acronym "is simply a catch-all for almost any type of automated geographic data processing" (Cowen, 1988, p. 1551). In fact, GIS are part of a larger constellation of computer technologies for processing geographic data.

Some of these technologies, like the *global positioning system* (GPS) and *remote sensing*, are used to collect geographic data. The GPS developed by the Defense Department in the United States relies on a series of 24 satellites in orbit and a network of satellite sensors or tracking devices located on the earth's surface. Portable receivers capture signals from the satellites and calculate very accurate surface positions from the measurement of satellite positions.

Remote sensing is the analysis and interpretation of data gathered by means that do not require direct contact with the earth. *Aerial photography* of the earth's surface, taken with an aircraft-mounted camera, is an important source of up-to-date data (Jensen, 2000). Aerial photographs can be scanned and rectified for printing or viewing on a display screen, as described in Chapter 3. In addition to aircraft, satellites also serve as platforms for devices that capture information about the earth's surface. *Digital image processing* for geographic data collection involves the use of satellites with sensors capable of detecting electromagnetic energy reflected off or emitted from objects on the earth's surface (Jensen, 1996). The data are then enhanced for viewing and analysis.

Computer technology also plays a part in the collection of secondary geographic data from existing maps. *Scanning* is a technique for capturing map data in digital form. Scanners use an optical laser or other electronic device to "read" a map and convert its features to a computer database of dark and light values. *Digitizing* requires use of a tablet and cursor to record coordinate locations of map features from a map placed on the digitizing tablet. It is also possible to construct a GIS data layer by screen digitizing, in which a cursor is used to record coordinate locations from a digital database or image file displayed on the monitor.

Remote sensing, GPS, scanning, and digitizing are the main methods for spatial data collection. One or more of these methods may be used, either by the person using the GIS or by the government organization or commercial vendor from whom a spatial database is purchased. The nature of spatial data and important issues related to scale, resolution, accuracy, storage, and retrieval of health and health-related data that must be considered at the data capture stage are discussed at length in Chapter 2.

Once spatial data exist in digital form, computer graphics software supports the creation of cartographic displays. *Computer-aided design*

(CAD) systems, as used with cartographic data, provide support for drafting features of interest like roads or land parcels. As they originally developed, CAD systems did not link these features to databases describing the features' attributes, so it was difficult to produce thematic or statistical maps using a CAD system. But developments in computer cartography have created systems for linking geographical and attribute databases to produce statistical maps. In computer mapping software systems, the ability to manipulate the geographical data—the location information—is usually quite limited.

The boundaries separating GIS from these other technologies are not rigid—in part because the technologies continue to evolve. Remote sensing, CAD, and the rest are valuable technologies that are related to GIS. But they are not, in and of themselves, considered GIS. Most efforts to define GIS as a technology emphasize the special nature of GIS software and the data structures on which the software is built.

These data structures and software functions are specifically designed to integrate and analyze data based on location. Spatial data representation and spatial analyses like map overlay have been developed without the use of computer-based systems like GIS (Poiker, 1985). People thinking about using GIS who are not familiar with basic geographic and cartographic concepts and techniques can benefit greatly from learning these concepts before and as they become GIS users. The data and modeling requirements of most GIS research applications, however, necessitate the use of computers.

We define GIS, as a technology, as computer-based systems for integrating and analyzing geographic data. The data structure of a GIS software system is not organized like a spreadsheet. Instead, the locations of features on the earth's surface are stored so that neighborhood relationships among features can be analyzed and so that groups of different features sharing the same locations can be identified (Figure 1.1). The following software functions distinguish GIS as a technology (Goodchild, 1995b):

- The ability to store or compute and display spatial relationships between objects (e.g., the house is adjacent to the toxic waste site, the school is connected to the water supply system).
- The ability to store many attributes of objects.
- The ability to analyze spatial and attribute data in addition to simply managing and retrieving data.
- The ability to integrate spatial data from different sources.

"The great interest in GIS would appear to reside in its technical basis for implementing integration methodologies" (Cowen, 1988, p. 1554). This interest is reflected in the wide range of GIS functions.

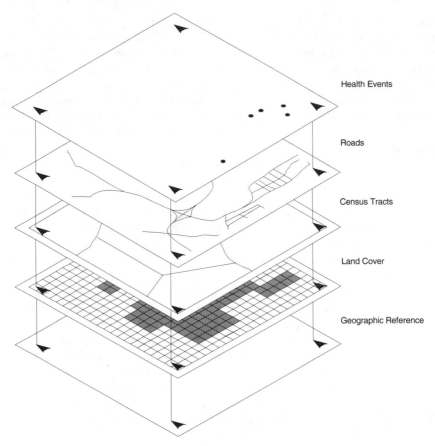

Health Events

Roads

Census Tracts

Land Cover

Geographic Reference

FIGURE 1.1. Digital geographic databases registered to a common geographic reference system. A composite of two or more layers can be produced because the geographic references match.

GIS FUNCTIONS

What are the main functions of GIS software? Some very detailed lists of integrated software functions that should be present in a GIS to support input, analysis, and output of data have been offered (Tomlinson & Boyle, 1981; Dangermond, 1984). The applications selected for discussion in this book were intended to illustrate how some of the most important generic GIS functions can be used to support public health research and policy analysis. The "toolbox approach" to defining GIS as a set of software functions is useful for comparing the hundreds of software packages on the market, but it says little about the software functions in relation to the spatial data they process (Cowen, 1988).

The approach taken here classifies GIS functions in user terms, that is, based on what people want to do with spatial data. Three broad categories emerge: spatial database management, visualization and mapping, and spatial analysis. As noted earlier, health analysts need and want to manage spatial databases. This includes creating databases of health events located on the earth's surface that can be processed and stored by computers, keeping track of changes by adding and deleting events from those databases, and editing the location and public health attributes of these events. Public health professionals and epidemiologists also want to visualize and map the spatial data they have acquired. This includes exploring visual representations of the patterns of health outcomes and risk factors and communicating information in the data to others in the form of maps. Equally important, public health researchers want to analyze the spatial relationships among the health events stored in the databases and to create new classes of health patterns based on those relationships. The development of the Internet has made it possible for some of these GIS functions to be supported in a network environment.

Spatial Database Management

One important function of GIS is managing spatial data. Identifying sources of, collecting, and preprocessing the spatial and health attribute data that would be managed in public health GIS are discussed in detail in Chapter 3. *Database management systems* (DBMS) are used to store, retrieve, and manipulate data in a database. A GIS software product, like other computer software systems, is built on an underlying data model. A data model is a detailed model that captures the overall structure of the data, independent of database management or implementation considerations (McFadden & Hoffer, 1994). A data model includes the relevant entities, relationships, and attributes, as well as constraints defining how the data are used. In the 1980s, a large body of research on the science of GIS explored the nature of spatial data models (Peuquet, 1984; Goodchild, 1992).

Spatial data embody complex and often hierarchical relationships that are not easily expressed in tables (Yearsley, Worboys, Story, Jayawardena, & Bofakos, 1994). As a result, GIS software packages are different from simple spreadsheets. Although a number of DBMS have been the basis for GIS software development, relational database designs were dominant by the early 1990s (Healey, 1991). *Relational database management models* organize data in the form of tables ("relations") where the rows represent units of analysis or objects of interest and the columns represent attributes (McFadden & Hoffer, 1994). Relational database management systems manage data as a collection of tables with data relationships represented by common values in related tables. In public health applications, the tables might includes individuals diagnosed with a particular type of health problem and listed in a disease registry, public drinking water lines, or hazardous waste sites (Figure 1.2). The associated attributes may be quantitative or qualitative, numeric or alphanumeric, and reported as nominal, ordinal, or interval/ratio data.

The geographic objects whose attributes might be described in a table can also be assigned spatial dimensions or topological properties (Laurini & Thompson, 1992). Objects represented as *points*, like public drinking water well locations, are 0-dimensional, that is, they have specific locations but no sizes. *Lines*—sometimes called arcs—are 1-dimensional objects, like the route of an emergency medical response vehicle; they have lengths but no specified widths. *Areas*—also called polygons—are 2-dimensional objects enclosing a space, like health planning districts. Some GIS are also capable of representing volumes, 3-dimensional objects. In a spatial database, the objects in the database have locations tying them as points, lines, or areas to the earth's surface (Figure 1.3). Thematic attributes, like reservoir yield or distribution line date of completion, are also stored and can be retrieved and analyzed.

In a relational database, data in different tables can be linked by matching values in a column in one table to values in another table until the data of interest have been retrieved from all tables (Worboys, 1995).

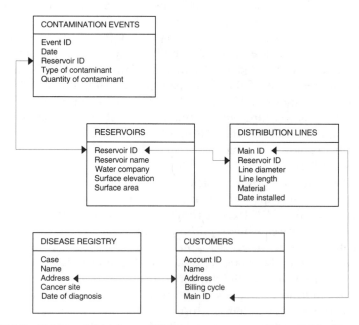

FIGURE 1.2. Tables of data from different sources containing fields that could be linked in a relational database to describe health outcomes associated with contamination events.

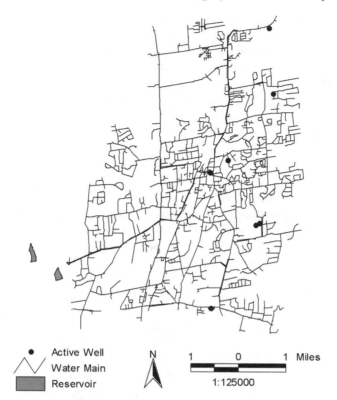

Active Well
Water Main
Reservoir

N

1   0   1 Miles

1:125000

FIGURE 1.3. Three spatial databases used to model a public drinking water system. Active wells are modeled as points. Water mains are modeled as lines. Reservoirs are modeled as areas. Produced by permission of the Connecticut Department of Public Health.

These relationships can be one to one, one to many, many to one, or many to many. One-to-one relationships occur when a record in one table links to exactly one record in another table. For example, one private well serves only one private residence and each such residence is served by only one private well. This kind of relationship is simple but rare. One-to-many and many-to-one relationships are more common. One water company serves many customers and vice versa. These relationships are relatively easy to model in relational databases.

Most spatial relationships are many to many. One point on the earth's surface can be enclosed in an infinite number of areas and those areas contain many points. Because spatial databases are so large, it is necessary to retrieve many rows of data in a matter of seconds for cartographic display of objects on the screen. To address problems with the relational model encountered to date, two approaches to GIS database management have been implemented.

The *"hybrid" model* (Healy, 1991) separates storage of the location information or digital cartographic data (the points, lines, and areas) from the storage of the attribute information. The attribute information is stored in a commercial relational DBMS, but the digital cartographic data are stored in direct access operating system files that speed input and output. The GIS software links the two during processing. Initially, GIS using this model relied on a single DBMS, but software producers are now moving to support multiple DBMS.

In the *"integrated" data model* (Healy, 1991), the GIS software processes queries of the database. The tables contain map coordinate data for points and lines and topological or neighborhood information identifying how these points and lines are connected. The attribute data can be stored with the coordinate data or in separate tables. The storage of location information in individual rows of the database slowed retrieval and processing in the early stages of GIS development, so most commercial GIS software opted for the hybrid model. The integrated data model, however, is receiving renewed attention as a model that facilitates the use of Structured Query Language (SQL) and object-oriented methods (Worboys, 1999).

The generic spatial database management functions of GIS currently in use include functions to create and maintain spatial databases. These functions enable users to add and delete records from databases, to edit information, to join databases, and to perform other functions familiar to most users of computer DBMS. The spatial database management functions of the GIS allow users to view and manipulate data in table format (Table 1.1).

This view of the data is useful for editing and for looking up information in a particular record. For example, a health researcher might need to edit information on a particular public drinking water main by modifying a field in a table (Table 1.1) to show whether the main was constructed before or after a particular year. The tabular view is not as useful for exploring the relationships among units of observation—for example, examining the spatial pattern of mains constructed before or after a particular year to identify patterns of water service at the time of a contamination event occurring at a particular location (Figure 1.4).

Visualization and Mapping

Once the spatial database has been created and can be retrieved, the graphical display and mapping functions of GIS come particularly into play. Visualization as a form of human cognition—"making things 'visible in the mind' " (Wood, 1994)—has been considered a key to many important scientific advances. Components of this process include visual exploration and confirmation of data ("visual thinking") and synthesis and presenta-

TABLE 1.1. Attributes of Public Drinking Water Mains

Main ID	Length (ft.)	Diam. (in.)	Date	Material
1	1097.51	12.00	Pre-1968	TR
2	2146.09	12.00	Post-1968	TR
3	1916.36	6.00	Pre-1968	DT
4	627.76	8.00	Pre-1968	DT
5	1913.46	6.00	Pre-1968	TR
6	538.11	12.00	Pre-1968	N-L
7	735.26	12.00	Pre-1968	N-L
8	554.65	12.00	Pre-1968	N-L
9	83.64	12.00	Pre-1968	N-L
10	47.63	12.00	Post-1968	N-L
.	.	.	.	.
.	.	.	.	.
1715	710.64	8.00	Pre-1968	TYT

tion of information ("visual communication") (MacEachren, Buttenfield, Campbell, DiBiase, & Monmonier, 1992).

Today's statistical graphics have their origins in the products of the late 16th century prepared as aids to abstraction in the research process (Tufte, 1983; Buttenfield & Mackaness, 1991). Like maps, other graphics were initially prepared and printed manually, with the data both stored and displayed in the printed product. The development of computers and computer graphics has made it possible to separate storage from display of large quantities of data. Computers have also made possible innovative cartographic and other kinds of displays that would be difficult or impossible to render by hand, including three-dimensional representations, animations, and scene generations. The development of GIS has coincided with an increased interest in scientific visualization in general, a major topic in computing since the National Science Foundation report on *Visualization in Scientific Computing* was published in 1987 (McCormick, DeFanti, & Brown, 1987). The links between the visualization functions of GIS and scientific visualization in general are an emerging area of interest (Hearnshaw & Unwin, 1994).

Graphs are increasingly recognized as essential to good statistical analysis, whether the analysis is spatial or not. This point is illustrated for attribute data by four fictitious data sets, each consisting of the same number of (x,y) pairs, presented in tables, statistics, and graphs (Table 1.2). Although statistical analysis of the four data sets yields the same standard

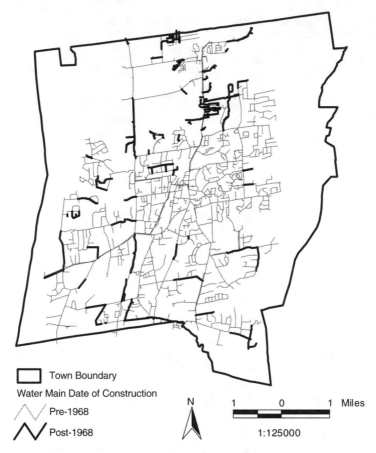

FIGURE 1.4. Mapping data on dates of water main construction to aid visualization. Produced by permission of the Connecticut Department of Public Health.

output (ignoring residuals), the graphs highlight the differences among the data (Figure 1.5). Admittedly, three of the small data sets were designed to represent a particular effect in an extreme form. But the illustration is still effective in demonstrating the different kinds of information that can be extracted from tables, statistics, and graphs, even though they represent the same data.

Similar illustrations highlight the importance of cartographic representation for statistical analysis. In this case, two pairs of attribute variables (X_1, Y_1) and (X_2, Y_2) having identical scatterplots and correlation coefficients exhibit distinctly different map patterns, even when the data are mapped using the same class breaks (Figure 1.6). The statistical correlations are the same but the geographical correlations are quite differ-

TABLE 1.2. Four Data Sets Each Comprising 11 (x, y) Pairs

Case ID	#1 X	#1 Y	#2 X	#2 Y	#3 X	#3 Y	#4 X	#4 Y
1	10.0	8.4	10.0	9.1	10.0	7.5	8.0	6.6
2	8.0	7.0	8.0	8.1	8.0	6.8	8.0	5.8
3	13.0	7.6	13.0	8.7	13.0	12.7	8.0	7.7
4	9.0	8.8	9.0	8.8	9.0	7.1	8.0	8.8
5	11.0	8.3	11.0	9.3	11.0	7.8	8.0	8.5
6	14.0	10.0	14.0	8.1	14.0	8.8	8.0	7.0
7	6.0	7.2	6.0	6.1	6.0	6.1	8.0	5.3
8	4.0	4.3	4.0	3.1	4.0	3.1	19.0	12.5
9	12.0	10.8	12.0	9.1	12.0	5.4	8.0	5.6
10	7.0	4.8	7.0	7.3	7.0	8.2	8.0	7.9
11	5.0	5.7	5.0	4.8	5.0	6.4	8.0	6.9

Number of observations = 11	Sum of squares = 110.0
Mean of X = 9.0	Regression sum of squares = 27.50
Mean of Y = 7.5	Residual sum of squares = 13.75
Regression coefficient of Y on X = 0.5	Standard error of b = 0.118
Equation of regression line $Y = 3 + 0.5X$	R-squared = 0.667

Note. Adapted from Anscombe (1973). Reprinted with permission from *The American Statistician.* Copyright 1973 by the American Statistical Association. All rights reserved.

ent. The maps for X_1 and Y_1 do not depict identical geographical distributions for the two variables, but they do point to an underlying geographic factor like proximity to a pollution source. Understanding the spatial distributions of X and Y is important for designing valid spatial sampling and spatial analysis strategies. These spatial distributions are not easy to see or likely to be revealed in tabular or statistical displays of the data.

The importance of the visualization and mapping functions of a GIS must be understood in context. Throughout the development of computer-assisted cartography, cartographic research has investigated how traditional map representations can be accomplished in an automated environment (Buttenfield & Mackaness, 1991; Kraak, 1999). Cartographers have criticized GIS software companies for "a lack of attention" to principles of graphical design and for failing to adopt graphical defaults based on perception research. These problems affect visual communication through other types of graphics too (Tukey, 1977; Tufte, 1983).

Setting aside issues related to the quality of the visual display, overreliance on visualization poses its own problems. "While the spatial perspective can be very powerful as a source of insight, it can also be

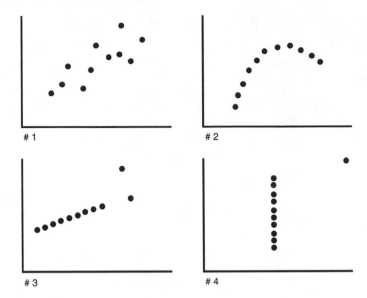

FIGURE 1.5. Scatterplots corresponding to the four data sets in Table 1.2. Adapted from Anscombe (1973). Adapted with permission from *The American Statistician.* Copyright 1973 by the American Statistical Association. All rights reserved.

highly misleading" (Goodchild et al., 1992, p. 409). Perceptions are context-dependent and change with experience. Some mechanism must be present for checking our perceptions and intuitions against other subjective and objective criteria. For example, the problems inherent in detecting and explaining meaningful spatial clusters of disease illustrate the ten-

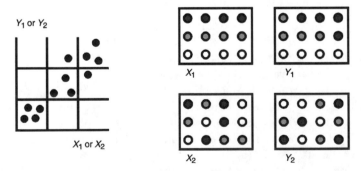

FIGURE 1.6. Two pairs of variables (X_1, Y_1 and X_2, Y_2) for 12 cases have identical scatterplots but very different spatial arrangements even when mapped using the same class breaks. Adapted from Monmonier (1996). Copyright 1996 by University of Chicago Press. Adapted by permission.

sions between visualization and analysis. A GIS offering only spatial database management and visualization capabilities would be incomplete. Despite these limitations, generic GIS visualization and mapping functions enable users to see the spatial relationships present in large and complex databases and to report the results of an analysis in cartographic and other graphic displays. Furthermore, GIS allows users to display available spatial databases quickly, easily, and interactively. These functions have provided spatial data analysts with a powerful mechanism for exploring spatial data.

Spatial Analysis

GIS software systems enable public health analysts to do more than simply manage and map data. GIS supports a range of spatial analysis functions. *Spatial analysis* refers to "a general ability to manipulate spatial data into different forms and extract additional meaning as a result" (Bailey, 1994, p. 15). Specifically, spatial analysis comprises a body of techniques "requiring access to both the locations and the attributes of objects" (Goodchild et al., 1992, p. 409). The results of a spatial analysis are "not invariant" when locations of the objects being analyzed are changed. As such, spatial analysis covers a broad range of numerical methods.

The spatial analysis functions of GIS fall into five classes: measurement, topological analysis, network analysis, surface analysis, and statistical analysis (Table 1.3). The *measurement* functions of GIS allow the user to calculate straight-line distances between points, distances along curved paths or arcs, and areas. Although the measurement functions are relatively few in number, they are extremely important. Distance as a measure of separation in space is a key variable used in many other kinds of spatial analysis. Distance is often an important factor in interactions between people and places.

Topological analysis functions include all the software functions used to describe and analyze the spatial relationships among units of observation. Most GIS can create buffers around points, lines, and areas, depicting all of the area within a user-specified distance of the objects. This category also includes spatial database overlay and assessment of spatial relationships across databases, including map comparison analysis. The public health analyst could identify the area within a specified distance of a public drinking water well or surface source, for example, and overlay the footprint of a proposed building to determine whether or not the building would be located far enough from the water source to meet legal requirements (Figure 1.7).

Network analysis is a branch of spatial analysis that investigates flows through a network. The network is modeled as a set of nodes and the links that connect the nodes. Once a network has been defined, it is possible to analyze the network and flows through it. These analytical models

TABLE 1.3. Spatial Analysis Functions of GIS

Function Class	Function	Chapters in which examples found
Measurement	Distance Length Perimeter Area Centroid Volume Shape Slope Aspect Measurement scale conversions	Chapters 5, 9
Topological Analysis	Adjacency Buffering Polygon overlay Point-in-polygon Line-in-polygon Dissolve Merge	Chapters 4, 5, 6, 8
Network Analysis	Connectivity Shortest path Routing Location-allocation	Chapter 10
Surface Analysis	Filtering Line of sight Viewsheds Contours Watersheds	
Statistical Analysis	Nearest neighbor Spatial autocorrelation Spatial interpolation Trend surface	Chapters 5, 6, 7

would be used, for example, to determine the shortest path through a street network for an emergency medical response (Figure 1.8).

Surface analysis techniques are often used to analyze terrain or other data that represent a continuous surface. Filtering techniques include smoothing and edge enhancement. Smoothing removes "noise" from the data to reveal the broader trends. Edge enhancement accentuates contrast and aids in identifying linear features like highways or fault lines. Line-of-sight analysis, viewshed, and watershed analyses apply to digital elevation models. Public health analysts who need to model environmental conditions related to terrain would make the greatest use of these GIS functions.

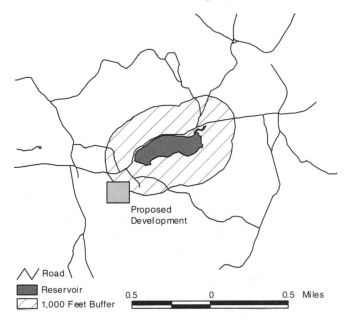

FIGURE 1.7. Buffering a polygon representing a public drinking water reservoir to show the area within 1,000 feet of the reservoir shoreline.

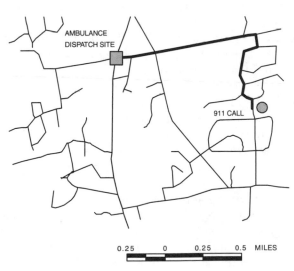

FIGURE 1.8. The shortest path through a street network from an ambulance dispatch site to the location of an emergency call.

Spatial data analysis is closely tied to spatial statistics and represents the fifth category of spatial analysis function that might be found in a GIS software package. Epidemiologists make extensive use of multivariate inferential statistics (Selvin, 1991), but in most instances these methods are not forms of *spatial* statistical analysis because they assume that the observational units represent independent pieces of information about the relationships being modeled and they focus on the attributes of objects and events rather than their spatial relationships.

Software for performing many spatial statistical analyses has been developed, but not as part of GIS software packages (Goodchild et al., 1992). The measurement, topology, and network functions—along with some simple aspatial statistical functions—are more commonly featured in GIS systems than functions to perform advanced multivariate inferential statistical or spatial statistical analysis. Some taxonomies of spatial analysis functions—particularly those developed by researchers with an interest in spatial statistics (Fotheringham & Rogerson, 1994; Bailey & Gatrell, 1995)—emphasize this last class of methods. Typical of this emphasis is the distinction between "spatial summarization" and "spatial analysis" techniques (Bailey, 1994). Relegated to the former class of techniques considered "prerequisite" to spatial data analysis are important GIS functions like projection, point-in-polygon and polygon overlay, buffering, contiguity analysis, and nearest neighbor search. Many of these techniques are based in the mathematics of set theory, topology, and geometry. Some taxonomies also set aside the location-allocation and network-modeling functions, either because these functions are seen as already incorporated into available GIS software packages (Bailey, 1994) or because they are normative and not concerned with statistical description and modeling of spatial data (Bailey & Gatrell, 1995).

Public health professionals may find that many of the multivariate statistical techniques they use have not yet been incorporated into GIS software packages, and that many spatial statistical and network analysis techniques with which they may be less familiar but want to apply are not available either. The measurement and topological analysis functions are generally present in all GIS software systems. Several options for integrating statistical analysis and network analysis software functions developed outside of GIS packages with the GIS software are available: freestanding, loosely coupled, closely coupled, and integrated software (Goodchild, 1992).

Under the *freestanding* approach, separate pieces of software are developed for individual spatial data analysis functions. One argument against this approach is that any spatial statistical analysis requires access to spatial data input, editing, management, and display functions, and it seems pointless to duplicate this functionality in stand-alone software. *Loose coupling* involves moving output from the GIS software analysis (e.g., a measure of whether a person is exposed or not exposed to an environmental contaminant based on residential location) into another software package where this input might be used to calculate and test the statistical significance of risk ratios. Close coupling involves developing software functions like the risk ratio calculation as a user-created modification to the GIS software. *Close coupling* obviously requires the user to have the necessary programming expertise. Full integration involves the GIS software developer, who must commit to expanding the set of functions available in the GIS package. *Full integration* makes the expanded set of functions available to all users of the software; the likelihood of functions being incorporated into commercial GIS packages is related to the number of customers who demand the particular function.

To the extent that many users of GIS are more interested in spatial database management than in spatial data analysis per se, loose coupling of GIS software with other statistical software packages is most likely for the immediate future. A number of the applications presented in this book illustrate this approach. The increasing emphasis on open systems in computing has affected the GIS industry. Many software vendors are developing products that make it easier for professional software developers or system users within an agency to create specially designed GIS applications with modified user interfaces and functions. These modifications can be made available to other users by fully incorporating them into a software update distributed by the vendor, marketing them as new software products, or distributing them for free to interested software users via the Internet. The "open GIS" movement has been particularly concerned with developing a standardized interface to ease data transfer among geographic information systems that use different, proprietary, approaches to managing spatial data (Phair, 1997).

GIS and the Internet

Maps and geographic data have been an important category of online content since the introduction and growth in popularity in the early 1990s of the World Wide Web (WWW) as a tool for accessing the Internet. In addition to the spatial database management, visualization and mapping, and spatial analysis functions that in-house GIS users call upon, publication and distribution of spatial data are increasingly important GIS-supported activities that enable organizations to share data, maps, and information as files or images sent over the Internet.

A more sophisticated model relies on a multitiered client–server design (Plewe, 1997). In this system design, the public health analyst sitting at a client computer uses a web browser and sends a request to one or more web server computers where a GIS application is running (Figure 1.9). This request is translated by programs connecting the web server to

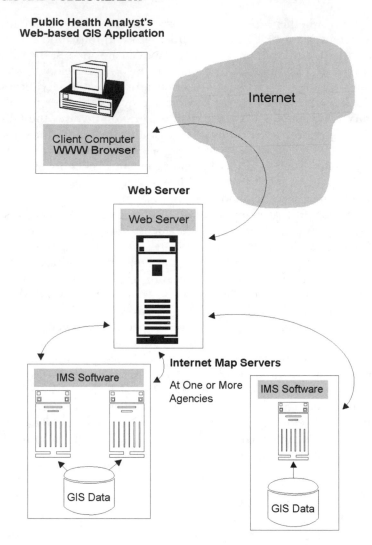

FIGURE 1.9. A client–server model for distributing geographic information over the Internet. This model is capable of providing real-time access to geographic data served by more than one agency and combined in one GIS application.

the GIS, which processes the request and returns a result in the form of a map, text, or data file. The result is reformated by the programs connecting the web server to the GIS into a format understood by the web browser and then returned to the public health analyst's client computer, where it is displayed. This pattern of requests and responses may be repeated many times during a single session.

The development of GIS on the WWW has broadened access to geographic data and GIS analyses because users do not necessarily need to have GIS software and databases resident on their own computers to access and use the information in a GIS application. Chapters 2, 3, and 4 reference a number of websites where maps, text, and databases of relevance to public health GIS are distributed. The greater access to health information made possible by delivering GIS over the WWW poses particular challenges for public health agencies and analysts because of the confidential nature of personal health records and concerns over privacy.

GIS enable public health professionals and epidemiologists to view and analyze the geographical distributions of health outcomes and to integrate information drawn from different sources based on location, so that the geographical distributions of health outcomes can be viewed and analyzed in relation to the geographical distributions of health risks and medical care resources. Public health GIS applications have built upon GIS developments in other fields.

TRENDS IN GIS APPLICATIONS

Although GIS have developed rapidly, the history of the technology "is little more than anecdotal" (Coppock & Rhind, 1991, p. 21). An overview of GIS applications in the United Kingdom, the United States, and Canada gives a sense of GIS developments in those countries up to 1989 (Bracken, Higgs, Martin, & Webster, 1989). A more formal history considers the many origins of GIS and the various influences affecting GIS development (Foresman, 1998). Some of the earliest systems were developed for environmental management, particularly of land-based resources like forests (Tomlinson, 1987). Many early adopters were large public or quasi-public institutions that had access to or were responsible for compiling extensive spatial data sets in the form of maps (Coppock & Rhind, 1991). These organizations generally also had access to the hardware resources needed to support storage and analysis of large databases in the mainframe era of the 1960s and 1970s. Remote sensing, automated mapping, and GIS are also important technologies in the military, although the literature on GIS does not emphasize these applications (Smith, 1992).

Adoption of GIS and related technologies also occurred relatively early, but selectively, at the local level in the United States. County and local governments are responsible for land registration, deed transfers, and property taxation. Local governments were interested in GIS for the opportunities they offered to create and manage *cadastral databases*, digital land parcel or property databases. Up to the 1990s, effective use of these systems to monitor property changes was primarily at the local level where the databases involved were more manageable in terms of size (Dale,

1991; Dale & McLaren, 1999) and directly related to urban and regional planning (Parrott & Stutz, 1991; Yeh, 1999).

At the state level in the United States, transportation and environmental management agencies were early adopters of GIS. In most states, one of these two departments generally took the lead in early GIS implementation. Public utilities (Mahoney, 1991; Meyers, 1999) and civil engineering firms were among the earliest nongovernmental adopters of GIS. Utilities, transportation, and telecommunication companies have also been leaders in the development of "mobile" GIS, which supports spatial data acquisition and attribute data entry in the field (Wilson, 1998).

The rapid diffusion of GIS technology to new application areas has depended on a number of developments in hardware, software, and spatial databases. Hardware has been recognized as one of the major "drivers" of GIS development (Dangermond & Morehouse, 1987). Larger memories for lower costs, workstations and desktop computers with high levels of graphics performance, network architecture as an alternative to multiuser host architecture, and low-cost, reliable output devices like the inkjet printer were among the most important hardware developments affecting GIS in the late 1980s and early 1990s.

The higher levels of graphics performance have also made graphical user interfaces possible in GIS software (Buttenfield & Mackaness, 1991). Many of the software packages initially developed relied on command- or query-based user interfaces that presented fairly steep learning curves for the software. Hardware and software developments and new operating systems have also forced GIS software companies to broaden their product lines to operate on a variety of platforms. Today, GIS software is a global industry with hundreds of products (Rodkay, 1995).

Although hardware and software developments have supported the diffusion of GIS technology over the last 2 decades, development of "foundation" spatial databases was a key to the rapid adoption of GIS technology by the business community. Most commercial enterprises sit on large databases containing location information (e.g., retail outlet locations, customer locations, supplier locations, shipment routes) and make decisions about how to manage business operations in a geographic context. The development of the U.S. Bureau of the Census TIGER/Line files (Callahan & Broome, 1984), a database covering the entire United States, for the 1990 census and their availability to the public at a relatively low price helped to create new markets for GIS software among census data users.

The *TIGER/Line files*, discussed in detail in Chapter 3, are a database containing line segments for streets and other linear features that can be used to create digital cartographic databases of census block, census tract, and other administrative and political boundaries (Marx, 1986). Address ranges on the street segments enable users to translate street addresses to locations on the earth's surface. The digital cartographic databases that could be created from TIGER could also be integrated with data from the Census of Population and Housing. New GIS-related businesses and products emerged as commercial vendors developed upgraded or customized versions of the TIGER/Line files. Within the research community, the availability of this database accelerated the expansion of GIS technology into the social sciences and public health.

PUBLIC HEALTH APPLICATIONS OF GIS

There are only a few examples of GIS applications in public health, epidemiology, or health planning from the 1980s (Bracken et al., 1989). Applications expanded rapidly during the 1990s and growth continues into the 21st century (de Lepper, Scholten, & Stern, 1995; Gatrell & Löytönen, 1998). The hardware, software, and database developments that have brought other new users to GIS partly explain this diffusion into the public health sphere. Like many other organizations, public health agencies and public and private providers or insurers of medical care services manage large databases that contain geographic information that can be meaningfully integrated based on location.

The primary impetus for the diffusion of GIS technology into the public health field in the United States was the federal government. A workshop on automated cartography and epidemiology organized by the National Center for Health Statistics in 1976 brought together representatives from federal agencies and the research community in response to an increasing awareness of computer-based mapping and geographical analysis (National Center for Health Statistics, 1979; Aangeenbrug, 1997). In addition to those agencies using computer-based systems for mapping and spatial data analysis at the national scale, other federal agencies began to adopt GIS technology.

The growing interest in environmental health, including risk assessment, created one "market" for GIS applications in public health (Stockwell, Sorenson, Eckert, & Carreras, 1993). Given that environmental management was an early GIS application area, GIS data layers describing environmental conditions were available to support these efforts. In 1994, the Agency for Toxic Substances and Disease Registry (ATSDR) held a workshop on GIS applications in public health and risk analysis to reinforce its commitment to GIS technology as a key tool for assessing "real risks to real people." The resurgence of infectious disease (National Science and Technology Council, 1995), particularly vector-borne disease, and the international efforts to address health problems like Lyme disease and rabies based on an understanding of the ecology of these diseases also led public health agencies to GIS.

Through the cooperative agreements that fund state and local health departments, these agencies stimulated the development of public health GIS applications at the state and local level and also brought the research community into collaboration with public health agencies at every level. By the mid-1990s, GIS sessions began to appear on the programs of public health conferences like the Public Health Conference on Records and Statistics and the annual meeting of the American Public Health Association (National Center for Health Statistics, 1995; American Public Health Association, 1996). Successful conferences focused solely on public health GIS, for example, the International Symposium on Computer Mapping in Epidemiology and Environmental Health held in 1995 (Aangeenbrug, 1997) and the Third National Conference on GIS in Public Health held in 1999 (Richards, Croner, Rushton, Brown, & Fowler, 1999), were supported by a wide range of sponsoring organizations at the national level.

In addition to organizing conferences, federal agencies like ATSDR and university-based researchers have taken the lead in developing GIS training programs specifically for public health professionals (Rushton, 1997; Richards et al., 1999). ATSDR, the Centers for Disease Control and Prevention, and the National Center for Health Statistics support a GIS lecture series, an online public health GIS newsletter, and a GIS list server (National Center for Health Statistics, 2000).

While federal leadership in supporting the development of public health GIS has continued, private-sector adoption of GIS for health is more difficult to track in the United States. The trends in GIS development described in the preceding section coincided with a period of increasing privatization of health insurance and health services delivery. Corporate concentration in the medical care industry itself and the movement of the insurance industry into managed care created a market for GIS technology (McManus, 1993). However, analyses of utilization and service organization conducted by private or nonprofit health care providers have rarely been shared in the published literature.

The development of public health GIS to date reflects, in part, lags in the availability of geocoded health data compared to other health-related GIS databases. Throughout the 1990s, "geocoded public health data have been in relatively short supply, limited to states with initiatives to geocode vital statistics data or to individual investigators who could geocode their own data" (Richards et al., 1999, p. 359). As of 1997, only 21 of 49 state directors of vital statistics who responded to a survey reported that their states used some type of automated geocoding of vital statistics records. Many local health departments do not have the trained staff, software, and hardware necessary to apply GIS technology. Organizations developing a GIS for public health analysis will not necessarily require access to the full range of GIS functionality. Even analysts with limited resources can acquire the hardware and software they need to geocode data and develop public health applications.

CONCLUSION

GIS as a technology is not the province of any single organization or group of users. Public health professionals and epidemiologists are becoming part of the GIS community. As they explore the potential of GIS in their own applications, the technology itself will continue to evolve in response to the needs of the many and varied groups within the GIS community.

GIS implementation involves organizing people to use a collection of computer hardware, software, and spatial databases to answer questions or solve problems (Kessler, 1992). A GIS application reflects—at least implicitly—how the GIS user views the world, including what are appropriate and meaningful ways to represent reality, what are the subjects of interest, and how and by whom information will be used. The technologies of GIS and the ideas they represent "are vitally embedded in broader transformations of science, society, and culture" (Pickles, 1995, p. 3). At present, these include the changes in how human beings communicate with each other through the use of electronic technologies and what the impacts of these changes will be for access to information, privacy, and individual and collective decision making. All of these changes have affected the collection and analysis of data on human health problems.

GIS implementation requires a significant commitment of time, money, and effort by the individuals and organizations adopting the technology. While the adoption of GIS technology will be advocated by public health professionals, epidemiologists, and medical care providers who see the value of geographical analysis of human health problems, the commitment of these resources may not seem justified to public health professionals and epidemiologists whose program activities and research are not primarily concerned with spatial analysis. Even for these public health professionals, however, GIS literacy and some GIS capability will become necessary because GIS have become the technology for managing and distributing spatial databases and most public health databases are spatially referenced. To the extent that the Bureau of the Census, the Environmental Protection Agency, vital statistics bureaus and disease registries, and medical care providers have adopted GIS technology, analysts who wish to access these data even for nonspatial analyses will become part of the GIS community.

CHAPTER 2

Spatial Data

Spatial data are observations with explicit locations. For geographers—and most people interested in studying human health problems—the relevant space is the surface of the earth. Geospatial data are obtained by observation and measurement of events or objects referenced to their locations in that space. GIS implementation requires access to geographic data. "The database is the foundation of a GIS" (Worboys, 1995, p. 45).

This chapter highlights some of the important attributes of geographic data that the GIS user must consider in developing an application. Because analysts use GIS to integrate data from different sources based on location, they need to have a clear understanding of the attributes of the data layers they are combining. Data at different scales and in different projections cannot be meaningfully integrated in a GIS without additional processing to bring the data layers into a common scale and projection. Because it is possible to overlay so many layers of data in a GIS display, the symbolization of data elements that will produce a legible display can be difficult to design.

In the first part of this chapter we consider the two broad models of geographic data, field and object, and how these models are expressed in raster and vector data structures. Next, we review the basic concept of location and how it is determined, either to define the set of locations that provide the spatial framework for field data or to georeference objects on the surface of the earth. Because an important source of geographic data is cartographic (existing maps), we also briefly review map scale, projections, and symbolization. We then consider the quality of geographic data, how it can be assessed, and its implications for GIS applications. We conclude with a description of the configuration of a simple PUBLIC HEALTH GIS incorporating various spatial databases that were used to prepare many of the maps and analyses presented in this book.

FIELD AND OBJECT DATA

There are two main approaches to modeling geographic information. From one perspective, we can think of phenomena that are continuously distributed just above, on, or below the surface. Precipitation, surface elevation, and soil are examples of *field data*. It is possible to visit any location on the earth's surface and ask "what is the elevation here?" or "what is the environmental quality here?"

Because these phenomena are continuous and can be observed everywhere, they are usually measured based on observations made at a set of regularly spaced sample sites on the surface. This network of sites creates a spatial framework for describing the distribution of the phenomenon. *Tessellation* is the geometric process of partitioning an area into smaller units that do not overlap but completely fill the entire area (Arlinghaus, 1994). Squares, triangles, and hexagons can be used as the basic units of a tessellation (Figure 2.1). When the units are the same shape and size, the tessellation is regular. Of the three, the regular square grid has probably been the most widely used because it can be represented easily in an array structure with row and column numbers identifying particular squares; furthermore, it is compatible with hardware devices used for capture of spatial data like remote sensing data or, like the line printer or inkjet printer, used for output (Peuquet, 1984).

Irregular tessellations in which the partitions do not have the same shape, size, or orientation can also be constructed. Perhaps the most commonly used irregular tessellation is the *triangulated irregular network* (TIN). A data value like elevation is observed at a set of sampling points on the surface. These points form the vertices of the triangles in the TIN. Each triangle in the TIN connects three neighboring points so that the plane of the triangle approximates the surface between the points and calculating the slope and aspect of the surface is straightforward (Figure 2.2).

In field-based GIS applications, the GIS database generally contains several layers to enable comparison and integration of the various fields of information. A public health analyst might want to look at land use in relation to soils to find where medium- and low-density residential development relying on septic systems is occurring in relation to soils that pose problems for septic system functioning. Because the spatial framework

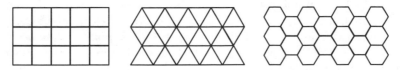

FIGURE 2.1. Regular square, triangular, and hexagonal tessellations.

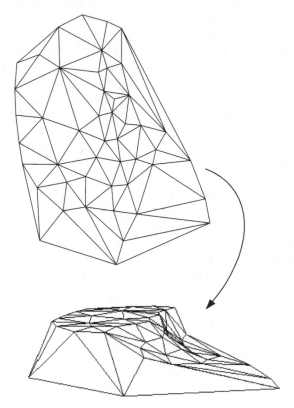

FIGURE 2.2. A triangulated irregular network (TIN) and the corresponding surface representation.

represents a set of locations on the surface, the observations made at these locations represent a sample of the phenomenon being modeled. Thus sampling error becomes a consideration in the GIS application.

From the other perspective, we can think of discrete objects that may be found on the earth's surface. A person, a hospital, and a public drinking water reservoir are examples of *object data*. Many health databases contain object data. *Objects* are entities that are identifiable, relevant to the particular public health problem at hand, and describable (Mattos, Meyer-Wegener, & Mitschang, 1993).

Each object of interest on the earth's surface has different types of attributes that are important for modeling purposes: textual/numeric, spatial, temporal, and graphical (Worboys, 1995). A public drinking water reservoir, for example, will have a set of textual/numeric attributes indicating its name, surface area, and other attributes (Figure 2.3). The polygon representing the shoreline or perimeter of the reservoir surface is a

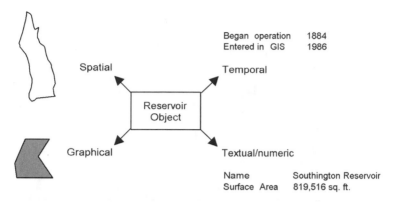

FIGURE 2.3. Attributes of a public drinking water reservoir as a spatially referenced object in a GIS.

spatial attribute. Attributes like the time the reservoir was developed as a public drinking water supply or the time it was first recorded in the database are temporal attributes. The symbol used to represent the reservoir as an object in cartographic displays is the graphical attribute of the underlying object. In this case, a solid filled polygon symbol of a particular hue is used to indicate that the polygon is a reservoir. If the reservoir had been represented using a line to show the shoreline, it would not be possible to "fill" the area corresponding to the reservoir's surface. It would only be possible to change the style, thickness, and color of the line.

RASTER AND VECTOR DATA STRUCTURES

The field and object views are expressed in the two main data structures used to implement GIS: raster and vector. These data structures have important implications for storage and processing of data (Worboys, 1995). In a *raster system*, every raster layer corresponds to a single attribute for a unit of space—for example, elevation or land use at a particular place or a value obtained by compositing two layers.

Stored in the computer, raster data are organized as an array of cells corresponding to particular places that are called "*pixels*"—shortened from "picture elements" (Arlinghaus, 1994). The GIS user defines the size of each pixel in terms of its area on the earth's surface to match the available data (Figure 2.4). A common ground dimension for remote sensing data in the United States is 30 meters × 30 meters, the pixel size of Landsat Thematic Mapper™ data (Jensen, 1996). The size of the pixel affects the size of an object that can be discerned in a digital image, thus determining

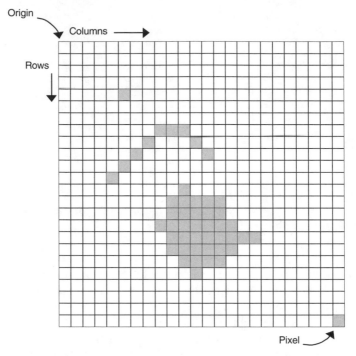

FIGURE 2.4. A raster data model.

the spatial *resolution* of the data. Some landscape features in an urban environment such as a single-family detached residence cannot be discerned in low resolution raster images like the 30-meter TM data because the features are smaller than the pixel size. On the other hand, such features would be discernable on a high resolution image that uses a small pixel size. Low resolution is useful for large geographical areas where only limited detail can be represented.

The GIS user can define the geographical extent of the data by specifying the number of rows and columns of pixels in the data layer. The location of each individual pixel in the raster is given by its particular row and column numbers. Raster data structures make it easy to overlay data layers as long as corresponding pixels are registered to exactly the same position on the surface of the earth.

In a *vector system*, every vector layer corresponds to a single class of objects that have the same dimensionality (point, line, or area), although data layers of different dimensionality can be used in a vector GIS application. A *vector* is a finite straight-line segment that can be described by the locational coordinates of its endpoints. In a vector data structure, a point such as a hospital location would be represented by a single ordered pair (*x,y*), a line or an arc such as a meals-on-wheels route by a sequence of straight-line segments, and an area or polygon such as a landfill by the vectors enclosing it. Every vector layer corresponds to a set of objects located in space and described by many attributes (Figure 2.5).

Vector data may or may not be topological. A vector database is topological if it contains information on the neighborhood relationships among objects (Figure 2.6). Specifying a "start node" and an "end node" for each arc indicates the direction of the arc. Areas to the left and to the right of a particular directed arc can then be identified.

In a vector system, "resolution" again refers to the smallest feature that can be discerned. The minimum length of a line object, the minimum separation required to display objects as separate and distinct, and the minimum size below which a long narrow area will be represented as a line and a small area will be represented as a point are affected by the scale of the database (Veregin & Hargitai, 1995). The extent of a vector data layer is described by a *bounding rectangle* within which all of the objects in the database can be placed.

GIS software systems can be identified as raster or vector depending upon the dominant approach taken to storing and processing spatial data. It is possible, however, to represent a range of spatial phenomena—field and object—with both data structures and to convert from raster to vector and vice versa (Figure 2.7). Raster/vector conversion is a function commonly found in both raster and vector GIS software systems.

However represented in the GIS, the field and object views of data are recognized as inverse ways of looking at geographic information (Peuquet, 1984; Worboys, 1995). The field view starts with a spatial framework over which the geographical domain of an attribute like precipita-

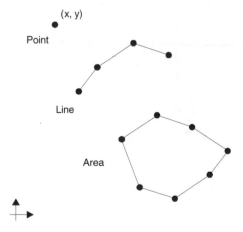

FIGURE 2.5. A vector data model.

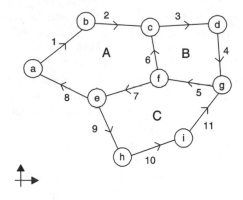

Directed Arcs, Nodes, and Areas

Arc	Start Node	End Node	Left Area	Right Area
1	a	b	X	A
2	b	c	X	A
3	c	d	X	B
4	d	g	X	B
5	g	f	C	B
6	f	c	A	B
7	f	e	C	A
8	e	a	X	A
9	e	h	C	X
10	h	i	C	X
11	i	g	C	X

FIGURE 2.6. A topological vector data model.

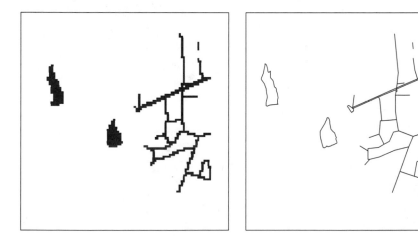

FIGURE 2.7. A raster database and a vector database representing the same situation of reservoirs and an adjoining network of water distribution mains.

tion or environmental quality is represented. The object view starts with objects that can be "embedded" in an otherwise empty space based on their locations. Both views require us to operationalize location.

MEASURING LOCATION

Location means position in space. Location is the basis for integrating geographic data in a GIS. *Absolute location* refers to position with respect to an arbitrary grid system like the geographic grid of parallels and meridians. Absolute location gives the position of a point so that its unique position on the earth is clear. "The burner stack is 41°48'N and 72°15'W" is a statement of absolute location. *Relative location* refers to position with respect to other objects in the geographic space. "The burner stack is 300' northwest of the intersection of Park and Broad Streets" is a statement of relative location.

Positional data in a GIS can come from several sources; these are discussed in detail in Chapter 3. Geodetic, photogrammetric, and digital image processing data are all primary sources for positional data because positions are determined by direct or indirect measurement of the earth's surface (J. Drummond, 1995). These primary sources of positional data provide an essential and accurate foundation for other spatial data. Maps and archival documents like gazetteers are secondary sources for positional data.

Geodesy is the science of observation and measurement of the shape, size, and dimensions of the earth as a whole and of the earth's surface (Arlinghaus, 1994). Position can be measured directly from the earth's surface by surveying (McCormac, 1995). With the development of satellite technology, *global positioning systems* (GPS) are now used to ascertain position (Van Sickle, 1996). GPS uses a series of 24 satellites of known position in space, together with satellite sensors or tracking devices located on the earth's surface. By recording the positions of the satellites with multiple sensors, very accurate coordinate locations can be computed for each sensor. The satellites and tracking stations are operated by the federal government.

Researchers working in the field can use the output from a GPS receiver to determine a latitude/longitude (lat/lon) pair describing position on the earth's surface. Signals from at least three satellites are needed to obtain horizontal positions (lat/lon) at a particular location; a signal from a fourth satellite is needed to obtain vertical position. Using GPS, a field researcher can obtain accurate locations for a variety of features in the landscape. A network of geographic coordinates can be determined by moving the sensors throughout an area and repeating the computations for mapping. Many GPS devices allow storage of the coordinates of the measured points, and these data can then be loaded directly into the GIS. The GPS has become a standard method for surveying. Individuals and organizations requiring this kind of positional data usually hire a surveyor or GPS technician to make the necessary measurements or develop an in-house capability to obtain the data.

Surveying and GPS involve collecting data directly from the surface of the earth. *Remote sensing* is the analysis and interpretation of data gathered by means that do not require direct contact with the subject. Aerial photography is a method of photographing the earth's surface from an aerial platform (Jensen, 2000). When the photo is taken directly above the surface in the image, the vertical photograph is known as an *ortho-photograph*. *Photogrammetry* is the measurement of aerial photographs to determine locations for mapping.

Digital image processing of geographic data relies on satellites with sensors capable of detecting electromagnetic energy reflected or emitted from objects on the earth's surface (Jensen, 1996). The energy detected is converted into a data value and telemetered to receiving stations either directly or via tracking data and relay satellites. The data are then enhanced for viewing and subsequent analysis by using digital image processing algorithms.

It is possible to obtain a variety of data from a single flight. Acquisition of photogrammetric and digital image data usually involves purchasing a database from a government or quasi-governmental agency that has means to produce these data.

In many GIS applications, positions are estimated from an existing map of the earth's surface created at a particular scale. For example, we could estimate the coordinates of a hospital by digitizing from an appropriately annotated topographic map. *Digitizing* requires use of a tablet and cursor to record Cartesian coordinate locations of map features from a map placed on the digitizing tablet or use of a cursor to screen digitize from a visual display. We could also estimate the coordinates by using a GIS to address-match geocode the hospital's address against a digital, address-ranged street network database (Figure 2.8) (W. J. Drummond, 1995). *Geocoding* is "the process by which an entity on the earth's surface, a household, for example, is given a label identifying its location with respect to some common point or frame of reference" (Goodchild, 1984, p. 33). Address-match geocoding as a GIS function is described in detail in Chapter 3.

Finally, coordinates for particular places like schools or toxic release sites are published in gazetteers and other archival sources in both paper and digital formats (Abate, 1991; Armstrong, 1995; Environmental Protection Agency, 1995). When using secondary sources of positional data, the GIS analyst should read the database documentation to understand the primary source of positional information for the published data and its accuracy. The scale and projection of the digital model or map and the

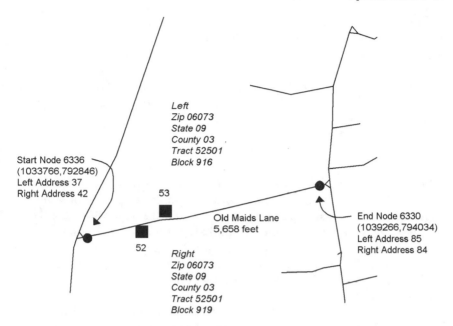

FIGURE 2.8. The locations of 52 Old Maids Lane and 53 Old Maids Lane in the Town of Glastonbury were determined by address-match geocoding in the PUBLIC HEALTH GIS. The segment length is 5,658 feet. A structure with Number 52 is estimated to be approximately 1,358 feet from the start node by interpolation because $(52 - 42)/(84 - 42) = 0.24$ and $0.24 \times 5,658 = 1,358$. A structure with Number 53 is estimated to be approximately 1,768 feet from the start node by interpolation because $(53 - 37)/(85 - 37) = 0.33$ and $0.33 \times 5,658 = 1,768$. The locations were geocoded with a 30-foot offset to represent the setback from the street centerline. The actual locations of structures numbered 52 and 53 (if they exist) would have to be verified from a field survey, air photo, or cadastral database. Because the TIGER/Line files are topological, the left and right zip, census state, census county, census tract, and census block identifiers are easily determined. The two structures are in the same zip, state, county, and tract but are located in different census blocks.

symbols used to represent objects affect the quality and accuracy of the positional data obtained from it.

SCALE, PROJECTION, AND SYMBOLS OF CARTOGRAPHIC DATA SOURCES

As models, maps are generalized representations of reality. Maps distort reality by simplifying the complex, three-dimensional surface of the earth for representation on a flat sheet of paper or video screen. The "cartographic paradox" is that "to present a useful and truthful picture, an accurate map must tell white lies" (Monmonier, 1996, p. 1). Scale, projection, and symbolization are three basic components of maps. Each is a potential source of distortion. Public health analysts using GIS need to understand these concepts and how to identify scale, projection, and symbols by reading the details of the description printed on a paper map or the data description supplied with a digital spatial database.

Scale

Map scale tells the user how much smaller the map is than the reality it represents. Map scale can be stated as a ratio, a simple bar graph, or a phrase (Figure 2.9). Ratio scales are particularly useful for comparison. A 1:5,000 map is a *large-scale map*, a map of a small area showing high detail. In contrast, a 1:1,000,000 map is a *small-scale map*, a map of a large area showing limited detail. The graphical scale is useful for representing scale on paper and in digital displays because the scale will be correct even if the map is enlarged or reduced during reproduction.

Scale is an important attribute of maps because scale affects the amount of detail that can be captured and represented. At the map scale in Figure 2.9, the locations of hospitals in Hartford, Connecticut, and the street network can be represented. When the map is compiled at a smaller scale to depict the state, the street network cannot be shown clearly. Similarly, meanders or curves in the Connecticut River are generalized as the scale decreases and areas like the Town of Hartford shrink to points and eventually disappear. It is important to understand that simply enlarging a small-scale map or zooming in the visual display of a spatial database does *not* enable us to see features that are not present in the database. Enlargement by zooming often aids visualization when features are clustered together, but it does not affect the level of generalization of the data.

When data layers are at different scales, the larger scale data should be recompiled to match the scale of the smallest scale data layer. This is accomplished through generalization of the larger scale data layers using techniques like line generalization. It is possible to develop GIS applications that call on different *scale* databases for the same region; in this case more detail can be observed as the user shifts through to higher scale data sets. Although scale can be constant at all points and in all directions on a globe as a true scale model of the earth, scale varies on a paper map because map projection stretches some distances and shrinks others.

Projection

Projection, a second basic component of maps and spatial databases, refers to the mathematical function that transforms locations from the curved, three-dimensional surface of the earth to a flat, two-dimensional represen-

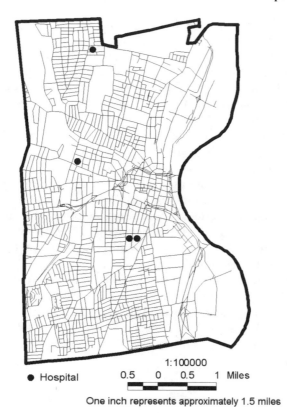

● Hospital

1:100000

0.5   0   0.5   1 Miles

One inch represents approximately 1.5 miles

FIGURE 2.9. A map of hospital locations showing different methods for representing map scale.

tation (Pearson, 1990; Maling, 1992). There is more than one system for describing positions of places such as environmental monitoring sites or objects such as hospitals. The network of meridians and parallels, which form a geographic grid, is used to reference locations on the earth's surface.

Meridians are true north–south lines connecting the poles. Each is half of a great circle, a circle created by passing a plane through the center of the Earth. They are spaced wide at the Equator and converge at the poles. *Parallels* are true east–west lines. They intersect meridians at right angles. The Equator is the only parallel that is a great circle. *Latitude* is the position of a place north or south of the Equator. It is measured as the arc of the meridian between the place of interest and the Equator. It ranges from 0° to 90°N or 90°S. *Longitude* is the position of a place east or west of the prime meridian. It is measured as the arc of the parallel between that place and the prime meridian. Longitude ranges from 0° to 180°E or

180°W. A parallel is all points having the same latitude; a meridian is all points having the same longitude.

Computer processing of lat/lon reported in degrees, minutes, and seconds and by direction poses some problems. For computer analysis of lat/lon data, the preferred measurement is the *radian*, a unit defined so that there are 2π radians to a circle, with one radian equal to approximately 57.296°. The computer functions used to generate trigonometric function values are based on radians and not on degrees. Most users of spatial data find it convenient to manage the conversion from degrees to radians by converting their data to decimal degrees. This enables storage of the lat or lon coordinate as a single real number rather than as separate integer values for degrees, minutes, and seconds. But it also retains relevance to the geographic grid so that users can easily conceptualize point locations and reference objects to paper maps. The GIS software converts the decimal degree lat or lon to its radian equivalent internally.

In addition, the computer cannot easily recognize "E" and "W" or "N" and "S" as directions. Instead, "+" and "–" are used to indicate directions, as in a Cartesian coordinate system (Figure 2.10). Thus, the lat/lon for the burner stack would be found in a digital spatial database not as 41°48'N 72°15'W but as (–72.25, 41.80) so that the longitude (east–west or "*x*" in Cartesian space) is given first (i.e., lon/lat rather than lat/lon), val-

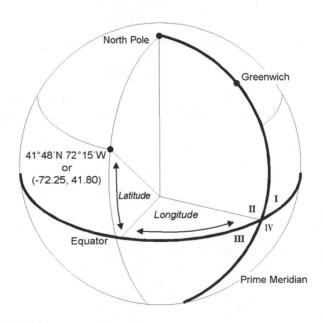

FIGURE 2.10. The geographic grid.

ues are in decimal form, and directions are correct. For most places in North America, longitude will be negative but latitude will be positive.

Because the surface of the earth is curved and not flat, lat/lon represents location in a three-dimensional space. Direct plotting of lat/lon coordinates results in an image that does not match what would be observed on the earth or a globe (Figure 2.11). Map projection provides a method for making the transformation from three dimensions to two. Most paper maps and many digital spatial databases represent projected spatial data. Map projection may be a more serious issue for users of small-scale maps and projected digital spatial databases than for users of large-scale paper maps. Distortion will not be as great on large-scale maps because the areas being mapped are relatively small, covering only a small portion of the earth's curved surface. Because one of the most important capabilities of GIS is integrating spatial data, however, a basic understanding of map scale and projection and their implications for geodata processing is essential. Databases cannot be properly overlayed or integrated if they are not in the same projection. Projecting spatial data from lat/lon or from one projection to another is a function commonly found in GIS software.

Three plotting surfaces have been used to develop practical map projections (Figure 2.12). Map projections based on these objects preserve different spatial properties of objects and their relationships. On a perfect map, areas on the map would be in correct proportion to corresponding areas on the earth, distances on the map would be true scale, directions and angles on the map would remain true to the corresponding directions and angles on the earth, and shapes of objects on the map would not be distorted. Not all of these properties can be achieved when we move from three to two dimensions. One way of classifying map projections is by the

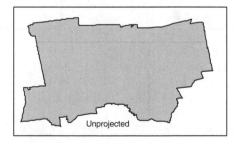
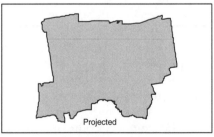

Unprojected

Projected

FIGURE 2.11. The importance of map projection is demonstrated by displaying a view of the unprojected boundary of a study area and a view of the projected boundary. At the latitude of the study area (around 41°N), a direct plot of latitude against longitude results in considerable distortion of the study area size and shape in the east–west dimension compared to boundary data projected in state plane coordinates.

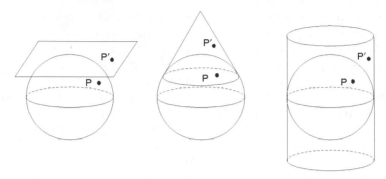

FIGURE 2.12. Three plotting surfaces used to develop practical map projections.

relationship they preserve. *Conformal* projections preserve shapes but not areas of land masses. *Equal area* projections preserve areas but may distort shapes. *Cylindrical* projections like the Mercator projection preserve true directions and angles but not shapes and areas.

The usefulness of the conformal projections is evident in the widely used State Plane Coordinate System in the United States. The *State Plane Coordinate System* provides a convenient means of locating mapping positions on a two-dimensional plane. The system is based on a rectangular grid defined for each state of the United States (Figure 2.13). The grids permit the methods of plane surveying to be extended over great distances at high precision.

In the continental United States, two conformal map projections are used for the state plane coordinate systems (Figure 2.14): the transverse Mercator secant and the Lambert conformal with two standard parallels (Pearson, 1990). The transverse Mercator secant projection defines a grid zone roughly 158 miles east–west (Figure 2.15). There are two true-scale lines running north and south in each transverse Mercator zone. Between these lines of secancy, the distances are less than true scale. Outside of these lines, the distances are greater than true scale. The distortion increases with increasing distance east or west from the secant lines. Within the zone, distortion is not a function of latitude, so north–south extension is unlimited. The transverse Mercator projection is well suited for states of major north-to-south extent like Illinois.

The Lambert conformal projection with two standard parallels defines a grid zone roughly 158 miles north–south (Figure 2.15). The parallels are two true-scale lines running east and west in each zone. Again, between the true-scale lines, distances are less than true scale. North and south of the lines, the distances become more than true scale. Within the zone, distortion is not a function of longitude, so east–west extension is

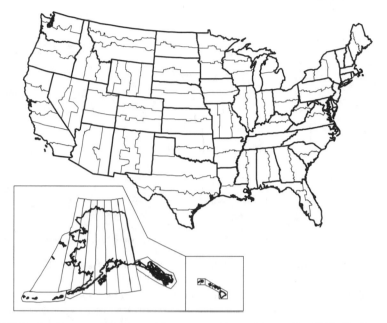

FIGURE 2.13. Zones of the State Plane Coordinate System for 1983. Each zone is defined by a projection system—central meridian and scale factor if transverse Mercator projection or standard parallels if Lambert projection—and an origin. Zones of the Universal Transverse Mercator projection system differ from the zones of other state plane transverse Mercator projections by only the zone-defining constants used. Adapted from Stern (1989). For additional information, see King (1999).

unlimited. The Lambert conformal is suited for states of major east–west extent like Tennessee. For each state plane grid, an origin is established to the south and west of all points so that the coordinates can be given as a *false easting* and a *false northing* (Figure 2.16). This means that none of the coordinates will have negative signs. Distance units in state plane coordinate systems are feet or meters depending on the datum plane and the data distribution practices in various states.

The planes produced by these projections are like tiles approximating parts of a sphere. Because they represent data on a plane, these systems support spatial analysis like the measurement of distance based in Euclidean geometry. Different states in the United States rely on different state plane coordinate systems for their paper and digital spatial databases (Warnecke, Johnson, Marshall, & Brown, 1992). A number of documents are available that describe the specifics of the systems used in each state (Stern, 1989; Snyder, 1987). To make a map of the entire state in a state

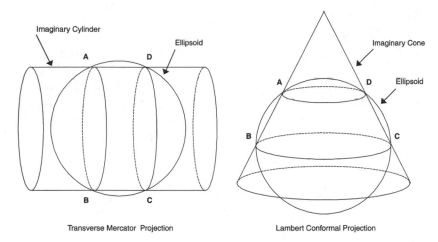

Transverse Mercator Projection

Lambert Conformal Projection

FIGURE 2.14. Surfaces used in state plane coordinate systems. The transverse Mercator secant projection provides the closest fit to the datum surface for a rectangular (*ABCD*) zone greatest in north–south extent. The Lambert projection provides the closest approximation to the datum surface for a rectangular (*ABCD*) zone greatest in east–west extent.

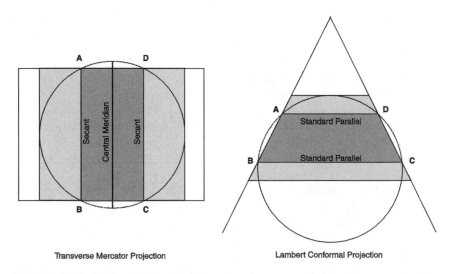

Transverse Mercator Projection

Lambert Conformal Projection

FIGURE 2.15. Scale relationships in state plane coordinate system projections. Along the standard lines of the projection (secants for transverse Mercator or standard parallels for Lambert conformal), scale is exact. Between the standard lines, distances are less than true scale.

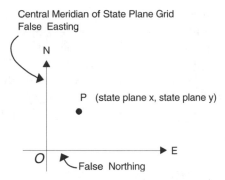

FIGURE 2.16. State Plane Coordinate System geometry. The central meridian is assigned a false easting. The origin *O* for measuring the state plane coordinates is located where the false easting intersects a false northing. The location of the origin *O* forces the eastings (state plane *x* coordinate values) and northings (state plane *y* coordinate values) to be positive numbers. The coordinates of point *P* are both positive.

with more than one state plane zone (Figure 2.13), analysts select one of the zones and project data for the entire state according to that zone or they select some other map projection.

In addition to the various projections used in data layers available at the state level, other map projections may have been used in the various map series published by the federal government. This situation poses problems for public health analysts who need to integrate data from both federal and various state sources. In order to use the GIS software functions to project or to change the projection of a digital spatial database, the analyst needs to know what projection the data are in to start. Because GIS software allows users to *display* data in different projections without actually reprojecting the data, an emerging strategy for dealing with these problems is to maintain all of the data in lat/lon. This approach facilitates data sharing. In a federal clearinghouse of digital spatial data, all of the bounding rectangles describing the geographic domain of the database are required to be given in lat/lon decimal degrees (Federal Geographic Data Committee, 2000). Techniques for integrating data layers are discussed in greater detail in Chapter 3, which describes foundation databases for public health GIS and how health data can be linked to them.

Symbolization

The visualization and mapping functions of GIS require data objects to be represented with some kind of graphical symbol. Bertin (1979) identified six dimensions of visual variability of map symbols: size, shape, value, texture, orientation, and hue (Figure 2.17). These aspects of symbolization can be and are manipulated to achieve certain objectives in cartographic communication (Monmonier, 1996). The range of symbols supported will vary from system to system, depending on software and hardware configurations. Standard cartography texts provide useful guidelines for map compilation and design. One body of cartographic research evaluates the impact of different symbolizations on the perceptions of map users (MacEachern, 1994).

GEOGRAPHIC DATA QUALITY

Because the database is the foundation of any GIS, the quality of the geographic data that goes into the system is paramount. The United States es-

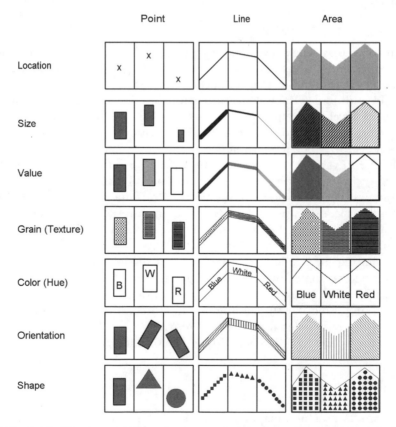

FIGURE 2.17. Visual variability of map symbols. Adapted from Bertin (1979). Copyright 1979 by United Nations Publications. Adapted by permission.

tablished the National Committee on Digital Cartographic Data Standards in 1982 (Morrison, 1995). Its draft report identifies five important aspects of spatial data quality (Moellering, 1987); these dimensions have since been accorded a degree of international consensus (Moellering, 1991).

Lineage is a "description of the source material from which the data were derived, and the methods of derivation, including all transformations involved in producing the final digital files" (National Institute of Standards and Technology, 1994b, p. 21). To an extent, lineage is not so much a measure of data quality as the information needed to assess data quality based on other factors. The contents of a lineage describe data at various stages in its existence. Development of standards for lineages is an ongoing process. The difficulty of developing useful lineages creates a problem for data suppliers, although the importance of lineages to spatial data quality assessment cannot be denied.

Accuracy, in general, refers to the level of error present in a database. An "accurate" database is one that is free from error. Because spatial databases contain both locational and thematic data (e.g., pixel and elevation, lat/lon and health outcome), users must be concerned with both positional accuracy and attribute accuracy.

Positional accuracy refers to the nearness of the values describing the position of a real-world object to the object's "true" position. Positional error may be introduced at the initial measurement of location. A second source of error is the chain of processing between the initial measurement or observation and its final "resting place" in a GIS database (J. Drummond, 1995). Because GIS analysis involves manipulations of databases like projection change and overlay, errors propagate.

The preferred test of positional accuracy is comparison to a data source of higher accuracy (Antenucci, Brown, Croswell, Kevany, & Archer, 1991). These tests are often made at the time of data capture, for example, when using a GPS receiver or digitizing or scanning an existing database. In this approach, positional accuracy is measured by comparing the final positional information to a known higher standard, perhaps a set of geodetically or photogrammetrically observed checkpoints. The standard database contains checkpoints whose (x, y) coordinate values are considered "true" coordinates, having been determined using a measurement system of higher quality. For each i of the n checkpoints available, the difference or error measured between the "true," or accurate coordinate (x_{ia}, y_{ia}) and the corresponding database coordinate (x_{id}, y_{id}) is recorded. The values are used to determine the *root mean square error* (RSME) as shown below:

$$RMSE = \sqrt{\frac{\left(\sum_{i=1}^{n}[(x_{id} - x_{ia})^2 + (y_{id} - y_{ia})^2]\right)}{n}}$$

GIS users are familiar with an aspect of RMSE in the digitizing process. At the start of the digitizing session, a set of control points whose coordinates are known in the map's projection grid system are marked. From these control points, the transformation constants used to convert all digitized coordinates to the projection coordinates are produced. The projection coordinates of selected control points can then be compared to their known coordinate values, and the differences used in the calculation of RMSE. In many GIS systems, the user will be presented with this value after digitizing and asked either to accept it or to repeat the process. Public health analysts can, then, be able to assess positional accuracy of spatial databases in the early stages of developing a GIS application, either from the description of positional accuracy accompanying a database acquired from another source or during the digitizing process.

Attribute accuracy is an aspect of data quality that considers the nearness of the values describing the real-world entity in the database to the entity's "true" attributes. In many public health applications of GIS, the attribute data for objects will already have been collected in a disease registry or surveillance system. The amount of information available about uncertainty or error in these attribute data will vary depending on whether the agency collecting the data has carried out and described procedures for determining the level of error in the data.

In public health GIS applications, consistent definitions of what constitutes a health event or a health service are needed to ensure attribute accuracy. As discussed in detail in Chapter 3, it is not always easy to define what is meant by a "case"; moreover, case definitions may change over time. Attributes of cases, like race, ethnicity, or ICDM diagnosis, also need to be coded consistently to meet standards for attribute accuracy.

When the attributes are measured as interval/ratio level data, the normal or Gaussian distribution and log normal distribution may be appropriate models of the relative frequencies of error. Sometimes these distributions are truncated to reflect maximum or minimum possible values. When the attributes are nominal, places or objects have been assigned to simple classes and differences, means, and standard deviations are not meaningful. Uncertainty may exist when the place or object is assigned to the wrong class, when two or more analysts do not agree on the assignment, or, in the case of remotely sensed data, when the class does not agree with the class assigned based on direct observation.

As with positional accuracy, attribute accuracy assessment relies on comparison with a source of higher accuracy. In remote sensing, for example, a sample of locations is selected and the class assigned in the digital image processing is compared to the directly observed "ground truth." The results can then be tabulated in a misclassification matrix where the diagonal represents correct classifications and the off-diagonal elements record incorrect classifications (Table 2.1). A number of indices can be calculated to summarize the overall level of accuracy (Congalton, 1991).

A major issue in the assessment of attribute accuracy is the degree to which errors are spatially systematic. *Spatial dependence* measured as *spatial autocorrelation* means that there is a correlation between errors for features located near each other. In health outcome data, for example, there may be geographically systematic variations in surveillance or diagnosis. These "errors" are *not* necessarily connected to *positional* errors in the data. "Unfortunately, we know very little about the spatial structure of uncertainty in geographic data" (Goodchild, 1995a, p. 76). Research investigating both the spatial structure of data errors and methods of visualizing uncertainty is ongoing.

Completeness as a measure of data quality refers to "the relationship between the objects represented in the data set and the abstract universe of all such objects" (Brassel, Bucher, Stephan, & Vckovski, 1995). Two types of completeness can be considered. First, are all of the relevant objects captured in the database? Health outcome databases derived from voluntary versus mandatory screening programs might have widely varying degrees of completeness in representing the true universe of all individuals with a particular health problem. Second, are all the records for an individual unit in the database complete? Completeness as a measure of data quality addresses presence and absence of data for the specified universe.

Finally, *logical consistency* is a measure of data quality that considers the "structural integrity" of a database (Kainz, 1995). A spatial database is logically consistent when it is compatible with the attribute data and when it complies with the requirements of the selected raster or vector data model. The health analyst would want to make sure, for example, that all

TABLE 2.1. An Example Error Matrix for Classification of Areas Based on Land Cover

Data classification	Ground truth classification				
	Deciduous	Conifer	Shrub	Barren	Row total
Deciduous	82	4	16	18	120
Conifer	6	23	6	5	40
Shrub	3	8	97	2	110
Barren	0	3	9	87	99
Column total	91	38	128	112	369

Overall accuracy 289/369 = 78%

of the health events in a database were modeled in the same way—as fields or as objects—and described by the same set of attributes. Consistency rules prevent invalid changes to the database and ensure consistency in data handling—for example, treatment of missing values—throughout a series of transformations.

Most GIS software systems can test for topological consistency in a spatial database. In a vector database, this would include checks for missing nodes, dangling arcs, duplicate centroids, and other inconsistencies in the node–arc–area relationships depicted in Figure 2.6. For a particular GIS database, the consistency checks would verify that each directed arc or line segment has exactly one start and one end node, that each node is a start or end node of at least one directed arc, that each area is bounded by one or more directed arc, and so on.

Logical inconsistencies present in a database may not prevent the health analyst from producing a graphic display or map of the areas, but would almost certainly affect any spatial analysis performed using the database. GIS applications that involve more spatial data analysis require higher levels of consistency in spatial databases. The topological consistency checks can be performed when spatial databases are created so that errors can be detected before the public health analyst incorporates the database into an application.

A GIS application involving multiple layers of data may meet the test of logical consistency for every layer but lack consistency across data layers. Data fields in vital statistics databases may change over time as fields are added or modified. Records from an earlier time period would not, therefore, be logically consistent with records from the later reporting period unless the earlier records were modified to reflect the new format with the added or modified fields. Two GIS databases collected at different scales or using different projection systems may be logically consistent as individual databases, but would cause serious problems if they were integrated without appropriate modification. Methods for performing logical consistency checks across data layers are still being researched and have generally not been incorporated into GIS software packages.

A final important issue in assessing the quality of a spatial database is the handing of *temporal* information (Guptill, 1995). Because GIS applications involve assembling data from many different sources, information about the temporal attributes of the data is extremely important. Even when each particular data layer represents the most current information available, the layers may not mesh temporally because census data, land use data, and data on other elements in the universe of geographic features are not updated on the same schedules.

An important approach to handling temporal information is to model it as an attribute (Table 2.2). Both positional information and attribute information can be assigned temporal attributes describing the

TABLE 2.2. Example of Temporal Description Attributes for a Public Drinking Water Well

Basic feature	Spatial object		Attributes	
Public drinking water well Well ID 101	101 *Feature observed:* *Feature expired:*	07/01/1989 Current	System value: *Value observed:* *Value expired:*	Manchester 07/01/1989 Current
			Status value: *Value observed:* *Value expired:*	Active 07/01/1989 10/13/1997
			Value: *Value observed:* *Value expired:*	Inactive 10/13/1997 Current

date when the data were observed and the date when the position or attribute "expired." In the Table 2.2, a public drinking water well changed from "Active" to "Inactive" status as a source of drinking water on October 13, 1997. The importance of historical information, as distinct from information just recording change as it occurs, is obvious in the case of process studies. Does the researcher need to reconstruct past patterns of land use or public drinking water supply as part of an epidemiologic investigation?

The characteristics of a spatial database can be described in *metadata*, data describing data. The Federal Geographic Data Committee (FGDC) issues metadata standards for spatial databases in the United States, and producers of digital spatial databases are expected to prepare metadata that complies with these standards (Federal Geographic Data Committee, 1998). According to the Content Standard, there are several categories of information covered in a metadata file for a digital spatial database (Table 2.3). The FGDC and other organizations have developed software to assist GIS users in preparing metadata files that meet standards. Some GIS software packages also provide support for metadata preparation. The FGDC also maintains a clearinghouse for registered, searchable metadata entries (Federal Geographic Data Committee, 2000).

Aside from the quality of the geographic data itself, there are additional desirable properties for digital geographic databases (Worboys, 1995). Secure databases prevent unauthorized access or allow different levels of access. Security is particularly important for many databases containing health records for individuals. The issue of confidentiality of health data and its implications for mapping is discussed in greater detail in Chapter 7. Reliability of a database (as opposed to reliability of measurement) means that systems and data will be up and accessible when us-

TABLE 2.3. Content Standard for Digital Geospatial Metadata

Metadata content area	Content	Mandatory
Identification information	Basic information about the data set, including citation, description, time period of content, status, spatial domain, keywords, and access and use constraints	Yes
Data quality information	General assessment of the quality of the data set, including attribute accuracy, logical consistency, completeness, and positional accuracy	As applicable
Spatial data organization information	Representation of spatial information in the data set, including direct spatial reference method and point and vector object information or raster object information	As applicable
Spatial reference information	Description of the reference frame for and means of encoding coordinates in the data set, including the horizontal and vertical coordinate system definitions	As applicable
Entity and attribute information	Information content of the data set, including the entity types, their attributes, and attribute domains	As applicable
Distribution information	Basic information about the distributor of the data set and options for obtaining it	As applicable
Metadata reference information	Description of the metadata information, including metadata date, standard, metadata access and use constraints, and identification of responsible party for metadata preparation	Yes

ers need information. Finally, use of the data is facilitated when technological change is transparent to the user. "Technology-proof" systems insulate users from the technical aspects of the database system so that databases are not required to change with each new technological advance in hardware and software.

SPATIAL DATABASES IN A BASIC GIS CONFIGURATION FOR PUBLIC HEALTH

Spatial databases are accessed through hardware and software in a GIS to support database management, visualization, and analysis. The configuration of the PUBLIC HEALTH GIS created to prepare many of the figures in this book illustrates one approach developing a GIS for public health. The PUBLIC HEALTH GIS covers a region in central Connecticut comprised of 16 towns in two counties (Figure 2.18). This region has an area of approximately 356 square miles. The 1990 population of the region was 604,553. The region encompasses a mix of urban, suburban, and rural areas, and thus illustrates the diverse contexts for using GIS in public health applications.

The PUBLIC HEALTH GIS is a stand-alone system that could be developed by a public health organization getting started in GIS. The system hardware includes the following:

- A PC with 128 megabytes of RAM and a 450 mHz processor, a 20 gigabyte hard drive, a floppy disk drive, a zip drive, and a CD-ROM reader.
- A 17" color monitor.
- A standard keyboard and mouse.
- A black-and-white laser printer capable of printing up to 11" × 17" format;
- A color inkjet printer capable of printing up to 8.5" × 11" format.

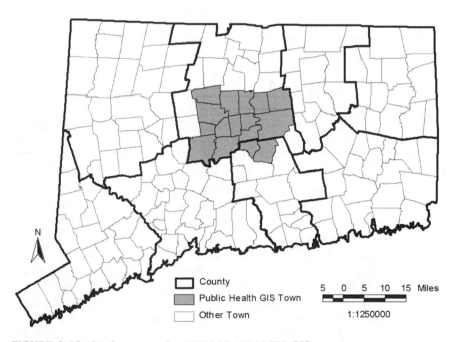

FIGURE 2.18. Study region for PUBLIC HEALTH GIS.

The system software includes the following:

- A vector GIS software system with limited raster capabilities that requires approximately 750 megabytes of storage.
- A standard package of word-processing and database management software, including relational database and spreadsheet packages.
- A statistical analysis software system.
- A graphics software system.

The system is configured with an ethernet connection and the necessary networking software to enable the computer to access information on an internal network and the Internet.

The PUBLIC HEALTH GIS database includes the full range of GIS data types assembled from a variety of sources. The GIS spatial and attribute databases used to prepare many of the examples in this book occupy approximately 500 megabytes on the hard drive. The organization of the data on the partitioned hard drive is an important part of the overall system design (Table 2.4). The c:\ drive on this system is a production environment for the GIS. The GIS software, the working applications, and the current databases are found here. The d:\ drive provides a development environment for applications that are being created, modified, and tested. Once ready for online use, these files can be moved to the c:\ drive. Foundation databases and image data, usually obtained from other agencies, reside in separate directories on the e:\ drive. The f:\ drive provides space for databases that are being edited and modified before they are ready to be moved to the c:\ drive.

All of the analyses, maps, and reports in this book from the PUBLIC HEALTH GIS were prepared using this system (Figure 2.19). This GIS can support a wide range of applications, as the examples demonstrate, but it has its limitations. On the input side, the system might be enhanced with the addition of a scanner and a digitizing tablet. In terms of processing, the main alternative to the PC would be a workstation. Different versions of the software would probably be required for the workstation platform. A larger monitor would also enhance the system. Users might find the stylus a more effective tool than the mouse for interacting with the system. On the output side, a large-format color printer or plotter capable of producing wall maps would be an important addition.

The PUBLIC HEALTH GIS described here would also need to be enhanced to support data distribution via electronic media or the Internet as an alternative to published reports and maps. A drive capable of writing data to CD would be useful, given the size of many public health databases. A more powerful processor with the appropriate software would be needed to serve data or GIS applications over an internal network or the Internet. This approach would also require additional personnel trained

TABLE 2.4. Organization of Data and Projects in the PUBLIC HEALTH GIS

Drive	Directory path				Description
c:\	data\	phgis\	attrib\	textfile\ spread\ database\	Attribute tables for health event databases in the PUBLIC HEALTH GIS (phgis); these can be organized in separate folders depending on whether the data are stored as textfiles, spreadsheets, or relational database tables.
			spatial\	vector\ raster\ other\	Spatial databases for health events in the PUBLIC HEALTH GIS (phgis); these can also be organized in separate folders depending on the data format. The attribute tables are joined to the spatial databases in the PUBLIC HEALTH GIS. Metadata files are stored with the data sets.
		othergis\	attrib\	textfile\ spread\ database\	Attribute tables for health event databases in another GIS project.
			spatial\	vector\ raster\ other\	Spatial databases for health events in another GIS project.
	projects\	phgis\	projects\ symbols\ icons\		Online PUBLIC HEALTH GIS applications and specially designed symbols and icons used in applications.
		othergis\	projects\ symbols\ icons\		Other online GIS applications and specially designed symbols and icons used in applications.
	docs\				Word-processing documents describing the GIS applications, databases, and system design, including database directories and user's guides for specially designed GIS applications.
d:\	gisvault\	data\	phgis\	attribute\ spatial\	Backup versions of the online data and versions used in creating, modifiying, and testing new or existing GIS applications.
		projects\	phgis\ othergis\		Backup versions of the online GIS projects and development versions used in creating, modifying, and testing new or existing GIS applications.
e:\	found\	doqq\ dlg\ TIGER\ cadast\ other\			Foundation data sets for the entire geographic domain of the public health organization. All or part of these data sets may be used in a specific GIS project.
f:\	working\	data\	phgis\ othergis\		Work space for preprocessing and editing data before they are moved to the d:\ drive for developing new applications or to the c:\ drive for online use.

in administering computer networks. Although it does not support the full range of GIS functions in a networked environment, the basic configuration of the PUBLIC HEALTH GIS reflects hardware and software trends over the last several decades that have affected GIS technology and provides a platform for developing GIS applications in public health.

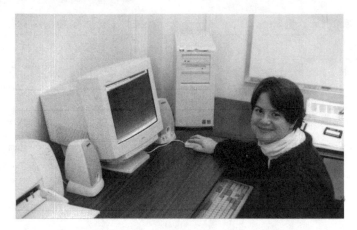

FIGURE 2.19. PUBLIC HEALTH GIS work area. Photograph by Kris White.

CONCLUSION

Many public health professionals and epidemiologists analyze databases that contain some geographic information, like a residential location. Use of these data in a GIS requires re-creating the database as a spatial database in a format that the GIS software can recognize. As GIS technology has developed, concern for the accuracy of spatial databases has grown and efforts have been made to develop standards for describing spatial databases that will enable users to assess the appropriateness and accuracy of the data and decide whether the spatial database can be used to answer the questions the user is asking.

GIS implementation involves creation, transformation, and analysis of potentially many spatial databases. In most GIS application areas, however, there are a number of "foundation" databases commonly used. The next chapter describes these databases and how they have been used in public health and epidemiological research.

CHAPTER 3

Spatial Databases for Public Health

Spatial data sets are fundamental components of GIS. The success of health-related GIS projects depends on having access to accurate, timely, and compatible spatial data. For organizations embarking on GIS projects, spatial data can be viewed as both a cost and a resource. Developing spatial data sets is expensive; it is estimated that well over half the cost of GIS projects goes to database creation, updating, and improvement. Yet database development is also an investment that creates long-term value for organizations and the people they serve. Spatial data sets are often useful for addressing a wide range of policy and planning issues. Their value extends well beyond the scope of the original projects for which they were created, and it increases as the data sets are used. This chapter describes the major types of spatial databases for public health GIS. We begin by discussing the concept of foundation data and summarizing major types of foundation data sets, including geodetic control, digital orthorectified imagery, and the TIGER/Line files. We then consider the diverse types of health data sets that can be incorporated in GIS. The final sections examine procedures for capturing health data in GIS and issues related to spatial data integration and sharing.

FOUNDATION SPATIAL DATA

In generating spatial databases for health GIS, the key linkage among data layers is the spatial linkage. Layers are tied together by their common geographical location. If a house is located a quarter-mile east of a park and adjacent to a hospital, these features should appear in the same relative positions in a GIS that connects data layers containing these features. In a GIS, we cannot link the locations of features directly to their positions on the earth since we are working at a scale much smaller than the earth. Therefore, spatial data layers must be connected to a foundation that makes spatial integration and linkage possible. Foundation data provide a geographical frame of reference to which other data layers are tied.

Foundation spatial data are "the minimal directly observable or recordable data to which other data are spatially referenced" (National Academy of Sciences, 1995, p. 16). We apply the term here to the spatial data layer to which other data layers are linked in a public health GIS project. As in constructing a building, the foundation supports the other data layers and defines the *footprint*, or geographical extent, of the GIS database. Many different types of spatial data can serve as foundation data, for example—digital imagery from aerial photographs or satellites, street centerline data, or property boundaries. These databases differ in their scale, resolution, degree of positional accuracy, and ease and cost of use. The choice of a foundation data set will be influenced by the scale of the analysis—for example, a study of health problems at the neighborhood scale requires foundation data at an equivalent spatial scale. This section explores the various types of foundation data for the United States and their characteristics.

Geodetic Control

Geodetic control is a system for registering location information to a set of well-defined points on the earth's surface. It includes a set of *survey monuments* on the ground and a *reference datum* that gives geographic coordinates for those monuments based on our knowledge of the size and shape of the earth. The reference datum is a key feature of geodetic control. In North America, the currently accepted reference datum is the North American Datum, 1983 (NAD-83). This datum is linked to the World Geodetic System, 1984, a geodetic control system for geographical coordinate use worldwide. The reference datum for North America has changed in recent years. For decades, the reference datum was the North American Datum, 1927 (NAD-27), replaced only recently by NAD-83. Spatial databases that were created before the mid-1980s often use NAD-27.

In developing GIS databases, it is critically important that all data layers use the same reference datum. Lat/lon coordinates based on NAD-27 versus those based on NAD-83 can differ by up to 100 meters in the lower 48 states, leading to positional errors and inconsistencies (Keating, 1993). When linking different spatial data layers, analysts should check the reference datums associated with each data set and, if necessary, convert all data sets to a common datum. Most GIS include commands for converting among NAD-27, NAD-83, and other common reference datums.

In most GIS applications, geodetic control is not used directly as a foundation data layer. Geodetic control is transparent, never displayed or connected with attribute information. However, understanding geodetic control and reference datums is vital for developing GIS data sets and ensuring consistent, accurate data linkage. In addition, the growing use of GPS receivers for generating coordinates heightens the importance of geodetic control because GPS coordinates are directly tied to geodetic control.

Digital Orthorectified Imagery

Digital orthorectified imagery (DOI) comprises pictures of the earth's surface that show the locations of features like roads, coastlines, and buildings. The pictures are raster images generated from aerial photography or satellites. Tied to geodetic control to permit matching with other spatial data layers, the images have the geometric properties of a map. DOI does not incorporate feature or attribute information: it simply provides an image of some part of the earth's surface. Identifying and recording features on the images requires image interpretation, field checking, or linkage with an attribute-based spatial data layer for the area. However, many significant landscape features are clearly visible on DOI.

An important kind of DOI for public health GIS is the *digital orthophotoquarterquad* (DOQQ). A DOQQ covers a "quarterquad," roughly a 4 mile × 4 mile area, at 1:12,000 scale. Produced by the U.S. Geological Survey in conjunction with other federal agencies, DOQQs depict roads, houses, trees, and other detailed features (Figure 3.1). With their high resolution and high degree of positional accuracy, DOQQs form a useful foundation data layer for localized, large-scale public health assessments, such as mapping individual exposures to environmental contaminants. Other data layers can be matched to DOQQs for detailed mapping and analysis.

Smaller scale DOI includes *satellite imagery* from systems like SPOT and Thematic Mapper. Sensors on satellites record energy reflected from the earth's surface for different wavelengths, or "bands," of the electromagnetic spectrum. Satellite images typically cover scales ranging from 1:50,000 to 1:100,000 at positional accuracies ranging from ±25 meters to ±70 meters (Keating, 1993). Although scale and positional accuracy vary widely across satellite imagery, generally the images show major features such as roads, rivers, fields, and water bodies (Figure 3.2). As in other forms of imagery, features are not labeled or identified; however, methods for digital image interpretation that distinguish land-use/land-cover features based on their distinct spectral characteristics are well developed and available in specialized computer software (Jensen, 1996). Some visible features in a satellite image vary seasonally because of changes in

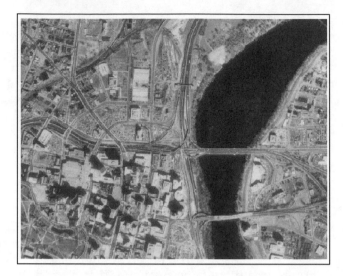

FIGURE 3.1. A portion of a digital orthophotoquarterquad for the area around downtown Hartford in the PUBLIC HEALTH GIS study area. The dark area running north–south just east of the center of the view is the Connecticut River. The town boundary between Hartford to the west and East Hartford is the center of the river.

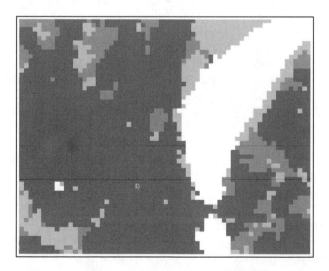

FIGURE 3.2. A portion of the land-use/land-cover database for the PUBLIC HEALTH GIS study area derived from Thematic Mapper imagery. The areas shaded dark gray were classified as commercial/industrial land. The areas shaded medium gray were classified as residential. The areas shaded light gray were classified as forest/turf. The areas shaded white were classified as deep or shallow water. This figure shows roughly the same part of the study area as Figure 3.1.

vegetation and precipitation. Cloud cover can also obscure features, complicating the interpretation of satellite images. In choosing a satellite image, the analyst should think through carefully the appropriate time of year for the image and the maximum allowable cloud cover. Detailed information is available for satellite imagery for the United States to aid the analyst in selecting useful images (U.S. Geological Survey, 2000).

Satellite images offer a useful foundation data layer for regional-scale health analyses covering states or parts of states. The images have been widely used in displaying and analyzing land-use, land-cover, and natural-resource patterns. In the public health field, the images have been utilized to analyze the geographic distribution and spread of vector-borne diseases such as Lyme disease (Glass et al., 1995).

Digital Line Graphs

Vector data also provide a foundation for regional-scale GIS development. *Digital line graphs* (DLGs) are vector databases that show transportation lines, water bodies, political boundaries, and elevation contour lines (Figure 3.3). Unlike imagery, DLGs include attribute information. Attribute codes describe the physical and cultural characteristics of points, lines, and areas on the DLG. DLGs are derived from the large- and intermediate-scale topographic maps created by the U.S. Geological Survey. They exist for all of the United States, excluding Alaska, at a scale of 1:100,000. Large-scale

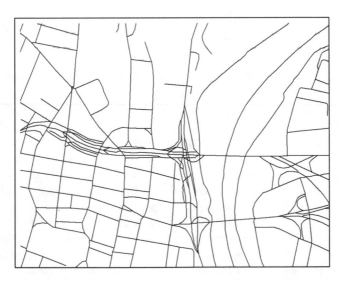

FIGURE 3.3. A portion of the 1:24,000 digital line graph database for the PUBLIC HEALTH GIS study area, including roads, streams, and town boundaries. This figure shows roughly the same part of the study area as Figure 3.1.

DLGs, generated from the 7.5-minute topographic maps, have been created for many areas of the United States (U.S. Geological Survey, 1998).

One concern in using DLGs is the accuracy and recency of attribute information. The sources of information for DLGs are topographic maps that themselves may be years out of date. The U.S. Geological Survey has updated its topographic map series through a procedure known as "limited update," focusing on those features that are most likely to have changed, such as roads and hydrography (U.S. Geological Survey, 1997). DOQs from aerial photography are the basis for limited-update revisions. The efficient, limited-update procedure will generate much more timely information for topographic maps and DLGs, but time lags naturally exist. For GIS, these issues are especially relevant in communities experiencing rapid population and commercial development where feature and attribute information changes frequently.

TIGER/Line Data

Another form of vector foundation data, compiled at 1:100,000 scale, is the *Topographically Integrated Geographic Encoding and Referencing* (TIGER/Line) data set (Marx, 1986). Produced by the U.S. Bureau of the Census, these files are used widely in population, health, political, and transportation mapping. TIGER/Line consists of *street centerline spatial data* in which street segments are represented as vectors to which attributes of the streets are attached (Figure 3.4). The TIGER/Line files differentiate the left- and right-hand sides of the street segment and include a wide range of attributes for each side: street name, address range, zip code, census and political units, and congressional district. In addition to street centerlines, the files also identify other important line features like railroads and water bodies.

The TIGER/Line files store spatial information for the geographical units the Census Bureau uses in tabulating and publishing census information. An understanding of census geography is important for any public health analyst who uses data compiled by the Census Bureau (U.S. Bureau of the Census, 1993). The smallest unit is the census *block*; each block is bounded by a set of connected street segments or other linear features such as rivers, railroad tracks, or municipal boundaries (Figure 3.5). A *block group* is a cluster of blocks, typically containing from 200 to 600 housing units. *Census tracts* comprise groups of contiguous blocks (and block groups) and have populations ranging from 2,500 to 8,000. TIGER/Line files also identify state, county, and local political boundaries, along with zip code boundaries. With this wide array of information, the TIGER/Line files are useful for creating polygons representing states, counties, census units, and other political/administrative regions that can

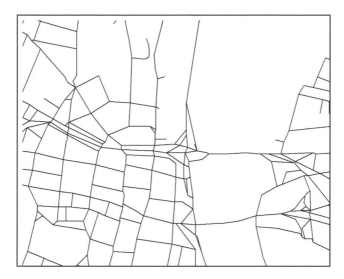

FIGURE 3.4. A portion of the TIGER/Line database of road features for the PUBLIC HEALTH GIS study area. This figure shows roughly the same area as Figure 3.1.

be joined to database tables describing the attributes of these areas. In fact, many vector GIS come bundled with TIGER-based spatial data to facilitate mapping of census data.

A major benefit of the TIGER/Line files is that they provide a connection between street addresses and locations on the ground. This makes it possible to locate or geocode address-based information such as hospital discharge records, birth certificates, and clinic locations. However, the TIGER/Line files do not record a precise location for each address, just an address range along a street segment; therefore, address locations can only be approximated by interpolation. This may pose few problems in urban and suburban areas where addresses are spread relatively evenly along street segments, but in rural areas TIGER/Line files must be used with caution for locating addresses if a high degree of positional accuracy is required.

TIGER/Line files offer detailed, large-scale, spatial data for urban and suburban areas. They cover all counties in the United States and were last released in 2000. Despite their wide coverage and applicability, the TIGER/Line files have several important limitations. First, street and address coverage is incomplete and in some cases inaccurate. Streets may be missing or misnamed. Address ranges may be missing, include incorrect values, or identify the wrong side of the street. These problems are espe-

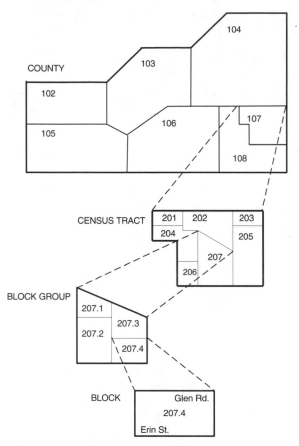

FIGURE 3.5. Geographic subdivisions for the U.S. Census. The smallest unit is the block. Each county is divided into census tracts, which are divided into block groups, and then into blocks.

cially relevant in rapidly growing communities where new residential development is taking place. Many local governments have enhanced and improved the TIGER/Line files for their local areas; this information was used to update TIGER for the 2000 Census (Sperling, 1995). Furthermore, commercial firms sell corrected and updated TIGER/Line files. In developing a TIGER database for a GIS, it is well worth seeking out the most accurate and updated version.

A second problem is that the positional accuracy of TIGER files is unknown and may vary from place to place. Positional accuracy is "no greater than the established National Map Accuracy Standards for 1:100,000-scale maps" (U.S. Bureau of the Census, 1992), although efforts were made to upgrade the positional accuracy of TIGER/Line for the 2000 Census. Thus, the files are logically consistent, but may be positionally inaccurate for large-scale mapping. This can affect health applications in several ways. It is impossible to pinpoint precise locations for large-scale mapping and analysis. Address locations are only estimated along street segments, and the segments themselves may be inaccurately located. Such positional inaccuracy may be irrelevant for a study of lead screening programs, for example; but in analyzing a problem like radon exposure, positional inaccuracy is extremely important. Also, TIGER data layers often do not match perfectly with layers generated from DLGs or DOQs. Rubbersheeting, discussed later in this chapter, is often needed to combine TIGER data with data from other sources. Despite these limitations, the TIGER/Line database remains one of the most important and widely used foundations for GIS-based health and socioeconomic analysis.

Cadastral Data

A second source of address-based spatial data, one that is generally more accurate than TIGER/Line for small geographic areas, is cadastral information. *Cadastral data* are data associated with land ownership. Cadastral features are not visible on the ground, but are legally defined to specify ownership and administration of land parcels (Huxhold & Levinsohn, 1995). Digital cadastral data files contain property boundaries and a wide range of attribute data, including land title, address, sale/resale information, and building type, size, and characteristics (Figure 3.6). Property boundaries are stored in a vector format, with property attributes attached. Because the files describe land ownership, they often have a high degree of positional accuracy and represent large spatial scales: 1:12,000 or larger. Address information is generally accurate and complete. Cadastral data also show street widths and thus better depict the built environment of a local area than does TIGER/Line.

Despite these advantages, cadastral data have important limitations. Although most communities collect and maintain cadastral spatial data, much of that data is not in digital form. Some communities still rely on paper maps and written descriptions of property boundaries, some of which are decades old. Furthermore, the quality and accuracy of cadastral data vary widely, depending on the recency and quality of the surveying or historical information on which it is based. Errors can creep into cadastral databases over time depending on how well the registry is kept as boundaries are resurveyed, landscape change occurs, and properties are subdivided. In addition, communities use different formatting systems for digital cadastral information, so conducting studies across community

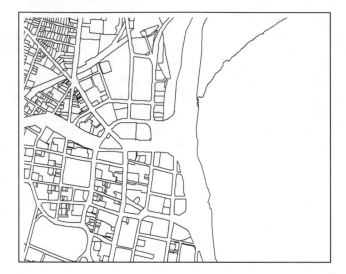

FIGURE 3.6. A portion of a cadastral database from the PUBLIC HEALTH GIS for the Town of Hartford. This figure shows roughly the same area as Figure 3.1. Property databases are generally maintained by local governments, so this database covers only Hartford and does not include properties in East Hartford.

boundaries can be challenging. Efforts are currently underway to develop common standards for cadastral information. Cadastral data files can also be large, unwieldy, expensive to create, and unnecessarily detailed for some kinds of spatial analysis. Network models (see Chapter 10), for example, require transportation routes to be represented as arcs, as in TIGER, rather than as double lines. Still, cadastral data offer an excellent foundation for address matching and mapping in small areas.

Choosing a Foundation Database

The foundation data sets described in this section each offer a unique set of advantages and disadvantages for public health GIS. They differ in scale, resolution, positional accuracy, and display of features, as well as in their raster or vector structure (Table 3.1).

The choice among foundation data sets depends on the scale and scope of the project, the resources available for data creation, and the types and scales of other data sets to which the foundation data will be linked. Projects that are national or regional in scope are more likely to utilize intermediate-scale foundation data, such as satellite imagery and DLGs. In contrast, studies of single communities or neighborhoods can take advantage of the detail and positional accuracy of cadastral data and DOQQs.

TABLE 3.1. Foundation Databases

Database	Scale	Source	Type
Digital orthophoto quadrangles	1:12,000–1:25,000	U.S. Geological Survey	Raster
Satellite imagery	1:25,000–1:100,000	Commercial	Raster
Digital line graphs	1:24,000 and 1:100,000	U.S. Geological Survey	Vector
TIGER	≥ 1:100,000	U.S. Bureau of the Census	Vector
Cadastral	1:200–1:12,000	Local government	Vector

HEALTH DATA

Foundation data create a platform for integrating spatial data layers that contain health, social, and environmental information. This section describes some of the major types of health information that can be incorporated in GIS for health planning, evaluation, and research. Our aim is here to introduce these data sets and highlight geographical issues that affect data use and integration in GIS; detailed discussion of the content of these data sources is available elsewhere (Halperin & Baker, 1992; Roper & Boorkman, 1994).

Vital Statistics

Local governments in the United States routinely collect information on all births and deaths that occur in their jurisdictions. These *vital records* are an important source of spatial data for public health GIS. Birth records document a wide range of conditions that affect newborn infants, including birthweight, gestational age, congenital malformations, and obstetric procedures, along with the mother's demographic and social characteristics and her use of prenatal services (Friis & Sellers, 1996). Information about the infant and the birth process is generally accurate, but data for the mother, especially that based on recall of timing and events during pregnancy, can have errors and inconsistencies. Still, birth data offer a nearly complete summary of basic maternal and infant health indicators for the population.

Birth records include the mother's residential address, a geographical identifier for GIS mapping and analysis. This information can be used to study environmental and neighborhood influences on maternal and infant health—for example, the effects of proximity to prenatal care services on prenatal care use and birth outcomes or the clustering of birth defects in relation to hazardous waste sites (Rushton & Lolonis, 1996).

Health departments also collect and report data on deaths in *mortality records*. Generated from death certificates, these data include demographic characteristics of the decedent and information about the cause of death, including the immediate cause and contributing factors (Friis & Sellers, 1996). Although demographic information is typically accurate, there are well-known problems with cause-of-death information stemming from errors and inconsistencies in diagnosis and difficulties in assigning causes when multiple causes are present (Garbe & Blount, 1992). Death certificates include two types of address-based geographic data: the actual place of death and the usual residence of the decedent. The place of death is often a hospital, nursing home, or other health care facility. This information can be used in analyzing health outcomes and service utilization by facility. In contrast, residential addresses provide a means for linking the residential environment to mortality outcomes.

Address-based vital statistics information presents several challenges to the GIS researcher. First, addresses may be incorrectly coded, making it impossible to identify geographical locations. In a study of birth defects in Des Moines, Iowa, 8% of birth records could not be geocoded because of errors in the addresses and "P.O. Box"– and "rural route"–style addresses (Rushton & Lolonis, 1996). Second, because of privacy and confidentiality concerns, many health departments do not release address information (Istre, 1992). They only provide data in aggregate form, by zip code, district, or census tract, making it impossible to analyze point locations. Third, even if current residential address information is correct, it may not accurately represent the environment of the person before and during pregnancy or prior to death because the relevant exposure may have occurred someplace other than the residence (see Chapter 5). This is particularly problematic for mortality data, given that the conditions that lead to death can result from lifelong exposures and behaviors.

Morbidity Data from Surveillance Systems and Disease Registries

Looking beyond life's vital events, morbidity data are an essential source of information for public health GIS. *Disease surveillance* involves monitoring distributions and trends in morbidity and mortality data collected for a specified population and geographical area. There are many kinds of morbidity data, ranging from information gathered by government agencies and health care providers to information from survey research projects. These data differ greatly in content, coverage of the population, and the geographic scale at which they are normally available.

Reportable disease data provide information on morbidity and mortality for certain "reportable" health conditions. Infectious disease has always been an important focus of public health surveillance in the United States (Centers for Disease Control and Prevention, 1997b). Authority to require notification of cases of disease resides in state legislatures. There is considerable variation in state provisions. All 50 states require physicians to report cases of specified notifiable diseases to state or local health departments. Notifiable disease reports and vital records are the two health data sources available at the local level in all states.

The National Notifiable Diseases Surveillance System is operated by the Centers for Disease Control and Prevention (CDC), in collaboration with the Council of State and Territorial Epidemiologists (CSTE). Reporting by the states to the national system is voluntary. States generally also report internationally quarantinable diseases (e.g., cholera, plague, yellow fever) in compliance with World Health Organization (WHO) International Regulations. There are approximately 50 infectious diseases designated as notifiable at the national level (Council of State and Territorial Epidemiologists, 1999). The list of nationally reportable infectious diseases and other conditions changes periodically, and reporting practices may differ from state to state (Roush, Birkhead, Koo, Cobb, & Fleming, 1999).

In addition to notifiable disease reports by providers such as physicians, hospitals, and laboratories, key data sources for infectious disease reporting in the United States include sentinel systems, hospital surveillance, school surveillance, special surveys at the state and local level, vital records, and vector/host surveillance for zoonotic diseases. *Sentinel* health events are cases of illness that signal a need for immediate public health intervention or serve as a warning of hazardous conditions or poor-quality medical care. A number of limitations of the current surveillance system have been described (Stroup, Zack, & Wharton, 1994). The fragmentation of the U.S. health system and voluntary reporting requirements affect the completeness of surveillance data. Generally, the reporting system is thought to work well for diseases that are serious, have clear symptoms, and require medical attention; however, coverage is incomplete for conditions that can be asymptotic (e.g., tuberculosis), that do not necessarily compel medical treatment (e.g., animal bite, gastroenteritis), or that carry social stigma (e.g., HIV/AIDS) (Friis & Sellers, 1996).

Underreporting of infectious disease conditions may be explained by a number of factors, including provider lack of awareness of reporting requirements. The level of public concern also affects disease reporting. Infectious diseases that carry some social stigma may be concealed. For many infectious diseases, symptoms are either too mild to prompt a person to seek medical care or they mimic flu-like symptoms associated with other common illnesses. For others, particularly emerging infectious diseases, the etiological definition may be incomplete or the case definition for surveillance purposes may be inadequate. "What is a case?" is not a trivial question. There may be differences of opinion about the criteria for defining a case of a disease. Sometimes case identification requires laboratory confirmation. In addition, case definitions change with changes in scientific knowledge. Changes in case definitions over time have an impact on what is included in the surveillance database. HIV/AIDS and Lyme disease, discussed in Chapters 7 and 8, illustrate these points.

Active surveillance systems obtain data by searching and periodic contact with providers. *Passive surveillance* systems rely on reports by providers themselves. Because of the costs associated with active surveillance, this type of system is often used strategically in limited areas or for limited time periods. Evaluation of active surveillance systems indicates twofold to fivefold increases in reporting of specified diseases and other conditions not subject to active surveillance (Vogt, LaRue, Klaucke, & Jillson, 1983; Thacker et al., 1986). Surveillance method, therefore, has implications for completeness of the data, an important dimension of spatial database quality. Active surveillance systems offer a mechanism for completing and correcting information from the reportable disease record, including address data used as geographical identifiers.

To protect privacy and confidentiality, federal agencies release reportable disease statistics only at the county level. Different policies exist in lower levels of government: some state or local health agencies will make information available for smaller geographical areas, or even by address, as long as the analyst agrees to maintain privacy and confidentiality. When address information exists, its accuracy can be problematic. Addresses may be missing or inaccurately coded. In an epidemiological study of reported rat bites in New York City, almost 40% of bite reports had missing or incorrect address information and could not be geocoded (Childs et al., 1998).

Disease registries are centralized databases for the collection of information on specific diseases, the best examples being the cancer registries managed by state and local health authorities (Friis & Sellers, 1996). Disease registries use a reporting system similar to that for reportable diseases, with health providers reporting occurrences to the appropriate state or local registry. Some disease registries actively seek out case information, while others simply gather reports. Furthermore, some registries keep longitudinal information, that is, they follow patients after diagnosis in order to track changes in health status and treatment regimes.

Cancer registries, the most extensive disease registries in the United States, offer a potentially valuable source of information for GIS analysis. Currently, 42 states and localities in the United States maintain cancer registries, some of which have existed for decades (Stroup et al., 1994). At the national level, the SEER program (Surveillance, Epidemiology, and End Results, of the National Cancer Institute) is an umbrella organization for a network of cancer registries that covers about 10% of the U.S. population. SEER includes active follow-up of living patients and is used to generate national estimates of overall cancer incidence and breakdowns by gender, race, age, and geographic location (Stroup et al., 1994).

As with the other types of health data, registries include residential address information, but that information is protected by laws governing privacy and confidentiality. Some states will release addresses for research studies as long as appropriate measures are taken to ensure confidentiality; however, once again, policies differ among states. Other problems with address information arise from changes and errors in the coding and formatting of addresses.

Surveillance systems and disease registries have been sources of data for many GIS case studies but very few statewide surveillance systems or registries have been fully linked to GIS (Devasundaram, Rohn, Dwyer, & Israel, 1998; Cromley, 2001). Implementation of a statewide or national surveillance system in GIS increases the likelihood that the case database will include cases identified using different case definitions and surveillance methods. To address this problem, case definition and surveillance method should be included as fields in a surveillance database.

Survey Data

To address a broader range of health issues than covered in standard vital statistics and morbidity data sets, public health researchers often turn to *survey information*. Surveys deal with a diverse array of health-related topics, topics that are beyond the scope of disease reporting systems and transcend biomedical concerns. Health surveys investigate health-related behaviors, psychosocial well-being, nutritional status, stress, and individual, family, and neighborhood circumstances that affect health. The major national surveys in the United States include the National Health and Nutrition Examination Survey (NHANES) and the National Health Interview Survey (NHIS). These surveys ask a detailed set of questions to a small, representative sample of the U.S. population. NHANES focuses on physiologic measures, measures of body weight and stature, and nutritional assessments. It has been conducted in three cycles since the early 1970s. NHIS, administered annually since 1957, collects information on health risk factors, chronic conditions, injuries, impairments, and health service utilization, based on household interviews (Stroup et al., 1994). These and other nationwide surveys offer a wealth of detailed health information that can be mapped and analyzed spatially.

Unlike other health data sets, surveys focus on a wide range of health-related issues such as disability, impairment, stress, and psychological well-being, and not just the presence of disease. They thus present a broader perspective on health than do standard public health databases.

Most surveys include residential address information because it is essential for contacting respondents; however, as with the other health databases, that information is not routinely released.

Surveys are also used to screen for problems like lead poisoning, PKU (phenylketonuria), and hypertension. *Screening surveys* are proactive public health activities that attempt to uncover health problems before symptoms appear and the problems are difficult and expensive to treat. Screening surveys differ in the range and nature of population covered. Some cover the full population, as in screening of newborns for PKU, and thus can be used to estimate incidence rates and create maps of geographic variation in incidence. By contrast, many screening surveys only target high-risk populations and people likely not to have been screened as part of their regular health care. Estimates and maps prepared from such surveys only pertain to the screened population. Reported incidence will naturally be higher in areas where more people were screened. GIS can be used to explore geographic variation in *screening penetration*, the percent of risk population screened.

Hospitals generate large quantities of spatial information on patients treated in their inpatient and outpatient facilities. These *hospital discharge data* provide an important base for examining hospital utilization and treatment patterns, though they are generally inadequate for population-based studies of morbidity because they are restricted to patients treated in hospitals. The large literature on small area variations in the rates of medical and surgical procedures relies primarily on hospital discharge data (Wennberg & Gittelsohn, 1982), and the data sets are widely used in health policy analysis and planning. Included in the data sets are: demographic information about the patient, primary and secondary diagnoses, diagnostic procedures, treatment procedures, length of stay, and insurance status. Hospital discharge data contain the patient's residential address, but that information is rarely released due to privacy considerations. Instead, hospital data can usually be obtained at the zip code level, because zip codes are part of the address and thus convenient geographical units for the release of hospital information.

This section has described several important, widely available health data sets that can be incorporated in public health GIS. The data sets address a cross section of public health issues and offer a framework for diverse geographical investigations. Increasingly these information resources are available on electronic media, including the Internet, and are readily accessible to users in a wide variety of settings (Friede & O'Carroll, 1996). Many other health data sets exist. We have not even mentioned the vast proprietary databases held by health insurance companies or the specialized data sets in areas such as occupational, veterinary, and environmental health (Weise, 1997).

Spatial Resolution of Health Data

Regardless of which data sets are used, the spatial resolution of the data is crucial for GIS applications. Although all health data sets deal fundamentally with individuals and usually include address information, none routinely release those detailed geographical identifiers because of important privacy and confidentiality considerations. Thus, the analyst is typically faced with using health data that are aggregated to predefined geographical units, such as counties, zip codes, or census tracts. This raises important substantive issues, as well as significant methodological issues as discussed in Chapter 5. Substantive issues concern the validity and usefulness of particular areal units for public health planning and analysis.

Most data from federal health agencies are available at the county level. Although counties are generally good geographical units for displaying health data at the national scale, they have important limitations (Croner, Pickle, Wolf, & White, 1992). Counties are administrative political units that bear little relationship to areas defined according to socioeconomic, demographic, or environmental criteria. Counties often encompass diverse physical environments and heterogeneous populations. Moreover, the areas differ greatly in population size and areal extent. Counties large in area visually dominate the national map, despite the fact that they may have tiny populations. Small urban counties can hardly be seen on a national map, though they have huge populations. Thus counties are not comparable to one another, and they have little in terms of population and environmental factors relevant to public health. By comparison, census tracts, defined by the U.S. Bureau of the Census for tabulation purposes, are more similar than counties in population size and follow moderately well the fuzzy boundaries of social, economic, and ethnic areas.

Zip codes, commonly used for the tabulation of health data, have problems analogous to those for counties. Originally, zip codes were devised by the U.S. Postal Service to facilitate mail delivery, with each zip code representing a collection of mail distribution points. The areas have little correlation with socially and environmentally defined areas. In cities, some zip codes encompass neighborhoods with highly divergent economic and social characteristics. For instance, one zip code in New York City includes census tracts whose 1990 median incomes ranged from $15,000 to $42,000, a threefold difference. A health statistic for such a zip code would represent an "average" of statistics for two very different population groups. Another problem is that zip code boundaries occasionally cut across political and census boundaries, making it difficult to overlay and integrate zip code data with other sociopolitical data (Kirby, 1996). Thus, while zip codes are convenient geographical units for the reporting of health data, they are by no means natural or rational units for GIS-based health analysis.

HEALTH SERVICES DATA

Health service information forms another valuable spatial data layer for public health GIS. Most health care providers—hospitals, physicians, clinics—offer their services from fixed locations and can be represented as point spatial data. A few health services, such as emergency medical services and mobile clinics, move from place to place and thus can be modeled as arc or network information. Beyond location, many other dimensions differentiate health services, including price, capacity, utilization, range of services provided, and the elusive quality of care.

Information about the locations and characteristics of health care providers is widely available. *Gazetteers* include geographical coordinates for major health facilities such as hospitals. These coordinates can be imported into GIS for mapping and display; however, one must make sure that the location coordinates use the same scale and projection system as the foundation data layer to which they will be linked. One shortcoming of gazetteers is that they do not include data on the characteristics of health service facilities. Such information must be brought in from other sources and linked to the facility sites.

Detailed information on health care providers comes from professional organizations like the American Hospitals Association (AHA) and the American Medical Association (AMA). The AHA publishes an annual directory of hospitals that includes statistics on utilization, personnel, services, and finances for hospitals in the United States (American Hospital Association, 1999). Included in the directory is each facility's street address, which can be geocoded to a point location. Similar kinds of directories exist for nursing homes and mental health facilities. For physicians, the AMA's Physician Masterfile offers analogous information and includes addresses that can be geocoded to identify point locations (American Medical Association, 1998). The Masterfile covers the vast majority of physicians, but certain important subgroups may be missing—for example, doctors who earned medical degrees outside the United States whose practices are often clustered in immigrant neighborhoods.

Data for other types of health care providers are often harder to come by. Health clinics, for example, are operated by federal, state, and local governments, as well as by voluntary organizations. Each type of agency maintains a list of its own clinics, but there may be no composite listing of facilities in an area. It may be necessary to piece together information from multiple sources or to conduct fieldwork to uncover all health service locations. Despite these challenges, creating spatial data layers for health care providers is generally easier than preparing health and foundation data layers. Health services are limited in number, exist at discrete locations, and change relatively slowly over time, making them more manageable to deal with in a GIS context.

MAKING HEALTH DATA MAPPABLE

In order to use health and health care data sets in GIS, the data sets must first be captured and linked to a foundation spatial database. Data capture is a complex process that draws on an ever-increasing array of tools including scanning, digitizing, downloading from the Internet, and entering data directly from the field via GPS. This section focuses on the two procedures typically used for capturing health information: address matching and joining.

Address Matching to Locate Health Events as Points

Health information is often georeferenced by street address. For example, we might have information on the residential addresses of people who died of breast cancer, or the addresses of hospitals, health clinics, schools, or workplaces. Using the process of *address match geocoding*, we can convert each address to a point on a map. The point is recorded as a pair of geographical coordinates that connect to the foundation database. At its simplest, address matching involves the comparison of two data sets: one containing the addresses of health events and the other a foundation database with its own address information. An address (street name, number) and zone (a town name or zip code) from the first database is compared against the full array of addresses in the second, and a "match" occurs when the two agree.

Address-match geocoding procedures differ slightly depending on the type of foundation spatial database used in matching. If it is a cadastral or property database, then the address associated with a health event is compared sequentially with the addresses in the property database. When a match occurs, the health event is assigned the geographical coordinates of the corresponding property. Up-to-date property databases form an accurate platform for address matching because each address is associated with a unique property on the ground. The downside is that such databases are typically very large and cumbersome to work with and they are compiled and maintained at the local level.

Street centerline databases, like TIGER/Line, are a more common foundation for address matching. Because street centerline databases do not include unique street addresses for specific structures, only address ranges along street segments, address matching relies on interpolation.

We match the particular address to a street segment (street name and address range) and estimate the location of the address along the segment by interpolating within the corresponding address range. For example, the street address "107 Oak Avenue" is assigned to the segment of Oak Avenue with address range 101–119 (Figure 3.7). By interpolation, the location of 107 Oak Avenue is estimated to be about one-third of the way along the street segment. GIS users can specify an offset to take into account the setback of the structure from the street centerline.

This form of address matching does not place points at the exact locations of the structures, but rather at estimated locations along street segments. In urban and suburban areas, where properties are spaced fairly evenly along segments, spatial accuracy is generally quite good. In rural areas, the uneven spatial distribution of properties can cause significant spatial error from interpolation.

Address matching is an iterative procedure in which we first attempt to match all addresses and then correct those that fail to match. Typically one-half to two-thirds of addresses match in the first attempt. We then examine the unmatched addresses for obvious errors or inconsistencies. Often there are simple errors in spelling or abbreviation that can be easily corrected. After correcting obvious errors, it is typical to achieve a "match rate" of over 90% in most parts of the United States. Anything less calls

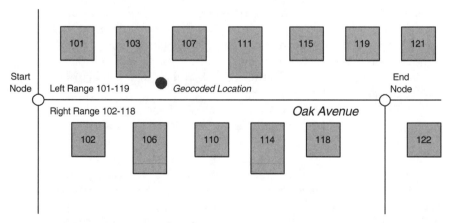

FIGURE 3.7. The TIGER/Line files include street centerline and address-range information that can be used in geocoding. This segment of Oak Avenue is represented by a start node and an end node, each with geographic coordinates. The address range for the left side of the segment contains odd-number addresses, while that for the right side contains even-number addresses. By interpolation, the location of 107 Oak Avenue is estimated to be approximately one-third of the distance along the corresponding street segment of Oak Avenue.

for an assessment of the quality of both the address list and the spatial database used in matching.

Addresses can fail to match because of errors in the address list, errors in the street or property database, or inconsistencies between them. Errors in the address list are common; they include misspellings and typographical errors in the street number, street name, or zone (Table 3.2). These errors can easily be corrected by carefully inspecting and editing the address list. Furthermore, most GIS provide the option of automatically correcting the most common types of errors using simple rules and conventions. One should approach these automatic correction algorithms with caution, however, because they may falsely change the original address data and generate a false sense of accuracy.

Errors in the street or parcel database, including missing street segments and incorrect address range information, also create problems for address matching. As the accuracy of spatial databases improves, it is less common today than in the past to find true errors in such databases. Rather, most errors result from the time lag between new residential development and database update. Addresses fail to match because they are located in newly developed areas that have not been mapped or entered into a spatial database. Since these addresses must then be geocoded or digitized by hand, it is well worth the investment to use the most accurate and up-to-date street or parcel database.

Finally, addresses can fail to match because of inconsistencies between the address list and the foundation database. These include differences in street-naming convention—for example, "6th Avenue" versus "Avenue of the Americas"—or in abbreviation—"St." versus "Str." Most GIS automatically correct obvious differences in abbreviation.

Although most analysts emphasize the "match rate," it is important to remember that a successful address match does not guarantee accuracy. Even if an address is successfully matched, it may not be assigned to the correct location. A field check of over 500 geocoded residential addresses to assess spatial accuracy uncovered a variety of errors (Cromley, Archambault, Aye, & McGee, 1997). The relative locations of 7% of the cases were incorrect. A few cases (less than 1%) had been geocoded to locations more than 500 feet away from the correct location. This type of error would be of particular concern in any study measuring distances from the geocoded location to another location because the true distance would be over- or underestimated. The remaining cases were estimated to be out of position by less than 500 feet. About half of these cases were on the wrong side of the street or on the wrong corner of an intersection. This type of error would be of particular concern in any study aggregating cases to an area like a census block or block group because census area boundaries often coincide with street centerlines so cases on the wrong side of the street would be aggregated to incorrect spatial units. For 1% of the ad-

TABLE 3.2. Sources of Error Affecting Address Match Outcomes

Record content	Street numbers	Street name	Street type	Zone (zip code example)	Address match outcome for perfect match
Correct address	16	Main	St.	13501	Match at correct location
Correct street segment	Left 2–20 Right 1–19	Main	St.	13501	
Error in address record					
Incomplete address		Main	St.	13501	No match
Error in street number	166	Main	St.	13501	No match
Error in street name	16	Nain	St.	13501	No match
Error in street type	16	Main	Rd.	13501	No match
Error in zone	16	Main	St.	113501	No match
Address does not correspond to a real structure	16	Main	St.	13501	Match represents a structure that does not exist
Error in street segment record					
Missing range	Left Right	Main	St.	13501	No match
Error in range	Left 2–14 Right 1–19	Main	St.	13501	No match
Range applied to wrong side of street	Left 1–19 Right 2–20	Main	St.	13501	Match represents incorrect location
Error in street name	Left 2–20 Right 1–19	Nain	St.	13501	No match
Error in street type	Left 2–20 Right 1–19	Main	Rd.	13501	No match
Error in zone	Left 2–20 Right 1–19	Main	St.	113501	No match
Incomplete street network database					No match

dresses, no residential structure could be found: either the structure had been removed or the street number was incorrect but fell within a valid address range. Such errors can have significant impacts on spatial analyses based on geocoded data.

These findings emphasize the importance of obtaining accurate address information and the need to look beyond the match rate in geocoding. Typically, the collection of addresses is decentralized. Addresses are entered at the source institution—for example, a hospital, doctor's office, or health clinic. From there, the institution transmits the information to a public health agency for mapping. Unless the addresses are used for billing or follow-up, the institution will have little stake in their accuracy and completeness. Errors emerge much later during address matching, and data editing and cleaning are performed by GIS personnel far removed from the source of data collection. Improving accuracy in geocoded address information requires not just better address-matching algorithms, but institutional arrangements that foster accuracy at the source.

The findings also emphasize the need for field checking of data, particularly when research findings are sensitive to the locations of cases in a few places. Researchers involved in GIS studies at a community scale can benefit from field trips to the study area before data collection and analysis to familiarize themselves with residential patterns and other landscape features of relevance to the particular study.

Joining Health Data to Geographical Areas

Many health and social databases only present information for geographical areas like counties, zip codes, or census tracts. They include the area name and/or identifier and a set of variables that describe the health events, population, or other attributes of the area—for example, the census tract number and number of diagnosed cases of AIDS by tract. Capturing area data in a GIS involves *joining*. We "join" the tabular data to a foundation spatial data set of area boundaries based on a common field like the census tract identifier. The data for each tract are attached to the corresponding geographical tract in the foundation database.

Joining requires that each geographical area have a unique identifier, either a name or a number. In the United States, state names are unique, as are zip code numbers. However, many widely used areal units such as census tracts or blocks have identifier numbers that are unique only within larger units of geography. Census tract numbers are unique only within counties, and block numbers are unique only within tracts. A project that cuts across these larger units must create a new field that uniquely identifies each small area. In a tract-level study that encompasses many counties in several states, for example, the state number and county number must be included along with the tract number to define each tract (Figure 3.8).

The Federal Information Processing Standard (FIPS) contains codes for states, named populated places, primary county divisions, and other entities (National Institute of Standards and Technology, 1994a). Familiarity with the FIPS and U.S. Bureau of the Census identifiers for geographical units within GIS databases is important for accurately joining and ma-

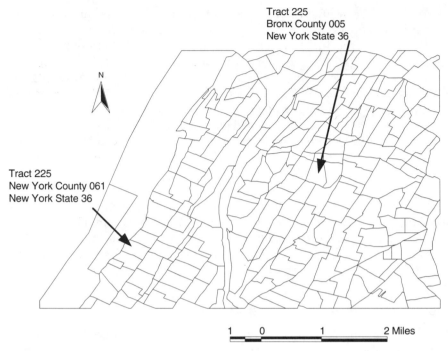

Tract 225
Bronx County 005
New York State 36

N

Tract 225
New York County 061
New York State 36

1   0   1   2 Miles

FIGURE 3.8. Census identifiers for tracts, block groups, and blocks are unique only in the context of the hierarchy of census units. Two tracts in New York City have the same tract identifier number, 225.

nipulating geographic databases produced by the federal government (Table 3.3). State governments may have developed additional numeric identifiers for geographical units within their states.

Typically joining links area-based health information to the corresponding geographical areas in a foundation spatial database. However, the procedure can also be used with address-based health data to find the area in which a health event is located. We match the address field in the health data set directly to the corresponding address field (street name and address range) in a foundation database table, like TIGER/Line, that contains area identifiers. Two tables, one for the health data set and the other for the foundation data set, are joined based on common address information. If this approach is used, the ability to map address-based health data as points is lost. As a consequence, the methods described in Chapters 4 through 10 for analyzing patterns of health data represented as points cannot be applied. Spatial information is lost when address-based health data are joined to areas rather than geocoded as points.

TABLE 3.3. Comparison of FIPS, Census, and State Identifiers for an Area

Area name	Hartford (City)	Hartford (Town of)
FIPS/Census state code for Connecticut	09	09
FIPS/Census county code for Hartford County	003	003
FIPS place code	37000	37070
FIPS class code	C1	T5
Census MCD code		070
Census place code	0970	
Connecticut state code	064	064

Note. These entries show that there are five different numerical codes for the same geographical area called Hartford. The FIPS and Census codes for the State of Connecticut and for Hartford County are the same. FIPS has two different place codes for Hartford: 37000 identifies Hartford as an active incorporated place, while 37070 identifies Hartford as a minor civil division. The Census minor civil division code for the Town of Hartford is 070; the Census place code for Hartford is 0970. Under a numerical coding system developed by the State, Hartford is 064. GIS users need to be aware of the coding systems that have been used to assign identifiers to geographical areas when joining and linking databases.

DATABASE INTEGRATION

The power of a GIS lies in its ability to link, integrate, and manipulate the diverse types of spatial data described in this chapter. Integrating such data sets can be challenging, especially when the data sets differ in scale, resolution, and geographic extent. Most GIS packages include a series of cartographic and geographic procedures for linking and integrating spatial data sets (Table 3.4).

A common data-integration problem arises when data layers that will be overlayed or linked in a GIS rely on different coordinate systems or different map projections. Typically this occurs when a health or environmental data layer is being integrated with a designated foundation data layer. Common in all GIS are procedures for transforming coordinates so that they are consistent with those of the foundation data layer. *Coordinate translation* involves computing new coordinates as a mathematical function of the original set. Linear transformations, for example, can be used to move, stretch, or twist the coordinate axes (Figure 3.9). These simple linear transformations are often necessary when integrating spatial data from a digitizing tablet or scanner with existing geospatial foundation data sets like DOQs or DLGs.

Sometimes geographical errors in overlaying data layers stem from positional inaccuracies that are unevenly or unpredictably distributed

TABLE 3.4. Spatial Database Collection and Preprocessing Operations

Function class	Function
Data collection	Scanning
	Digitizing
	Address-match geocoding
Data conversion	Importing/exporting
	Edgematching
	Clipping
	Raster/vector conversion
Geometric transformation	Translation
	Rotation
	Map projection
	Rubbersheeting
Generalization	Line thinning
	Line smoothing

across the map. In this case, matching data layers requires nonlinear coordinate transformations that stretch or shrink different parts of a map until features align correctly with those on the foundation data layer. *Rubbersheeting* is the process of geometrically adjusting features to force a digital map to fit the designated foundation data layer (Antenucci, Brown, Croswell, Kevany, & Archer, 1991). Rubbersheeting changes the relative locations of features, thus distorting the original map. Therefore the process should be used judiciously to make relatively small changes in map coordinates. Of course, when the map is being linked to an up-to-date, planimetrically correct foundation data set, rubbersheeting can partially compensate for positional errors in the source map. Distorting an inaccurate source map may be a good thing. Rubbersheeting is often required in order to integrate data with low or unknown positional accuracy with more accurate foundation data layers—for example, in linking the TIGER/Line files, with their variable positional accuracy, to a DOQQ base.

Another kind of coordinate transformation is needed when data layers are based on different map projections. *Map projection transformation* is the change in coordinates from one map projection to another. Data that come from different sources often utilize different map projections, so that coordinates must be reprojected for the data to overlay properly. All GIS have built-in functions for converting among common map projections.

Another common problem in creating and linking spatial data sets involves changing the geographical extent of the data set. The analyst may

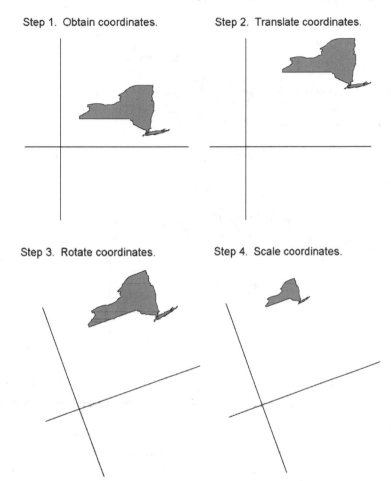

Step 1. Obtain coordinates.

Step 2. Translate coordinates.

Step 3. Rotate coordinates.

Step 4. Scale coordinates.

FIGURE 3.9. Coordinate translation of a spatial database of New York State.

want to focus on one portion of the mapped area—for example, one municipality within a county—or to join maps together to create a map layer that covers a larger geographical area. In GIS, one can extract a portion of a mapped data set by cutting out the portion from surrounding areas and saving it in a separate file (Figure 3.10). These *clipping* or *windowing* procedures are easy and efficient in GIS, where they can be done by using the cursor to define a rectangle or irregular shape.

Edgematching is a procedure for joining maps together by matching common features along the shared map boundary. For example, a particular road appearing at the edge of one map is matched to its counterpart at the edge of the adjacent map (Figure 3.11). Most edgematching proce-

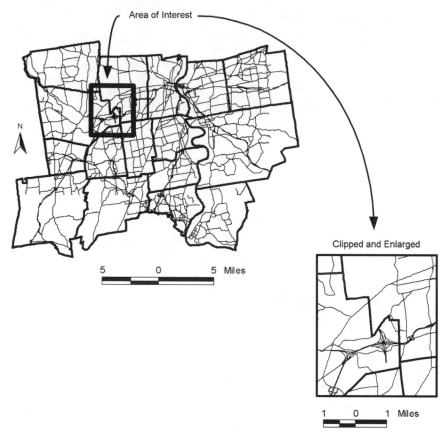

FIGURE 3.10. A window created around an area of interest can be used to "clip" the features of interest for viewing and analysis and for creating new databases containing just the clipped features.

dures also adjust features located in the area of overlap between the two adjacent maps to create a seamless map. For the procedure to work correctly, the maps being joined must have the same scale or resolution and contain comparable features. It is important to realize that edgematching creates a new topology for the database as, for example, two line segments are joined into one. The new topology enables new geographical analyses that address issues within the larger area.

DATA SHARING

Assembling diverse spatial data sets and linking them with foundation spatial data is a time-consuming, labor-intensive, and expensive process. The

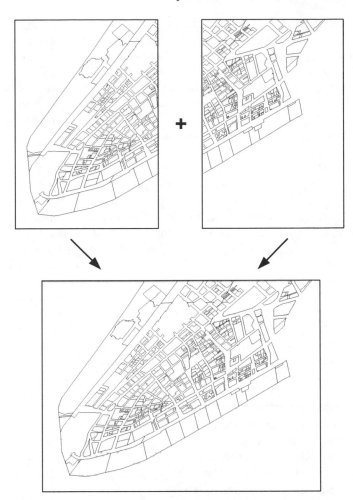

FIGURE 3.11. Two spatial databases of information for adjoining areas are joined by "matching" common features along the boundary to create a single seamless database.

final product—an integrated ensemble of health, environmental, social, and foundation data—represents not only a major investment, but also a major resource, with value to other users analyzing issues in the same geographical area. *Data sharing*, the transfer of data between two or more organizations, offers many important benefits to the developers and users of geographic information (Onsrud & Rushton, 1995). The value of spatial data derives from its use, so enabling diverse groups to draw on the same data creates value by stimulating use. Data sharing is also a means for spreading the costs of database creation among multiple users and avoiding needless duplication of effort. Finally, there are often synergies in multiple use and analysis of a common spatial database. One group's insights spark another's, resulting in greater value overall.

Organizations at the regional, state, and national levels are increasingly recognizing these benefits and taking steps to promote spatial data sharing. In some parts of the United States, regional consortiums are developing integrated spatial databases for their regions by combining foundation data with environmental, social, and transportation information. States are also taking the lead by creating spatial data clearinghouses or unified state-level spatial databases. Most of these efforts involve extensive participation by local governments who provide spatial data and draw upon it for local and regional planning purposes. At the national level, efforts are underway to develop a *national spatial data infrastructure* (NSDI) that consists of environmental and foundation data for the entire United States (National Academy of Sciences, 1993). This project involves extensive cooperation among various levels of government and the use of explicit metadata standards that permit data integration and sharing. In the long run, the NSDI will form a national resource for planning and policymaking in many arenas, including health.

Despite the many advantages of data sharing, technical and institutional barriers often get in the way. Sharing requires networked systems and agreements and common data formats that permit electronic exchange of information among users. Differences in hardware, software, and metadata standards impede spatial data sharing. For example, some local governments resist participating in the NSDI because of the cumbersome metadata standards. More fundamentally, sharing requires cooperation among diverse institutions and branches of government and a shared sense of purpose. Differences in organizational needs, cultures, and interests make cooperation among organizations challenging at best (Obermeyer, 1995). Organizations often operate autonomously, emphasizing their particular needs and missions. According to Craig (1995, p. 108), "Agencies could share data, but they choose not to do so." Thus, data sharing is an inherently political process reflecting power, inertia, and access to resources. These political and institutional factors far outweigh the technical barriers to data sharing (Onsrud & Rushton, 1995).

An important barrier to sharing health data is the need to protect the privacy and confidentiality of health information. Many state and federal agencies gather health data on individuals and are involved in data sharing. A study conducted in Wisconsin identified 30 units in 13 different state agencies that collected and maintained health information on identifiable individuals (American Civil Liberties Union of Wisconsin, 1999). These activities were carried out under specific statutory and regulatory authorizations for gathering, using, and releasing health information, in recognition of the many valid reasons for agencies to collect and rerelease medical data. Nevertheless, advances in computer technology, including GIS, raise new questions about transfers of identifiable encoded data without safeguards to ensure that patients have authorized the release of information and that data integrity is maintained. "The dilemma is how to balance demands for data to serve some real or perceived greater good with demands for personal privacy and patient autonomy" (American Civil Liberties Union of Wisconsin, 1999). The basic elements of the NSDI have been suggested as a model for establishing an effective process to catalog, make accessible, and protect geographically referenced health data (Neibert & Reichardt, 2000).

CONCLUSION

This chapter has examined spatial data resources for public health GIS in the United States and geographical, technical, and institutional concerns in data integration. Investing in a GIS means investing in spatial data. Given the wide array of data sets available and the high costs of new database development, organizations need to carefully assess their spatial data needs and view development as a long-term investment rather than a short-term expense. As developers and users of spatial data, it is essential that public health organizations participate in the emerging efforts to create open, accessible, and integrated spatial data resources. Agencies need to plan how spatial data will be used internally, how to make it accessible to others, and how to promote spatial data sharing in partnership with other organizations.

CHAPTER 4

Mapping Health Information

Preparing and displaying maps of health information are two of the most important functions of public health GIS. GIS offer a flexible, computerized environment that facilitates new forms of data exploration and analysis. One can easily pan across a map, zoom in on areas of interest, or query a database to examine areas or events of special concern. Health information can be linked with social and environmental features to examine geographical associations. The map, then, is just one product of a process of exploring, viewing, and analyzing spatial information. There is no perfect map; rather, each map is one of an almost infinite array of possible representations of spatial information. This chapter describes the procedures for displaying spatially referenced health information and preparing maps in GIS. After offering a general introduction to the mapping process, we discuss strategies for mapping health information. The next section considers how we can move beyond the map to view and explore health information. The final section addresses map design, creating a map for presentation or publication.

THE MAPPING PROCESS

Advances in computer technology and GIS have fundamentally changed the process of mapmaking. Traditionally, maps were viewed primarily as tools for communication (DeMers, 2000). The main goal was to communicate information most effectively by carefully preparing a "finished" map. Issues of design and composition were paramount. Today's GIS and computer technology have turned this perspective on its head. The mapping process now emphasizes the representation and analysis of information rather than the preparation of a finished map (Tobler, 1959; MacEachren, 1995).

The mapping process brings together four key elements: the *spatial data* that is stored or entered into the GIS, as discussed in Chapters 2 and 3; the *representations* of that information on maps or computer screens; socially defined *queries* about the spatial data; and the *analysts* who create maps and respond to queries (Figure 4.1). The activities associated with mapping exist in and are shaped by the social and economic contexts in which maps are made (Chrisman, 1997). People and organizations involved in the mapping process decide what information will be analyzed, the types of queries to be made, and how the information is represented on a map.

The elements in the mapping process are interconnected. Queries, the questions asked about geographical issues and associations, play a central role. They define the kinds of data and information that are collected and analyzed, and shape how the analyst represents that information on a map or computer screen. Viewing the data spatially often leads to new and revised queries, and thus to new maps. Viewing data spatially may even provide an impetus for collecting new spatial data. Thus, the mapping process links data, representations, queries, and people in an iterative and fluid way. It has no clear starting point, results in no necessary "finished" product, and thus can lead to many different representations of the same information.

The use of mapping to examine the high rates of breast cancer in

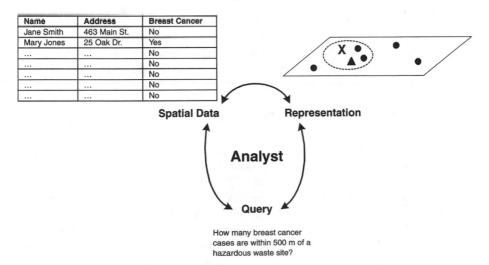

FIGURE 4.1. The mapping process.

Long Island illustrates well this new mapping process (National Cancer Institute, 2000). In the 1980s, many women in Long Island expressed concern about the high rates of breast cancer in their communities. Taking matters into their own hands, the women formed breast cancer coalitions, conducted surveys of breast cancer prevalence in their communities, and created simple "pin maps" of breast cancer prevalence. Their maps generated a host of hypotheses about the links between environmental and social factors and breast cancer (Grimson, 1999). Some community groups plotted the locations of environmental features on their pin maps of breast cancer cases. At the same time, the New York State Health Department conducted a GIS-based investigation into the connections between breast cancer risk and exposure to hazardous industrial facilities and high traffic density (Lewis-Michl et al., 1996). Data from a case–control interview study of breast cancer were overlayed on maps showing the locations of industrial facilities and major traffic corridors and then the relationships between health and environmental factors were analyzed statistically.

These investigations did not produce conclusive findings, but they laid the groundwork for a much larger GIS and epidemiological study of breast cancer and environment on Long Island sponsored by the National Cancer Institute. An Internet-based health GIS that will give community groups and researchers access to a diverse array of health, social, and environmental data sets for the region is currently being developed (National Cancer Institute, 1999, 2000). For those investigating high rates of breast cancer on Long Island, mapping and analysis have been closely intertwined. Many different groups, including grass roots community groups, researchers, local and state health departments, and federal agencies, have viewed and analyzed spatial health data. They have explored hypotheses, prepared maps, and created queries to represent their diverse perspectives. Mapping and GIS analysis continue, drawing upon more accurate data covering a range of social and environmental risks.

REPRESENTING HEALTH INFORMATION

A key component of the mapping process is the representation of spatial information. *Representation* is the process of creating symbols to portray objects, quantities, or events. Maps are representations, as are the views on a GIS computer screen (MacEachren, 1995). Representations both illuminate and hide information. The symbols included on a map or display reveal features and associations; meanwhile, other features not represented by symbols are hidden from view. No map could possibly represent the richness of the earth's surface and its inhabitants, so, as Monmonier (1996, p. 1) writes, "the map must offer a selective, incomplete view of reality."

Representing health information on maps and map displays requires the intelligent use of symbols. Symbols convey information. They reveal what is important, show contrast, and identify patterns. As discussed in Chapter 2, the six *visual variables*—size, shape, orientation, texture, color hue, and color value—differentiate symbols on maps (Bertin, 1979). The symbols and mapping strategies used in representing health information vary according to the type of spatial information that is to be displayed. Point data are often shown on dot or point symbol maps, area data on choropleth maps, and linear data on network or flow maps. These are not rigid choices, however. A single map or view can combine all three types of information to show complex features and patterns—for example, point symbols can effectively show certain kinds of area data. These different mapping approaches are discussed in the sections that follow.

Representing Point Information

Much health information consists of point locations—for example, hospitals, residences of people who experience particular health problems, accident locations, and hazardous facilities – that can be represented effectively on dot or point symbol maps. On a *point symbol map*, point symbols correspond to one or more events, and concentrations of point symbols reveal clusters of events (Figure 4.2). As the number of points varies across the map, the viewer senses the general pattern of density change. Point maps are useful devices for viewing health information. As noted earlier, many community-based breast cancer groups in Long Island, New York, have gathered data on the residential locations of all women diagnosed with breast cancer. Point symbol maps of geocoded locations have been used to search for clusters of breast cancer and to generate hypotheses about links to environmental hazards.

A challenge in using point symbol maps to represent spatial patterns of disease is that differences in dot density may simply reflect differences in risk population. A cluster of breast cancer cases may coincide with a cluster of women whose age and sociodemographic characteristics place them at risk for breast cancer. One way to address this problem is to display the locations of both people diagnosed with a disease and those at risk by using contrasting point symbols. Differences in density reveal clusters of one group relative to the other (Figure 4.3).

Creating point maps involves the careful choice of symbols. Symbols differ in size, shape, hue, and the other visual variables. Varying symbol size is one way to create contrast and to show quantity. In a *proportional symbol map*, symbol size is proportional to the number of events at a place. Large dots are highly visible, representing large concentrations of events. Shape also distinguishes symbols, making them easier to perceive and understand. Symbols can be *geometric*, involving simple geometric shapes like

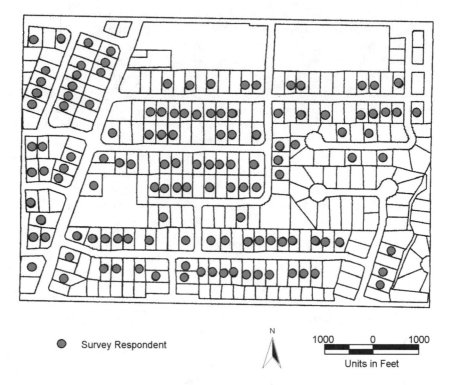

● Survey Respondent

N

1000   0   1000

Units in Feet

FIGURE 4.2. A point symbol map showing residential locations of survey respondents.

circles or squares, or *pictorial*, involving simple pictures such as houses or churches (Fry, 1988). Geometric symbols are generally easier to read and distinguish on maps, but they are not as interpretable as picture symbols.

Color hue and value are also important devices for differentiating symbols and other map features. A recent collaborative research project between the National Center for Health Statistics (NCHS) and geographers at Pennsylvania State University examined the effectiveness of color for representing public health data on maps (Brewer, MacEachern, Pickle, & Herrman, 1997). The researchers concluded that "color is clearly worth the extra effort and expense it adds to map making because it permits greater accuracy in map reading" (p. 434).

The map in Figure 4.3 combines shape and color value to create contrast. Small, circular gray dots represent women over age 25, and black stars identify women diagnosed with breast cancer. The darker shade and contrasting shape draw the eye to the places where women diagnosed

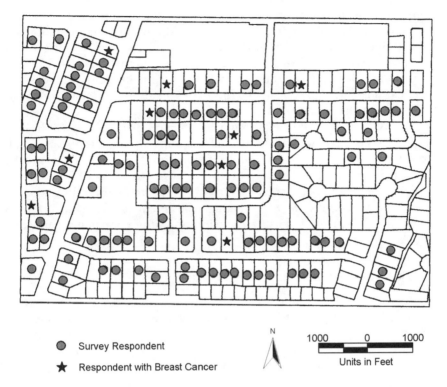

● Survey Respondent

★ Respondent with Breast Cancer

N

1000   0   1000

Units in Feet

FIGURE 4.3. Use of contrasting point symbols to differentiate respondents.

with breast cancer live, while the smaller dots form an almost continuous distribution in the background.

When the density of dots is high, dot maps become cluttered and difficult to interpret. Dots hide other dots, obscuring differences in density. In these situations, the analyst can use proportional symbols to distinguish areas of high and low concentration. But proportional symbols maps themselves can become cluttered, and large symbols are not geographically precise. In these cases, the analyst can use a density estimation method, like kernel smoothing, discussed in Chapter 5, to create a continuous representation of point density. Another strategy is *area conversion* in which points are grouped into geographical areas and these areas are shaded according to the number of events within them.

Some kinds of health events, such as motor vehicle collisions, are clustered along roads or other line segments. In displaying this kind of information, policymakers often want to know the density of events by line segment—for example, which roads or street segments have the most collisions. To represent such information, we can shade line segments based on number of events. Varying the color or width of the line segment highlights differences in number or density of events. Figure 4.4 shows a conventional point symbol map of motor vehicle collisions in part of Connecticut and a corresponding shaded line segment map of the same information. The second map clearly reveals roads and intersections with high collision frequencies.

The GIS analyst must experiment with combinations of symbol size, shape, and color, as well as the overall mapping strategy, to create an effective map representation of point information. Most GIS systems make this experimentation relatively easy by offering an array of options for symbol design. One can create alternative layouts in the GIS and view them on the computer screen, making adjustments as needed. The map or map series is printed in its final version only after choosing the most effective design.

Representing Area Data

Health information is often available for areas—zip codes, counties, states, or countries—that form a template for representation. In representing area information, we fill areas with symbols, colors, or patterns to show the intensity or number of events within the area. *Dot density maps* use point symbols within areas to depict numbers of events in the corresponding areas.

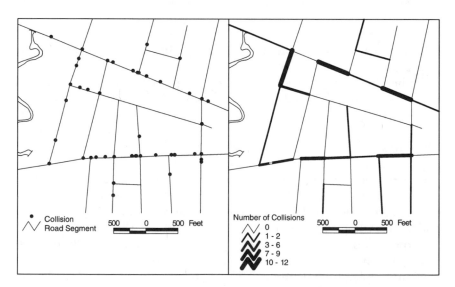

FIGURE 4.4. A point symbol map of motor vehicle collision locations on the left above was converted to a line symbol map as shown on the right.

In *choropleth maps*, areas are shaded with different colors, patterns, or intensities to display place-to-place variation. These kinds of maps are widely used in health mapping for several reasons. First, much health and demographic data is only released by area. Second, by not showing precise locations, such maps avoid concerns about privacy and confidentiality. However, area-based maps cannot display the detailed geographic patterns that emerge from point symbol maps, or maps that show the underlying spatial organization of street networks, residences, and other landscape features. They give the impression of uniformity *within* areas and show sharp changes *between* areas, when in fact the underlying distribution may change gradually or continuously. They often therefore arbitrarily partition the underlying distributions of cases and population, affecting the validity of rate calculations for the mapped areas.

The appropriate mapping approach depends on the type of area data being represented. If the data refer to counts of events, people, or facilities by geographical area, dot density mapping is generally the preferred approach. Dots are arranged within areas, and the viewer perceives differences in numbers in the changing patterns of dot density (Figure 4.5). The number of dots is proportional to the number of events, say, one dot representing 300 people. Typically dots are arranged randomly within areas to avoid sharp breaks in the dot pattern at area boundaries.

Choropleth Mapping

More commonly, area health data refer to rates or ratios or other statistics that apply to areas. In these situations, choropleth mapping is the preferred approach. In a choropleth map, the data values that fall within a specific class interval are assigned a unique color, shade, or pattern. Differences in intensity are visible in the varying colors or patterns across the map.

A key issue in choropleth mapping is the choice of class intervals. Changing the class interval scheme can fundamentally change how the map looks and the message it sends. Most GIS offer the mapmaker a range of options for defining class intervals. A common one is *equal interval classification*, in which the range of the data values (maximum value–minimum value) is divided into a fixed number of classes (Figure 4.6). Each class represents an equal interval of possible data values. Although this method often works well, if there are extreme values in a highly skewed data distribution, the vast majority of areas will fall into one or a few classes, while other classes remain empty. The map will show little spatial variation in such instances because the majority of observed values are very similar. The fact that there are empty classes may be important in understanding the data distribution. The equal interval approach was suggested by Becker (1994) as a suitable approach for developing classifications to facilitate comparison of maps.

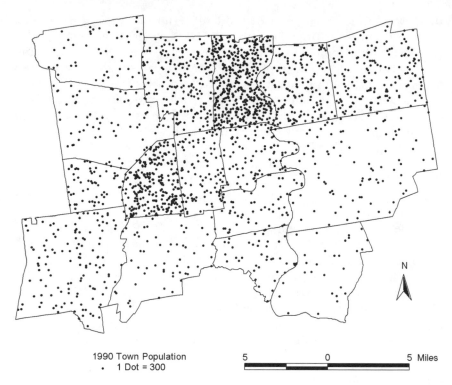

FIGURE 4.5. A dot density map of population distribution by town in the PUBLIC HEALTH GIS study area.

Alternatively, the *n-tile classification* method creates an equal *frequency* of values in each class. This method ensures that each class is equally represented on the map, but it can be misleading because areas that have very similar data values may be assigned to different classes. These areas will appear quite different on the map, even though their actual data values are quite close. The *n*-tile method tends to perform better than the equal interval method for highly skewed data distributions because it differentiates values in the bulge of the data distribution. However, the method typically does not produce intervals that are similar in size. The first class might include data values ranging from 0 to 2, the second from 3 to 24, and the third from 25 to 110. Logically one would infer that the classes represent similar data ranges when in fact they do not. *N*-tile maps can be highly misleading unless the viewer carefully consults the map legend. If the data distribution is uniform or normal, there will be no difference between the equal interval and n-tile classifications.

The *natural breaks* method searches for *breaks*, natural divisions

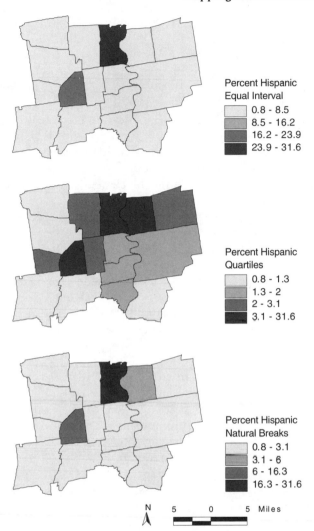

FIGURE 4.6. Choropleth maps of the same data created using different methods for determining class intervals.

among groups of data values, in the data distribution. Classes represent real clusters of data values, and class breaks divide the clusters. The advantage of this method over the previous one is that it does not arbitrarily divide observations that have similar values into different classes. However, it produces class intervals neither of equal width nor with equal numbers of observations, so the results are unpredictable and totally dependent on the data. In some GIS software, natural breaks are determined statistically as breaks that minimize within-class variation (Jenks & Caspall, 1971; Jenks, 1977). For a fuller discussion of the strengths and limitations of the many methods that exist for defining class intervals, we urge the reader to consult a cartography reference book (Muehrcke & Muehrcke, 1992) or to visit the "Choropleth Advisor" website (Rushton & Armstrong, 1997).

Why does the approach to data classification taken matter to the public health analyst? Monmonier (1996) points out that many, many choropleth maps can be made from the same data simply by changing the class intervals. It is possible to manipulate map readers' impressions of spatial patterns of health events simply by changing class intervals (Figure 4.6).

An innovative method for choropleth mapping that addresses the problem of defining class intervals is the "classless" choropleth map (Tobler, 1973). Instead of defining a fixed number of class intervals, the mapmaker shades areas on a continuous value scale, with shading intensity or value proportional to the actual data value observed for the geographical unit (Figure 4.7). These maps are visually effective, but difficult to produce. In addition, a detailed legend would be required to show the actual data values associated with each shade. As GIS and computer graphics technology advance, classless maps may become easier to construct and more readily available for health mapping.

The classless map attempts to address one of the major drawbacks of choropleth map classification schemes like the equal interval, n-tiles, and natural breaks methods. The drawback is that these classifications are derived from the univariate distribution of values and ignore spatial relationships among the units for which data are being mapped. As a result, statistical "cliffs" in the data distribution may not match with visual "cliffs," or differences between places on the map.

Methods for defining optimal class intervals that take into account statistical distribution and spatial relationships have been developed for interval/ratio and for ordinal level data (Cromley, 1996; Cromley & Mrozinski, 1999). Cromley and Cromley (1996) developed a classification method that maximizes spatial similarity among contiguous units in the same class interval and applied the method to data published in the *German Cancer Atlas*. Although the ability to generate a matrix that describes spatial contiguity of the mapping area is important in implementing these methods, and while GIS systems can produce this type of matrix, most GIS systems as yet have not incorporated these approaches to map classification in their standard options for classifying data for choropleth mapping.

Another important issue in choropleth mapping is the choice of area shading. Generally speaking, the best practice is to use a single color and

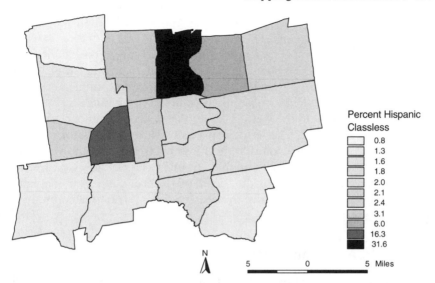

Percent Hispanic
Classless

	0.8
	1.3
	1.6
	1.8
	2.0
	2.1
	2.4
	3.1
	6.0
	16.3
	31.6

N

5   0   5 Miles

FIGURE 4.7. In a classless choropleth map, continuous shade tones of a single hue correspond monotonically to unique data values within the distribution being mapped.

vary its intensity. Less intense (lighter) hues typically represent areas with low data values and more intense (darker) hues those with higher values.

In some health mapping projects, the goal is to show values in relation to some average or population value—for example, mortality rates above or below the national norm. For these types of maps, a diverging color scheme is often highly effective. One color is used to represent values above the norm and another color to indicate values below the norm. For each color, differences in intensity reveal the difference from the norm. The work of Brewer et al. (1997) provides an excellent guide to the use of diverging color schemes in choropleth mapping.

When a series of maps is being prepared for publication, the analyst should also consider how well the class intervals selected will work over time. Using the same class intervals might facilitate comparison of maps for different points in time or for different diseases. The analyst will also need to plan the symbology very carefully. When the same number of class intervals and shades are used in a series of maps that display rates for male and female lung cancer across the same geographical areas, map comparisons may be misleading. For example, map viewers may develop the impression that the disease rate associated with the "red" area on the map displaying female lung cancer rates is as high as the rate associated with the "red" area on the map displaying male lung cancer rates, when in fact the highest rates among females are much lower than the highest rates observed among males (Becker, 1994).

To summarize, health data analysts using GIS to prepare choropleth maps need to investigate how data are distributed through their range, how data are distributed spatially across the choropleth units, and which class breaks have particular substantive value from an analytical point of view for the analyst and the viewer. Analysts can take advantage of the relative ease of developing a series of maps using different classification and symbolization approaches to evaluate the impacts of these choices on the message the map conveys. GIS enables public health analysts to produce multiple views of the data in the form of different types of maps and charts to support more effective analysis of data and better communication of results.

Modifiable Area Unit Problem

The nature of areas themselves present several challenges for mapping. In one sense, there is no "true" choropleth map. The map's appearance and the message it conveys vary depending on the size, number, and configuration of area units. This is the *modifiable area unit problem* (Openshaw, 1984).

One important aspect of this problem is the location of area boundaries in relation to the underlying distribution of health events and population. Depending on where boundaries are located, the area units can divide clusters of health events or concentrate them in a single zone. For centuries, politicians have exploited this situation to "gerrymander" electoral districts, purposely drawing boundaries to achieve a desired electoral outcome. Monmonier (1996, p. 158) demonstrates how this works with an example based on John Snow's famous map of cholera in London (Figure 4.8). When Snow's point data are aggregated to areas, the geographical pattern of cholera varies greatly depending on the area units used. On some maps, the cluster of cases around the Broad Street pump disappears. This issue is discussed in relation to vector-borne disease in Chapter 8.

Choropleth maps vary with the number and sizes of area units. Small areas are more likely to capture the underlying pattern of health events, showing fine-grained variation over space. In contrast, large areas conceal local differences, reducing the variation in values over space. A county-scale map cannot show differences among towns and neighborhoods, for example, and state-level data hide disparities across counties. The scale of areal units affects our perceptions and understanding of health patterns (Figure 4.9).

Choropleth maps can also mislead the viewer by giving a false impression of equivalence among areas. The fact that each area has a data value associated with it implies that the areas are comparable in size and significance. A choropleth map by state gives equal significance to the health sta-

Snow's Dot Map

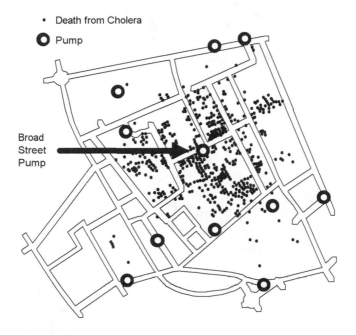

Areal Aggregations and Density Symbols

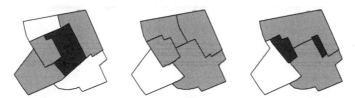

FIGURE 4.8. A reconstruction of John Snow's map of cholera cases in London and three choropleth maps produced by different areal aggregations. From Monmonier (1996). Copyright 1996 by University of Chicago Press. Reprinted by permission.

tistics for Wyoming and California despite the vast difference in their respective state populations. Furthermore, less populated areas are often larger in size, which causes them to attract attention when they are shaded on the map. On a state map, Montana looks much more prominent than Rhode Island though its population is less. To tackle this problem, one can create a *cartogram* in which the sizes of areas are proportional to their populations. Places with large populations are expanded in size and ap-

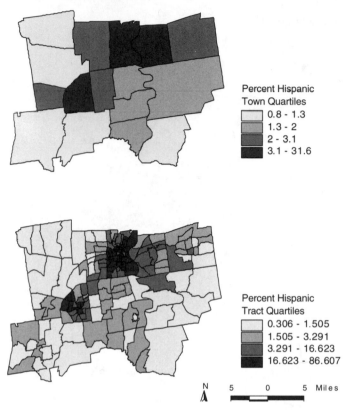

FIGURE 4.9. The same number of class intervals and the same method for determining class intervals reveals greater spatial and numerical variation in the census tract map than in the town map.

pear large on the map. Because they distort traditional geographic space, cartograms are often difficult for viewers to understand and interpret. Note, however, that when areas differ greatly in population size, standard choropleth maps also distort.

When mapping area data, it is essential to analyze the effects of the modifiable area unit problem on maps and results. By using small-area data, one can always show finer-grained and more detailed spatial patterns than can be shown with large-area data. It is often the case, however, that the analyst only has access to large-area information. How can this problem be addressed? One approach is to use ancillary data to estimate variation within large areas. *Ancillary data* describe geographic features that constrain the distribution of risk population or health events. As discussed in Chapter 6, ancillary data can be used to allocate events within large areas to subareas in which the events are most likely to occur.

Another approach is to apportion data for large areas based on related data for smaller areas. This is the problem of *areal interpolation*, of estimating values for areas (Goodchild & Lam, 1980). For example, assume that we know from hospital discharge data the number of children by zip code who were hospitalized for asthma. Data on risk population, in this case the number of children, are available for much smaller geographic units, census blocks. If the blocks nest perfectly in zip codes, we can apportion the asthma data for a given zip code to blocks within that zip code based on the proportion of children residing in each block. This method assumes that the risk of hospitalization for asthma is constant within a given zip code. If the small areas do not nest perfectly, the most common approach is to allocate the population of split blocks to corresponding zip codes based on the area of overlap (Goodchild & Lam, 1980). More complex methods that rely on additional ancillary information are discussed in Flowerdew and Green (1994).

By using ancillary data, we can move from small-scale data to a larger scale, more detailed representation of spatial variation. GIS greatly facilitate the use of ancillary data and the matching of data across geographical scales. Defining areas of overlap and allocating data from one layer to another are standard operations in most GIS.

Despite their advantages for representation, small-area health data pose "large statistical problems" (Diehr, 1984). Often there are few health events in each small area, making maps and estimates unreliable. This is especially true if the data cover a short time period or a rare disease. This "small numbers problem" is discussed further in Chapter 5.

VIEWING HEALTH INFORMATION

The ability to visualize and explore health data interactively is a main advantage of GIS in public health analysis. A *view* is a graphic representation of data. It is the part of the computer display board that one can see on the computer screen. The extent of the view is always less than or equal to the addressable space in a data set. Simply put, one cannot display a larger geographic area than one has data for. In GIS, the spatial objects in the view and the tables of attributes describing them can be directly linked. The analyst can access the two together and explore the relationships among attribute data in the table and the spatial representation of that data in the view.

Public health analysts will typically approach a database with two types of questions: What are the health problems of interest and where do they occur? Where are the places of interest and what kinds of health problems occur there? Many public health organizations are organized functionally to address specific kinds of health problems—for example, maternal and child health, infectious disease, or injury. GIS users in these settings will have already established what kinds of health problems are of interest to them and may want to use GIS to gain a better understanding of the geographical distribution of these health problems. For example, we might ask, "Where are the residential locations of all children born with birth defects in Arizona?" Here the attribute (children born with birth defects) is given, and we want to know where the events that have these attributes occur. We call this method "viewing by attribute."

On the other hand, we might be concerned about health events at a particular place. The environmental health analyst might wish to study a variety of health outcomes in an area affected by a contamination event. Individual citizens and community groups are often interested in understanding a variety of health problems experienced in their own neighborhoods or communities. In these cases, the GIS users have already established a place of interest and want to understand the health status of the population in that place. We call this method "geographical viewing." For example, we might ask, "How many cases of Lyme disease and associated tick-borne disease occurred in Fairfield County, Connecticut, last year?" Interacting with spatial databases displayed in a GIS view enables public health analysts to answer the basic questions of what and where.

Viewing by Attribute

Viewing by attribute starts with the characteristics of events, as described in the table, and identifies those events on a map. In the simplest case, we identify the location of a single event. For example, assume that we have a database showing the locations of all motor vehicle collisions in Connecticut. One particular collision that resulted in a fatality is of interest. We can select that collision record in the table and its corresponding location will be highlighted in the display (Figure 4.10). Some systems enable users to pan and zoom to the selected collision even if it is not currently in the view at the time the collision is selected.

A more complex operation is to select by attribute, identifying multiple records based on their common attributes. We select events that have particular characteristics and display their locations on the view. For example, policymakers may want to know the locations of all motor vehicle collisions that involve pedestrians. We query the table for all collisions involving pedestrians, select those collisions, and their locations will be identified on the view (Figure 4.11).

It is also possible to select events by attribute and location simultaneously. For example, we might want to identify all motor vehicle collisions that occurred in Hartford, Connecticut, that involved pedestrians. The geographical query is to select the town of Hartford, and the attribute query is to select only collisions involving pedestrians. We need to

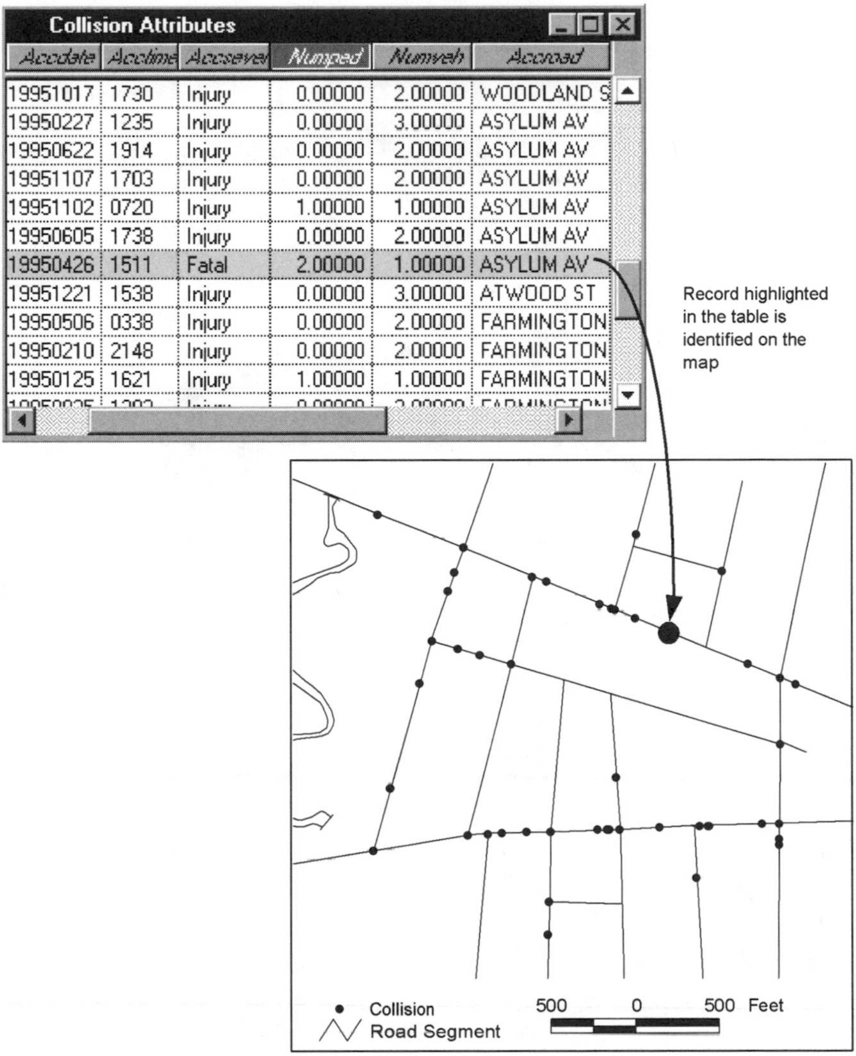

Collision Attributes						
Accdate	*Acctime*	*Accsever*	*Numped*	*Numveh*	*Accroad*	
19951017	1730	Injury	0.00000	2.00000	WOODLAND S	
19950227	1235	Injury	0.00000	3.00000	ASYLUM AV	
19950622	1914	Injury	0.00000	2.00000	ASYLUM AV	
19951107	1703	Injury	0.00000	2.00000	ASYLUM AV	
19951102	0720	Injury	1.00000	1.00000	ASYLUM AV	
19950605	1738	Injury	0.00000	2.00000	ASYLUM AV	
19950426	1511	Fatal	2.00000	1.00000	ASYLUM AV	
19951221	1538	Injury	0.00000	3.00000	ATWOOD ST	
19950506	0338	Injury	0.00000	2.00000	FARMINGTON	
19950210	2148	Injury	0.00000	2.00000	FARMINGTON	
19950125	1621	Injury	1.00000	1.00000	FARMINGTON	
19950005	1202	Injury	0.00000	2.00000	FARMINGTON	

Record highlighted in the table is identified on the map

• Collision
/\/ Road Segment

500   0   500 Feet

FIGURE 4.10. Viewing by attribute allows the user to highlight a motor vehicle collision with the attribute "Fatal" from a table of data and find the location of the collision in the GIS display.

find the *intersection* of these two queries, that is, events that satisfy both conditions. Depending on how the data set is structured, there are several ways to perform these queries. One is first to select Hartford in the view, then query the data set for collisions involving pedestrians. Alternatively, if the name of the city where the collision occurred is included in the data

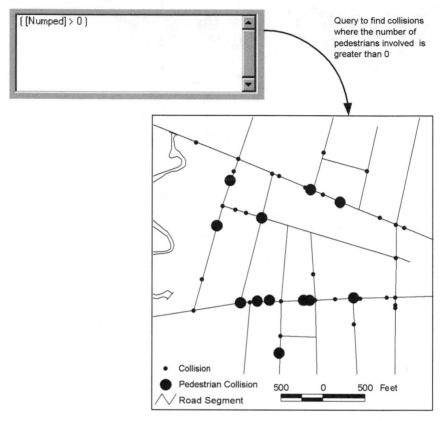

[[Numped] > 0]

Query to find collisions where the number of pedestrians involved is greater than 0

- Collision
- Pedestrian Collision
- Road Segment

500   0   500 Feet

FIGURE 4.11. Viewing by attribute allows the user to query a database table to identify all collisions that satisfy a set of criteria and to highlight the locations of these collisions in the GIS display.

set, it would be possible to query the database to select events where the accident town is Hartford and the collision type is pedestrian.

Most complex queries involve Boolean operations (Table 4.1). *Boolean operations* are operations that are applied to sets and logical propositions. In GIS queries, these operations define how the attributes of events are to be combined. Two common Boolean operations are AND (intersection) and OR (union). The AND operator finds the intersection of two attributes. It identifies events that satisfy two conditions simultaneously.

In the above example, we selected collisions based on an AND query. A sequence of AND operations finds events that satisfy more than two conditions simultaneously. To identify collisions that occurred in Hartford, involved pedestrians, and also involved a school bus, we would cre-

TABLE 4.1. Boolean Operators

Boolean operator	Notation	Definition	Example
Equality	S = T	A relationship between two sets when the sets contain precisely the same elements.	If S is the set of collisions obtained by using the GIS to find all collision points within the polygon of the Hartford town boundary and T is the set of collisions obtained by using the GIS to query the collision attribute table to find all collisions with AccTown=HARTFORD and there are no errors in the spatial or attribute information, then the two sets would have the same collisions as members and the sets would be equal.
Subset	T ⊆ C	A relationship between two sets where every element of S is an element of the second set T.	If C is the set of collisions occurring in the state of Connecticut and T is the set of collisions occurring in Hartford, then T would be a subset of C. C would not be a subset of T.
Intersection	P ∩ T	A binary operation that takes two sets and returns the set of elements that are members of both the original sets.	If P is the set of all pedestrian collisions in the state of Connecticut and T is the set of all collisions in Hartford, then the intersection of P and T would be the set of all pedestrian collisions in Hartford.
Union	B ∪ H	A binary operation that takes two sets and returns the set of elements that are members of at least one of the original sets.	If H is the set of all pedestrian collisions in Hartford and B is the set of all collisions in Hartford involving a school bus, then the union of B and H would be the set of all collisions in Hartford involving *either* a school bus *or* a pedestrian or both.
Empty or Null	∅	The set contains no elements.	No motorcycles were involved in collisions in Hartford that also involved a pedestrian. A query to find the intersection of pedestrian and motorcycle collisions in Hartford would return an empty set.
Difference	B\H	A binary operation that takes two sets and returns the set of elements that are members of the first set but *not* the second set.	The difference of B and H would be the collisions in Hartford that involved school buses not including any school bus collisions in Hartford that involved pedestrians.
Complement	P′	A unary operation applied to a set that returns the set of elements *not* in the set. The complement is always taken with reference to a universal set.	The complement of P, the set of all pedestrian collisions the state of Connecticut, would be the set of all other collisions in Connecticut.

ate the following query to find every record where the accident town is "Hartford," the collision type is "Pedestrian," and the vehicle type is "School Bus."

The OR operator finds the union of two attributes, that is, events that satisfy at least one of the two attributes. To select collisions that involved a pedestrian or a school bus, we would create the query to find every record where the collision type is "Pedestrian" OR the vehicle type is "School Bus." The collisions identified in this query would include any collision involving a pedestrian, any collision involving a school bus, and any collision involving both. Queries can combine Boolean operators to identify detailed subsets of events for display, as shown in Table 4.1.

The ability to perform complex queries, both geographical and attribute-based, is an important feature of GIS. In a real-world setting, the challenge is to move from verbal queries like "Show me the fatal collisions that occurred on two-lane roads and involved people who were driving while intoxicated (DWI)" to the precise logical and geographical statements that are needed to perform these queries in GIS. This query looks for events that satisfy three conditions: fatal collisions, location on two-lane roads, and DWI. In addressing the query, we need to satisfy all three conditions and find the intersection among them. Creating queries calls for a skilled GIS analyst who can translate verbal statements into logical ones and then perform the GIS operations needed to satisfy them.

Geographical Viewing

Geographical viewing starts with geographical areas of interest and asks about the attributes of events located within those areas. In a GIS view, the analyst can select locations, or pan and zoom to particular locations, and then examine the attribute data in the table for those selected events. The map is the starting point and the analyst links back to attribute information in the table.

Using standard query tools in GIS, one can select features according to their point or area locations. Figure 4.12 contains a view of point data showing the locations where people were bitten by rats in the Bronx, New York City, in a certain year. We can click on one of those points to view the attribute data associated with the particular cases at that point: age of person, the location of the bite on the person, activity, and so on. GIS users can also select by area. To determine which rat bites occurred in the borough of Staten Island, we select that borough by "turning on" the borough data layer in the display and clicking on the borough of Staten Island, then selecting cases occurring within the selected borough. This operation gives access to the attribute information for cases in that borough. Tables, charts, and statistics can be generated to describe the aggregate characteristics of those selected cases, such as median age, gender, and location (home, work, park) where the biting incidents took place.

Another kind of geographical viewing is a type of "windowing" in which we select events within a user-defined area. Most GIS include a tool that allows users quickly to draw a rectangle, circle, or irregularly shaped polygon in the view. Events located within the polygon are selected so that one can explore and summarize their characteristics (Figure 4.13). By

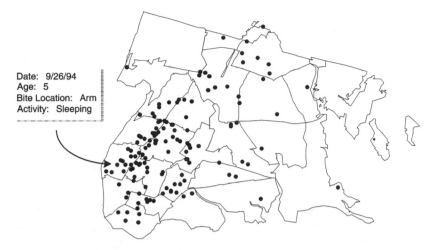

Date: 9/26/94
Age: 5
Bite Location: Arm
Activity: Sleeping

FIGURE 4.12. The geographical viewing capabilities of a GIS enable users to access the attributes of an event like a rat bite that occurred at a particular location.

drawing a window around those cases and selecting them, the analyst can generate summary statistics that compare events inside and outside the window.

Geographical viewing offers a powerful means of exploring data based on geographical location. The map, and the viewer's knowledge and perceptions of places on the map, stimulate queries about what types of health problems exist in particular areas and why the problems cluster geographically.

Changing the View

Views are not static. Within the limits defined by the scale and extent of the data set, one can change the view by moving across the map or by focusing in on areas of interest. *Pan* refers to movement across a map, bringing new areas into the view. Often the view includes just part of the geographical extent of a data set. Using the pan function, we move across that geographical extent to bring another part of the map into the view. We can also change the view by zooming in or out. When we *zoom in* to an area, we move toward it, keeping it in focus in the view. Zooming in is useful for getting a closer look at areas of special interest. By zooming in to a cluster of health events, we reveal the detailed geography of the disease cluster. Drawing upon other data layers, we can observe the concentration of events along roads, or in relation to parks, landfills and other features. To *zoom out* is to move away from the map, bringing a larger geographical area

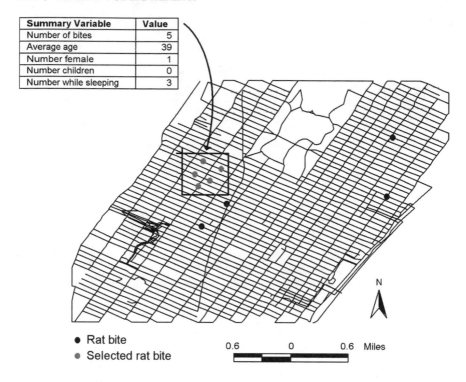

Summary Variable	Value
Number of bites	5
Average age	39
Number female	1
Number children	0
Number while sleeping	3

• Rat bite
• Selected rat bite

0.6   0   0.6   Miles

N

FIGURE 4.13. Selecting rat bites within a user-defined rectangular window. At-tributes of bites inside the window are summarized in tabular form.

into the view. Zooming out is useful for examining regional differences, for getting a "wide-angle" view of broad spatial patterns.

An important point to remember about changing the view is that the scale and extent of data in the GIS limit the view. If our foundation data encompass only the state of Iowa, we cannot pan beyond the state to see neighboring areas of Minnesota or Nebraska. Similarly, if our original foundation data is at a scale of 1:24,000, by zooming in to the map we will not see more detail than exists at the 1:24,000 scale. This is one reason why it is so important to think carefully at the beginning of a GIS map-ping project about the scale and extent of the foundation data to be used.

Viewing and Analyzing Geographical Associations

Another way to change the view is to add or remove features visible on the view. Known as *cartographic overlay*, such procedures involve the overlay of data layers to show geographical associations. In most GIS, cartographic overlay requires a simple click of the mouse to make data layers visible or not visible in the display. For example, we might begin with a crime map that shows locations where assaults occurred. To identify places where schoolchildren might be at risk of assault, we activate the schools data layer, overlaying the school locations on the view of assaults (Figure 4.14). The overlay reveals that school *A* is in an area with a greater number of assaults than school *B*, which may mean that students who attend school A are at greater risk of assault. By adding and removing data layers in this way, we can begin to visualize and explore geographical associations.

Spatial queries are procedures for creating new information about the geographical relationships among data layers that are visible in carto-graphic overlay. For example, we might want to know how many homes are located in a protected watershed region. To answer this question, we need to overlay the point data layer showing the locations of homes with the area (polygon) data layer depicting the watershed. The spatial query counts the number of homes that fall within the watershed. Spatial que-

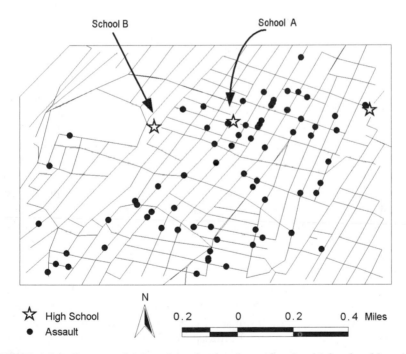

FIGURE 4.14. Cartographic overlay of a data layer showing high school locations with another data layer showing the locations of assaults. The overlay reveals that high school *A* is located in an area with a higher number of assaults than high school *B*.

ries are similar to the queries described earlier, except that they (i.e., spatial queries) are based on the relative locations of features rather than on their attributes. While cartographic overlay offers a picture of the relationships among layers, spatial queries provide a quantitative or qualitative summary of those relationships.

Spatial queries depend fundamentally on the type of spatial data—raster or vector—that one is working with. Raster layers that are registered together and have the same pixel size will overlay perfectly. Under these circumstances, spatial queries can be performed on a pixel-by-pixel basis using *map algebra* (Tomlin, 1990), which consists of Boolean and algebraic operations to combine and relate pixel values. All of the operations described in Table 4.1 can be performed to create new raster images based on combinations of data layers. If the pixel values are measured on an interval or ratio scale, they can be combined via algebraic operations. For vector-borne diseases, like Lyme disease and hanta virus, such operations have been used in estimating vector density as a function of elevation, land cover, and vegetation density, as discussed in Chapter 8.

When using vector data, spatial queries are based on comparisons of relative location as defined by geographical coordinates. The types of spatial queries depend on the types of features—point, line, or polygon—being compared. Queries that compare two point data layers typically involve calculating distances between points. One can determine both average distances between points on different layers and numbers of points in one data layer within a given distance of points in the other data layer. These types of queries have many potential applications in public health GIS, but they are especially important in analyzing locations of health care services and geographical accessibility to those services, as discussed in Chapters 9 and 10. For example, health service planners often want to know: How far is each town from its nearest hospital? This spatial query involves comparing two point data layers, one showing the locations of towns and the other the locations of hospitals.

Spatial queries involving point and polygon vector data are also common in public health GIS. In this case, the queries involve identifying the areas where points are located, or the numbers of points within areas, or the numbers of points within a distance radius of an area. One of the most common types of queries is to determine the area in which a point is located, for example, the political district or block in which a residence is located (Figure 4.15). The point data layer is superimposed on the polygon data layer that shows area boundaries. Then, a *point-in-polygon* operation is performed to identify the particular area that contains the point. Although the human eye can easily visualize and respond to a point-in-polygon query, such queries are complex from a technical and computational standpoint and are based on polygon topology. After completing the query, the analyst can add the polygon name or number as a new at-

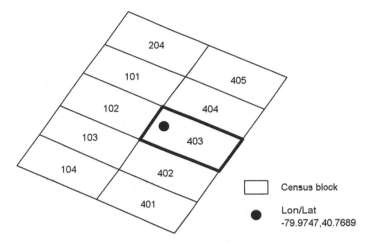

FIGURE 4.15. Point-in-polygon operation to find the block in which a point is located. The operation involves comparing the geographical coordinates of the point, in this case (lon/lat) coordinates, to the coordinates of the vertices of the polygon to determine if the point is "inside" the polygon.

tribute in the point data layer. Alternatively, one can use point-in-polygon operations to identify and characterize the points that fall inside particular polygons. The watershed example, mentioned above, exemplifies this type of point-in-polygon query. Note that the number of homes located within the watershed becomes a new attribute of the watershed polygon.

Another class of spatial queries addresses the associations between linear features and point and area features. Line-point queries involve distance relationships; for example, we might ask, How many homes are located within 500 meters of a highway? To respond to this query, the GIS computes distances from each home to the highway, and counts the number of homes that have a distance less than 500 meters. Line-polygon queries ask which linear features fall within a particular polygon, for example, Which highways pass through the Williamsburg neighborhood? A *line-in-polygon* operation, similar to the point-in-polygon operation noted above, is used in solving these types of spatial queries.

The final class of vector spatial queries involves comparing two or more polygon data layers. One can overlay the polygon layers and use Boolean or algebraic operations to create new information. For instance, we might want to find all census tracts that are located in the service area for Saint Francis Hospital and have a median household income under $25,000. We overlay the hospital service area data layer with the layer containing census tracts with incomes below $25,000 and use the Boolean AND operator to find tracts, or parts of tracts, that satisfy both criteria.

Polygon overlay can be a time-consuming process, especially when it involves large numbers of polygons, because it works from the detailed topological relationships among the polygons (DeMers, 2000). To save time in polygon overlay, we can often preprocess the polygon data layers to remove polygons that are not of interest. In this example, we could eliminate census tracts with incomes above $25,000, using only the remaining tracts in performing the spatial query.

Spatial queries are an essential component of all GIS systems, enabling the user to create new information based on geographical relationships between various layers of spatial information. Chapters 5 through 10 consider the use of different types of spatial queries in diverse public health GIS applications, including environmental health, communicable and vector-borne disease, and health services access and location.

GIS AND MAP PUBLICATION

The mapping process as implemented in a GIS emphasizes the representation and analysis of information. Nevertheless, finished maps remain an important product of GIS to support the various stages of compilation, exploration, and analysis of data and to present results. A single map or a series of maps may be prepared for publication, either in traditional printed format or in digital form for display on the Internet. These maps are finished products that may be viewed and referenced by a diverse audience. There are a number of design elements worth considering in preparing maps for publication.

Key Elements of Thematic Maps

Thematic maps typically contain certain key elements (Table 4.2). These elements define the nature and source of a map's contents. They also assist the map reader.

The *title* of the published map describes the major theme of the map. Carefully written titles are important for communicating that theme. The *legend* of a thematic map identifies and defines the symbols used on the map. *Neatlines* define the borders of the map and areas within it, including insets and legends. They can be used effectively to partition the document and draw the viewer's eye to different map elements.

Published maps should also include a north arrow and a scale. The *north arrow* indicates map orientation. As discussed in Chapter 2, map *scale* is important because it affects the degree of detail that can be portrayed.

Some cartographers have suggested that these are not essential ele-

TABLE 4.2. Elements of Thematic Maps

Element	Description
Title	Describes major theme of map
Legend	Defines map symbols
Neatlines	Define borders of the map sheet and areas within it, including insets and legends
North arrow	Describes map orientation
Scale	Describes map distance in relation to earth distance
Source	Describes source, date, and reliability of mapped data
Agency	Identifies agency responsible for preparing and/or publishing the map

ments for thematic map design (Slocum, 1999). Given a map of the United States, for example, readers will likely recognize the map domain and have a sense of the orientation and scale even if they are not explicit. Many public health GIS applications, however, deal with localities or regions that may be less familiar to map readers. A north arrow should be included, particularly if the orientation of the map on the page is different from north and if direction is important in interpreting the map content. This might be the case in mapping the plume from a point source of emissions into the atmosphere.

The scale of the map is information that should also be clearly presented. Maps have traditionally been compiled at a series of standard scales (1:24,000, 1:50,000, 1:200,000, etc). The scale element assists the reader in placing the published map along this series. Furthermore, published maps are documents that are acquired by libraries and research institutes, catalogued, and made accessible to a potentially large audience. Inclusion of a map scale assists in cataloguing and helps individuals find maps that might reveal the spatial patterns of interest to them because the maps were prepared at a scale that can display the necessary detail.

Printed maps may also include the *source* of the data that are the theme of the map. The information might include the date of the data and pertinent information about the reliability of the data. Finally, the *agency* responsible for preparing and/or publishing the map should be included.

GIS software packages include a range of functions that help users take the information from a cartographic display of data and compose a map document for printing or storing in common graphics formats. Text, charts, tables, photographs, and other elements like the date the map is printed can often be incorporated into the map document. Layouts can be stored as templates to preserve the standard elements in the design.

Map Publication on the Internet

Increasingly, maps, like other documents that have traditionally been printed and distributed on paper, are being published in digital form on the Internet (Kraak & Brown, 2000). In the criminal justice field, some police departments are posting maps of crime occurrence on the Internet to give citizens access to the information for their communities. Although public health departments have been more cautious than other organizations and agencies about posting maps of health data on the Internet, such distribution is bound to increase in the future.

There are three main types of map that can be published on the Internet: static maps, dynamic maps, and on-demand maps. *Static maps* are maps that can be viewed as documents on the Internet (Peterson, 1997). These maps can be created by scanning existing paper maps or by saving map layouts in one of a variety of common graphics formats like JPEG (Joint Photographic Experts Group) or GIF (Graphics Interchange Format). The viewer can access the map by clicking on a link that references the graphics file. Basically, static maps can be located and viewed, but viewers cannot interact with these maps and cannot modify them.

Dynamic, or interactive, maps are maps that allow the user to interact with the map in some way. These maps may allow viewers to display the map in a different projection or to separate map data layers (Peterson, 1997). Viewers may be able to click on an element in the view or pass the mouse over an element to obtain further information (Swanson, 1997). In other cases, functions may enable the user to change class intervals on the thematic map.

On-demand maps are maps that are generated from databases according to requests made by the viewer. A common example of this type of map is a street network locator map that is generated when the user enters an address. The Internet mapping application processes the user's request and returns a response to the browser.

Map publication on the Internet raises additional issues for cartographic design and map distribution. These include map design issues for the computer screen as a medium. But online map publication involves much more than just design questions related to screen versus paper because the map image now has a *front end*—the user interface for the mapping application displayed within the browser—and a *back end*, the digital databases accessed to respond to queries and requests and to produce the resulting map. These issues affect the design of static, dynamic, and on-demand online maps.

The size and resolution of the computer screen are major factors affecting map design (Plewe, 1997). The portion of the map that can be viewed will be determined by the size of the screen and the area inside the web browser. If a map is larger than the available space, viewers will have to scroll to see every part of the map. On a standard 14" monitor, the window for viewing the map will probably be roughly 10" × 6.5".

Computer screens are raster devices. Screen resolution is generally much lower than the resolution of many desktop printers, which are capable of 300 dots per inch (dpi) as a minimum. Viewers' monitors may have resolutions ranging from 60 to 100 dpi. This sets a maximum size for raster maps of roughly 550 pixels by 300 pixels. The lower resolution also limits geographic detail, text size, and shade patterns.

It may be less expensive to publish maps in color online than in printed form. However, not all colors are browser-independent. Viewers who do not have color printers will only be able to print black-and-white versions of the maps.

In addition to the design of the map, publication of maps online requires design of a user interface. The user interface provides the viewer with access to the tools for map navigation, map display, and map querying and analysis. In intranet applications that provide access to maps within organizations, interface design can be very simple. For Internet applications where maps will be accessed by a potentially large and unknown group of viewers, interface design may be more challenging.

The greater the number of functions available to the user for interacting with the map, the greater the number of controls there will be in the interface and the more complex it will become. Map images, graphical icons and buttons, text with and without hyperlinks, and forms supporting various types of input can all be used in interfaces supporting mapping applications (Plewe, 1997). The arrangement of elements in the interface is also important. Controls that will be used more frequently may be placed in different areas from those that will be used only rarely. Map navigation controls for panning and zooming are generally placed close to the map image.

As the number of functions increases, processing requirements increase. There is a tension between how much of the processing occurs on the server versus on the client machine. Generally, more functions result in more processing on the client. These functions can usually only be supported if the client has or can obtain the necessary plug-in or software to support the function.

In addition to designing the front end of an online mapping site, organizations choosing to publish maps on the Internet need to think about map and database issues. Computer processing and the Internet have blurred distinctions among traditionally defined formats of published materials and have spurred the development of new formats. Online mapping raises the graphics versus data issue. A site that provides access to static maps will be storing graphic images on the server and making them available through webpages. A site that provides access to dynamic or on-demand mapping applications will be storing and maintaining digital spatial or other databases on a server and will manage requests for information from those databases.

In the earliest stages of the World Wide Web, hypertext markup language (HTML) became the standard for formatting and maintaining documents to be shared over the Internet. HTML is a tag-based language. The tags are used to determine how the document will appear, that is, to encode information for graphical presentation on pages within web browsers. The growth of the Internet and the potential for transferring very specific kinds of data over it have given rise to the need for a language that can describe data and the relationships between data. XML is emerging as a language that can apply tags to identify information content—what an object is—in addition to presentation—how it should be rendered on the page. By focusing on content, languages like XML can be used to manage data transactions over the Internet, including the transfer of metadata. These developments in the Internet as a whole are also affecting the distribution of spatial data.

What are the implications of these developments for GIS applications in public health? GIS clearly support preparation and publication of maps as a form of information on health status and health services. The growing trend toward distributing information on the Internet means that public health organizations need to plan for data distribution. Will maps or data or both be provided? If publication on the Internet is important, the institutional requirements for a successful GIS application increase. In addition to staff who can maintain the databases used in-house and design GIS applications, staff are needed who have expertise in webpage and interface design. Staff are also needed who can administer and maintain the servers and software that support the Internet mapping and data distribution applications. Even if the GIS is operated in a self-contained environment and used to print paper maps for distribution, public health analysts will need to become familiar with online mapping because much of the foundation and other data they will need to access to develop their GIS applications will be distributed over the Internet.

CONCLUSION

GIS has revolutionized the process of mapmaking. From obtaining data to developing maps, to creating on-demand images on the Internet, the process can be accomplished in a fully automated, digital environment. Technological developments are stimulating a new mapping process that emphasizes displaying, analyzing, and viewing health information in new and innovative ways rather than creating a finished map. But the ease of operating GIS makes it even more imperative that users have a firm understanding of the basic principles of geography and cartography. Maps can lie. They can mislead just as easily as they can lead (Monmonier, 1996). Successful mapping depends on the knowledge and skills of analysts who use the systems and the integration of those systems in decision-making processes at the state, local, and community levels. As the links between the GIS and public health communities expand, mapping, viewing, and analyzing geographically based health information will occupy an even more central position in efforts to improve performance of essential public health activities and to promote community health and well-being.

CHAPTER 5

Analyzing Spatial Clustering of Health Events

Public health professionals are often faced with the task of investigating disease *clusters*, unusual concentrations of health events in space and time. Clusters can come to the attention of public health departments when concerned citizens perceive an excess of ill health in their communities, or through surveillance systems that detect an unusual concentration of health events by searching for patterns in routinely collected data (Neutra, Swan, & Mack, 1992). Whether the analysis is confirmatory, verifying that a perceived cluster exists, or exploratory, searching for patterns, GIS can play a crucial role in analyzing spatial clusters. As GIS technology develops, innovative spatial statistical methods are being linked with GIS to analyze the spatial clustering of disease in populations and to assess changes in health status and disease prevalence over time.

This chapter discusses methods for analyzing spatial clustering of health events and the use of GIS to implement these methods. We cover a representative set of methods for analyzing area- and point-based health information and explain the procedures and concepts that underpin the methods. The emphasis is on GIS operations and applications rather than on statistical issues.

Spatial clustering methods can help provide answers to an array of fundamental public health questions. Do any unusual clusters of health events exist in an area? What places have unusually high or low prevalences of disease? Where are the risks of ill health highest or lowest? Spatial analysis methods offer a means of filtering health information in order to describe geographical patterns and identify unusual occurrences of health events.

Figure 5.1a shows the residential locations of children who have leu-

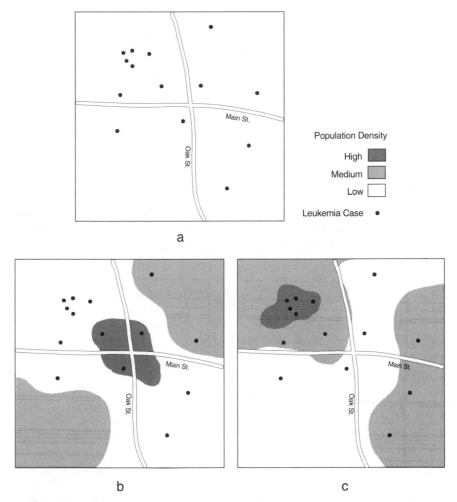

FIGURE 5.1. A hypothetical distribution of leukemia cases in relation to two different spatial patterns of risk population.

kemia in a hypothetical city. A geographical cluster of cases appears in the northeast section of the city. Does this area have an unusually high rate of childhood leukemia? Answering this question requires several important bits of information. First, we need to examine the number of cases of leukemia in relation to the population at risk. The *population at risk* is the set of people who, because of their age or gender, can contract the health problem of interest. As discussed in Chapter 1, the larger the risk population, the larger the number of cases one would expect to find. By definition, childhood leukemia occurs in children, so the risk population comprises all children living in the city or some part of the city. Because population is distributed unevenly over space, the density of health events will vary even when the underlying rate of ill health is uniform. Figures 5.1b and 5.1c depict two alternative spatial distributions of risk population for the leukemia example. In Figure 5.1c, the leukemia cluster occurs in an area of high-risk population density, thus population accounts for the disease cluster. In Figure 5.1b this is not the case.

A second issue in analyzing clustering is to define the geographical extent, or *scale*, at which clustering occurs. A cluster of cases within a 5-square-mile area has a very different meaning than a cluster of cases within a 2,500-square-mile area. The first indicates a highly localized cluster of disease, whereas the second identifies a large region with an elevated disease rate. All clustering methods focus on one, or in some cases a few, spatial scales. Sometimes the analyst can control the choice of spatial scale; however, often the analyst will find scale dictated by the scale of the underlying population or health data. The leukemia example addresses clustering at the intraurban scale, that is, it searches for clustering within small neighborhood areas, rather than across cities or regions.

Scale critically affects the kinds of inferences that can be drawn from cluster studies. Clustering within cities or communities reflects localized factors such as point sources of environmental contamination. In contrast, elevated disease rates for states or regions result from regionwide factors like climate or culture. The scale at which a health problem is studied should reflect an understanding of the disease process and likely causative factors. Furthermore, patterns at one geographical scale can conceal patterns at other scales. A state's "average" rate of disease may result from having some communities with unusually high rates and others with unusually low rates. These disparate rates are lost in the statewide average. Analyses below the state scale are needed to reveal such high-rate communities.

Third, analyzing clustering requires a set of *criteria* for judging how much clustering exists. Does an excess of one or two cases constitute a cluster? Where do we draw the line in defining "significant" clusters? There is no perfect answer to these questions, but geographical and statistical methods can help analysts and policymakers make scientifically informed decisions. Many clustering procedures rely on statistical criteria that describe the likelihood that clusters could have arisen by chance in a given population. Such criteria may utilize a known probability distribution such as the Poisson distribution, or they may utilize Monte Carlo simulation methods which involve generating a large number of random possible outcomes. Some procedures also emphasize the arrangement of health events, not just in relation to population at risk, but also in relation to potential sources of contamination or environmental hazard—for instance, do the events cluster near a toxic waste facility, or are they arranged along roadways or power lines? These methods are discussed in Chapters 6 and 8.

The types of methods used in analyzing disease clustering depend fundamentally on whether the analyst has access to area data or point data. The sections that follow describe spatial clustering methods for area and point health data.

ANALYZING CLUSTERING USING AREA DATA

The most common way of analyzing clustering in area health data is to prepare choropleth maps of disease incidence or prevalence rates, as discussed in Chapter 4. When the areas differ in population size, however, as is typically the case, the calculated rates of disease for those areas have different degrees of reliability. Rates for small areas—areas with small populations—vary more and are less reliable than those for large areas. For small areas, a difference of one or two cases can make a huge difference in incidence or prevalence rates. This is known as the *small numbers problem*.

Figure 5.2 illustrates the small numbers problem with data on low birthweight (percent of babies born weighing less than 2,500 grams) for two areas that differ in population size. Area 1 averages under 200 births per year, while Area 2 averages over 1,600 births per year. Note the large variability in low birthweight in Area 1 from year to year. The low birthweight rates fluctuate from 5% to 16% and appear unpredictable. In Area 2 the rates are more stable, ranging from 12% to 16%. A choropleth map of low birthweight rates by area for a single year does not represent their varying degrees of reliability. For small areas like Area 1, the map can give a false picture of the level of health depending on which year's data happen to be selected for mapping. Area 2's mapped value is likely to be closer to its "true" underlying value.

Probability Mapping

Probability mapping is a well established statistical method for addressing the small numbers problem (Choynowski, 1959). In probability mapping we map the statistical significance of rates rather than the rates themselves. Statistical significance is measured by probability values that show the likelihood of a rate occurring given the normal rate of disease in the corresponding national or regional population. We refer to this rate as the *population rate*, p. The probability value for an area indicates the likelihood that the rate observed in that area would occur by chance if the underlying risk of disease was equal to p. Probability values close to 0 or 1 indicate rates that are significantly different from the population rate.

There are many statistical methods for computing probability val-

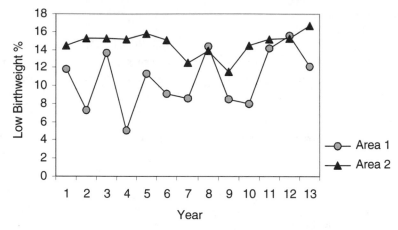

FIGURE 5.2. The small numbers problem illustrated with data on low birthweight over time for two health areas in New York City. Area 1 is a "small" health area, averaging 200 births per year, and its low birthweight rates fluctuate greatly from year to year. Rates are much more stable in Area 2, a "large" health area with 1,600 births per year on average.

ues. One of the most common is the *Poisson test*, used for modeling the probability of rare binary (present/absent) events in large populations. Many health problems (e.g., cancers, birth defects) fit this definition because they are rare, occurring in only a small fraction of the population, and binary, either present or absent in an individual. Consider a small area containing a population, n, and k cases of disease. We want to find out whether the presence of those k cases in a population of size n is unusual. In other words, is the actual number of cases significantly higher than expected based on the national or regional prevalence rate?

If the national or regional rate is p, the expected number of cases in the study area, lambda, is the study area population, n, multiplied by the national or regional rate:

$$\lambda = np$$

For example, if the study area contains 40,000 people and the national prevalence rate is 1 per 10,000, we would expect 4 cases in the study area because $\lambda = 0.0001(40,000) = 4$.

If we know the number of cases, k, occurring in a study region population, we can use the Poisson distribution to determine the probability, $P(k)$, that the observed number of cases would occur in a population of the study region's size. The Poisson distribution states that in a population of size n, the probability of x cases occurring is $P(x) = e^{-\lambda}(\lambda^x/x!)$. In this example, the probability of one case would be 0.073 (Table 5.1). From this calculation, we can determine the probability of k or more cases occurring by chance, $P(x \geq k)$, if the true rate of disease in the population were p. That probability is calculated as:

$$P(x \geq k) = 1 - \sum_{x=0}^{k-1} P(x)$$

For example, if there are 6 cases of disease in the study region where only 4 cases were expected based on national or regional rates, the corresponding probability value would be $1 - 0.785$, or 0.215. This means that there is a 21% chance of 6 or more cases occurring by chance if the underlying prevalence is 1 per 10,000. The closer this value is to zero, the smaller the likelihood that it would arise by chance alone. In this case, since the probability is not particularly small, we infer that the rate of disease is not unusually high. In general, probabilities less than 0.05 or 0.01 are considered to indicate significantly high prevalence rates.

Comparing choropleth and probability maps of low birthweight rates for Manhattan in New York City that were produced with a GIS illustrates the differences in these approaches (Figure 5.3). The map of actual rates shows considerable variation among neighborhoods, with an area of high rates in northern Manhattan. In the probability map, some of the areas with exceptionally high or low rates disappear. These are typically small

TABLE 5.1. Poisson Probabilities, $\lambda = 4.0$

Number of cases (x)	Probability $P(x)$	Cumulative probability $P(\leq x)$
0	.0183	.0183
1	.0733	.0916
2	.1465	.2381
3	.1954	.4335
4	.1954	.6289
5	.1563	.7852
6	.1042	.8894
7	.0595	.9489
8	.0298	.9787
9	.0134	.9919
10	.0053	.9972

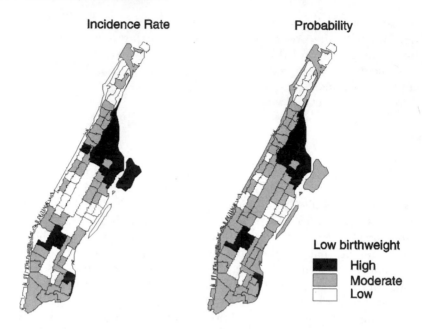

FIGURE 5.3. A map of incidence rates and a probability map of the same low birthweight data for Manhattan show different patterns. On the probability map, areas in the high and low categories are places that have rates significantly higher or lower than the overall rate. Compared to the incidence rate map, the probability map shows fewer areas in the high and low categories. Many areas with small populations drop out of those categories on the probability map.

unpopulated areas, whose rates are unstable due to the small numbers problem.

Probability mapping is a useful way of addressing the small numbers problem when mapping area health data, but it has two limitations. First, it does not preserve the content of the original data. Instead of mapping health incidence rates, it shows probability levels whose only connection to the rates themselves is through a statistical computation. Second, probability mapping tends to overemphasize the significance of rates in areas with large populations, because statistical significance is directly related to sample size. For an area with a large population, a rate that is slightly higher than the expected rate will often be statistically significant because the size of the population increases statistical power. This means it is easier to reject the null hypothesis that there is no difference in rates. Thus, a statistically significant difference may not be substantively meaningful. Analysts need to look beyond statistical significance by examining the raw diseases rates, the locations of high-rate areas, and any additional information that might assist in interpreting high-rate areas. GIS support this more comprehensive view of statistical significance.

Empirical Bayes Smoothing

Empirical Bayes estimation is a method for addressing some of these issues while dealing with the small numbers problem (Clayton & Kaldor, 1987; Cressie, 1992; Langford, 1994). It represents a compromise between probability mapping and simple choropleth mapping of rates. In empirical Bayes smoothing, rates are adjusted upward or downward, or *smoothed*, according to the size of the population on which they are based. The smoothing process pulls rates toward the national or regional rate, making the rates more stable and less variable. The rates for small areas are smoothed more than those for large areas, reflecting differences in reliability linked to population size.

Three assumptions underlie empirical Bayes methods (Langford, 1994). The first is that the smoothing process should not affect the overall rate for the study area. We assume that this overall rate is reliable and unbiased. Second, as noted earlier, rates for small areas are adjusted more than rates for large areas. Finally, we assume that the incidence rates for all areas in the study region follow a known probability distribution, called the "prior distribution." Some common distributions are the gamma, beta, and log normal distributions.

The mathematical details of empirical Bayes smoothing are well beyond the scope of this book, but by using these three assumptions we can describe the conceptual basis for the procedure. Many prior distributions used in empirical Bayes smoothing have two parameters, α, which describes the shape of the distribution, and β, which indicates the scale of the distribution. These are estimated statistically to "best fit" the distribution of actual health rates. The incidence rate across all areas is β/α.

Now consider a small area i with population P_i and k_i cases of disease. The actual incidence rate for area i is k_i/P_i. Having estimated alpha and beta from the prior distribution, the smoothed incidence rate for area i is calculated as:

$$(k_i + \beta)/(P_i + \alpha)$$

When area i is small in geographical size, k_i and P_i are often small and the smoothed rate approaches the overall incidence rate. Conversely, when k_i and P_i are large, they dominate the smoothing process and the smoothed rate for area i is very close to the actual rate, k_i/P_i.

As a consequence, empirical Bayes smoothing greatly affects rates for small areas. Figure 5.4 shows a map of actual death rates from fire by county for the United States and a map of smoothed rates for the same

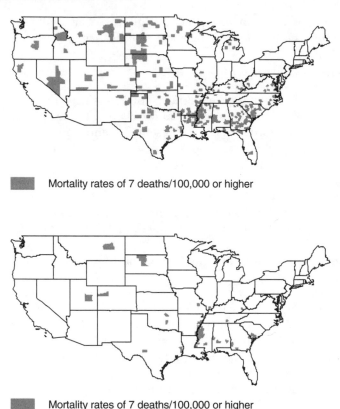

FIGURE 5.4. The top map is a choropleth map of U.S. counties with observed fire- and burn-related mortality rates of seven deaths per 100,000 population or higher, 1979 to 1987. The bottom map shows the empirical Bayes fire- and burn-related mortality rates of seven deaths per 100,000 population or higher, 1979 to 1987. The choropleth map and the smoothed map show different patterns. From Devine and Lewis (1994). Copyright 1994 by John Wiley & Sons, Ltd. Reproduced by permission.

data (Devine & Louis, 1994). Counties with rates above 7.0 are shaded on the maps. The map of actual rates shows spatial clustering of high rates in the sparsely populated counties of the western states. More than 200 counties have rates above 7.0. In contrast, the smoothed map shows only 50 counties with high rates. Many of the less-populated counties in the West moved out of the high-rate category. Because of their small populations, their rates were adjusted down toward the overall mean. Despite their high actual rates, these counties have such small populations that we cannot confidently categorize them as "high-rate" places.

An important issue in empirical Bayes estimation is to define the overall rate to which other rates are smoothed. For many kinds of health problems, using the same rate for all areas "washes out" the geographical variation and dependence that we know exists. Neighboring areas often have similar rates because of similarities in their social, economic, and environmental characteristics. A localized rate for the region in which an area is located would serve as a better benchmark for smoothing.

Cressie (1992) and Marshall (1991) describe procedures for performing regionalized empirical Bayes smoothing. These procedures recognize and model the spatial dependence that characterizes virtually all health information. Generally the procedures work by computing for each area the localized rate of disease in its neighborhood. Then the disease rate for area i is smoothed toward this neighborhood rate rather than the national rate. There are several approaches to defining the neighborhood of an area within the larger study area.

Defining Neighborhoods

Defining each area's "neighborhood" involves spatial operations that can easily be accomplished in GIS. One way to identify neighborhoods is based on *adjacency*, that is, whether or not areas share a common boundary (Figure 5.5a). If two areas border each other, they are considered to be in each others' neighborhood. GIS systems often include operations for identifying adjacency among areas.

Another criterion for identifying neighborhoods is *proximity*, the distance between areas. If area j is located within a certain critical distance of area i, it is in i's neighborhood (Figure 5.5b). There are two ways of defining proximity with area data. One is to determine the *centroid*, or central location, for each area, and then calculate the distance between area centroids. Most GIS include built-in functions for defining area centroids. Using this approach, area j is in area i's neighborhood if the distance between the two centroids is less than the critical distance. Alternatively, we can define proximity based on the fraction of area lying within the critical distance of i's centroid. Area j lies within i's neighborhood if a large proportion of j's territory falls within the critical distance radius. GIS can be used to automate these spatial operations and compute locally smoothed empirical Bayes estimates.

Local Measures of Spatial Autocorrelation

Another important class of methods for exploring area health data includes localized measures of spatial dependence such as Anselin's (1995) local indicators of spatial autocorrelation (LISA statistic) and Getis and Ord's (1992) G^* statistic. These measure the association between a value at a particular place and values for nearby or adjacent areas. The statistics are

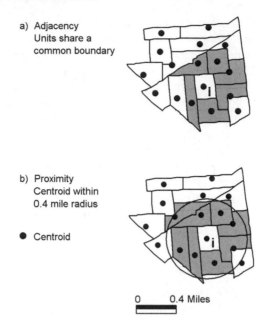

a) Adjacency
   Units share a
   common boundary

b) Proximity
   Centroid within
   0.4 mile radius

● Centroid

0   0.4 Miles

FIGURE 5.5. Defining the geographical neighborhood for area i based on (a) adjacency and (b) proximity. Note how the neighborhoods differ depending on the criteria used.

useful for finding disease clusters based on area data. A *cluster* is a region that has abnormally high rates, that is, a local concentration of high rates.

Getis and Ord's G^* statistic illustrates well the structure of these localized measures of spatial dependence. Consider an area divided into m subareas. x_i refers to the value of the health indicator (e.g., incidence or prevalence rate or standardized mortality ratio) for area i. w_{ij} defines the nearness of area i to area j, either based on adjacency or proximity, as discussed above. Given these definitions, the standardized G^* statistic is:

$$G_i^*(d) = \frac{\sum_j w_{ij}(d)x_j - W_i^* \bar{x}}{s\{[(nS_{1i}^*) - W_i^{*2}]/(n-1)\}^{1/2}}$$

where

$$W_i^* = \sum_j w_{ij}(d) \text{ and } S_{1i}^* = \sum_j w_{ij}^2$$

$$\bar{x} = \sum_j x_j / n$$

$$s = \{\sum_j (x_j - \bar{x})^2 / n\}^{1/2}$$

G^*_i is positive when high rates of disease cluster in i's local neighborhood. This indicates a disease cluster or geographical grouping of high prevalence rates.

Although G^* is a statistical measure, calculating it involves several common GIS operations. GIS can be used for determining adjacency or proximity and creating choropleth maps of the G^* values. Figure 5.6 shows a map of G^* statistics for data on sudden infant death syndrome (SIDS) by county in North Carolina (Getis & Ord, 1992). High G^* values indicate geographical clusters of SIDS among counties. The map reveals a high concentration of SIDS in the south central portion of the state, a concentration that was not clearly evident on the map of actual SIDS rates.

This section described a diverse set of methods for analyzing area health data. The methods provide valuable ways of modeling spatial dependence and addressing the small numbers problem, issues that plague traditional mapping of area health data. But area health data have limitations that cannot be solved by more sophisticated methodologies. As noted in Chapter 4, the locations of area boundaries may fundamentally affect the results of the analysis. Boundaries can split apart geographical clusters of health events so that clusters are not apparent in the separate area statistics. In addition, the statistics generated vary with the size and configuration of the areas. One way to overcome these problems is to work with point-based health information.

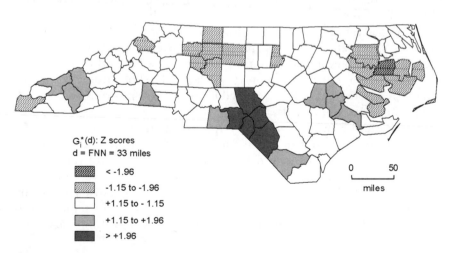

FIGURE 5.6. A map of standardized values of the G^* statistic, a local measure of spatial autocorrelation, showing spatial patterns in SIDS rates in counties of North Carolina for 1979 through 1984. The furthest nearest neighbor distance, d, is 33 miles. From Getis and Ord (1992). Copyright 1992 by Ohio State University Press. All rights reserved. Reprinted by permission.

METHODS FOR ANALYZING POINT DATA

A wide range of methods exist for analyzing spatial clusters of disease with point data. This section considers a representative, but not exhaustive, set of methods. For more information on the full suite of methods, the reader can turn to several excellent reviews of the literature (Marshall, 1991; Kulldorff, 1998; Gatrell, Bailey, Diggle, & Rowlingson, 1996). Point-based cluster detection methods can be divided into three groups: those that assess overall clustering in a study area; those that seek to identify cluster locations; and "focused" tests that assess clustering around a point source like a hazardous facility. The latter two are of more direct interest to GIS since they can take full advantage of the display and analytical capabilities of GIS. We discuss one method for detecting overall clustering and then consider a more varied set of procedures for identifying cluster locations. We do not address focused tests here; the interested reader can find useful information in Bithell (1995) and Lawson and Waller (1996).

Tests of Overall Clustering: Cuzick and Edwards's Method

For public health analysts, a first step in analyzing point-based maps of ill health is to evaluate the overall tendency toward clustering. Cuzick and Edwards's (1990) method addresses this question when geographic coordinates are available for both cases and controls. The method examines the k nearest neighbors to each case. If cases are geographically clustered, most of those k nearest neighbors will also be cases. The test statistic, T, represents the total number of k nearest neighbors that are cases. Clearly, a large value for T indicates that cases are spatially clustered in relation to the underlying geographical distribution of controls. The method includes a significance test for T that determines if the actual level of clustering is significantly greater than would be expected if cases and controls were randomly assigned (Cuzick & Edwards, 1990).

Cuzick and Edwards's method requires geographical coordinates for each case and each control in the database. Euclidean distances between points are calculated to determine nearest neighbors, and then significance tests are performed (Jacquez, 1996). GIS do not have an essential role in this method, since the operations are primarily statistical, not spatial. However, GIS are useful for geocoding addresses to generate the coordinates and for storing and managing the case–control information.

Identifying Cluster Locations

More directly tied to GIS are methods for visualizing and exploring geographical evidence of disease clustering. The goal is to provide innovative ways of viewing and analyzing point health data that enable public health analysts to identify places that have elevated disease rates, to gain insights into the likelihood that such rates would occur by chance, and to prioritize areas for further investigation. From a GIS standpoint, the methods described in this section loosely follow the field and object data models, discussed in Chapter 2, in analyzing cluster locations. The first four cluster methods search a continuous field for evidence of clustering, whereas the last method searches around the health events modeled as objects. This classification is based on how the clusters are originally modeled. Once identified, clusters can be analyzed as either field or object spatial data.

Kernel Estimation

Kernel estimation is not a cluster detection method per se, but a method for exploring and displaying spatial patterns of point health data. It is a method for generating a map that shows the density of health events modeled as a continuous field (Gatrell et al., 1996). Although health events occur in particular human or animal hosts, at distinct locations, the risk of ill health exists almost everywhere. Thus, we can view health risk as being distributed continuously over space, with "peaks" representing areas of poor health and "valleys" areas of better health. Kernel estimation is useful for generating such a continuous surface from point data.

In kernel estimation, a "window," or kernel, is moved across the study area, and the density of events is computed within this window (Figure 5.7). Typically, the window is a circle with a constant radius, or *bandwidth*. Events within the window are weighted according to their distance from the center of the window, the point at which density is being estimated (Bailey & Gatrell, 1995). The *kernel function* describes mathematically how those weights vary over distance. Events located near the center have a greater weight than those distant from the center. In this way, kernel estimation reflects the underlying geographic locations of events within each window.

After computing kernel estimates of the density of health events within each regularly spaced window, one can generate a map of density using standard map contouring procedures. The smoothed surface may be displayed as a contour map, a three-dimensional surface, or as a continuously shaded map with gray or color tones representing density levels (Figure 5.8).

Smoothed maps of health events are useful for showing variation in disease intensity, but they do not assess clustering in relation to risk population. However, we can use kernel smoothing for cluster detection by creating a spatially smoothed map of risk population similar to the smoothed map of health events. At each grid point we compute the difference be-

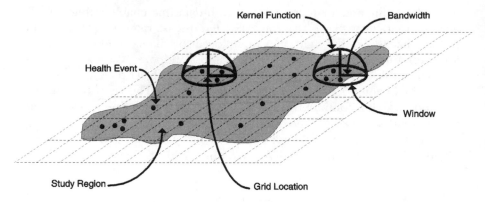

FIGURE 5.7. A schematic of the kernel smoothing method.

tween the disease intensity and the intensity of risk population (Kafadar, 1996). Clusters exist when the disease intensity greatly exceeds the population intensity.

A key issue in implementing kernel estimation is selection of the bandwidth. Larger bandwidths smooth the data more, removing local variation. In contrast, small bandwidths result in very little smoothing, producing an irregular bumpy map. Generally we seek a compromise between these two extremes. One approach is to experiment with different values of the bandwidth and choose the one that gives the best balance be-

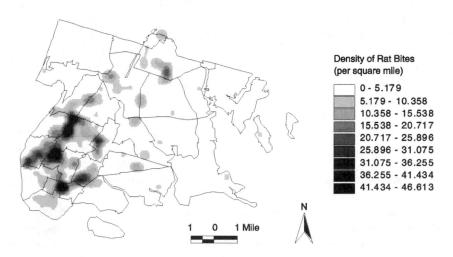

FIGURE 5.8. A contour map, generated by kernel estimation, showing the density of rat bites per square mile in the Bronx, New York. Data provided by the New York City Department of Health.

tween smoothing the data and depicting local variation. Algorithms for finding the optimal bandwidth are also available. Another promising approach is to use different bandwidths over different parts of the study area. For more detailed discussions of these and other issues, see Gatrell et al. (1996).

Geographical Analysis Machine

Another "field" method for analyzing spatial clustering is the geographical analysis machine (GAM) developed by Openshaw, Charlton, and Craft (1988). Unlike kernel estimation, the GAM includes a test of the statistical significance of disease clusters, that is, the likelihood that the observed number of cases in an area would have arisen by chance if the underlying risk of disease was not elevated. The GAM is an exploratory tool that searches for circles containing a significantly high prevalence of disease. It is a data- and computationally intensive method that evaluates health outcomes in circles of varying sizes spread densely across the study area. Significant circles, that is, those with high prevalence rates, are displayed on a map to show the locations and intensities of possible clusters.

The first step in GAM is to lay a fine grid over the study region. The grid points form the centroids of circles in which clustering is assessed. Around each grid point, different-sized circles are drawn (Figure 5.9). The circles should be at least large enough to encompass adjacent grid points. Next we determine if the incidence rate within each circle is higher than expected based on the overall "typical" rate of ill health in the population. This requires estimating the population at risk and the number of health events or cases within each circle to give the incidence rate. If possible, the rates should be age–sex adjusted to reflect demographic differences in risk population.

The next step is to determine which of the many circles around each grid point contains a significantly high rate of disease according to the Poisson test or some other statistical criterion. The actual number of health events within the circle is compared to the "expected" number of events based on the total risk population inside the circle. Circles that have significantly high rates are drawn on the map. We repeat this process for all grid points to examine all possible locations and sizes of clusters. The final map that shows all significant circles provides a visual representation of spatial clustering. The clusters appear as dense concentrations of significant circles.

GAM involves a logical sequence of GIS and statistical operations, from generating grid points to mapping significant circles (Table 5.2). It is really a hybrid GIS that incorporates standard GIS functions in a single-purpose analytic system.

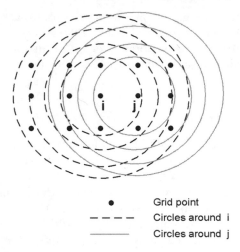

Grid point
Circles around i
Circles around j

FIGURE 5.9. A geographic analysis machine (GAM) computes the numbers of health events within circles of different sizes around each grid point.

GAM was originally developed to study clustering of certain cancers, especially childhood leukemia, around nuclear facilities in England. During the 1970s and 1980s, several widely published reports noted elevated rates of cancer near nuclear facilities. Of particular concern was the British Nuclear Fuels plant at Sellafield. A nearby village had reported what appeared to be an unusually high number of cases of childhood leukemia during the past decade. In this volatile context, GAM was used to explore and assess spatial clustering near Sellafield and other nuclear facilities. The analysis revealed a dense concentration of significant circles near Sellafield, pointing to an excess of cases around the nuclear facility (Figure 5.10). Another cluster appeared near a similar facility at Dounreay. However, other nuclear facilities had no clusters nearby, and several concentrations of significant circles were uncovered in places where no nuclear facilities were located.

TABLE 5.2. GIS Operations in GAM

Generate grid points

Generate circles of varying radii around each point

Count the number of cases within each circle

Determine the risk population within each circle

Apply statistical test to determine if the number of cases is high relative to the risk population

Draw the circle if the number of cases is high

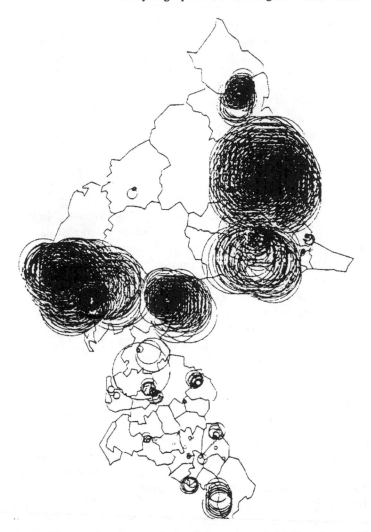

FIGURE 5.10. The results of an analysis of clustering of childhood acute lympho-blastic leukemia in a study region in England using GAM. From Openshaw, Charlton, and Craft (1988). Copyright 1988 by Regional Science Association International. Reprinted by permission.

The apparent cluster at Sellafield stimulated detailed epidemiological studies of cancer prevalence in the area, along with alternative spatial analyses of the same data. While most evidence confirmed the Sellafield cluster, some questioned whether the cluster was necessarily caused by the direct impact of radiation. A detailed case–control study found an excess risk among children whose fathers worked at the nuclear facilities, especially those fathers who were exposed to a high dose of ionizing radiation before the children's conception (Wakeford, 1990). Others hypothesized that the cluster was viral in origin and that the leukemia epidemic was triggered by in-migration of workers to the region (Thomas, 1992). Clearly, the kinds of spatial analyses that are embedded in GAM cannot directly address these hypotheses. Yet, by sifting through large amounts of data and displaying patterns that might not otherwise be apparent, GAM provided a platform for more detailed investigation.

Despite its innovativeness and important role in the Sellafield study, GAM was widely criticized on statistical grounds. The main problem is that GAM lacks a clear statistical yardstick for evaluating the number of significant circles that appear on the map. Because the circles overlap, many significant circles often contain the same cluster of cases. As a result, the Poisson tests that determine each circle's significance are not independent. This is the problem of multiple testing (Kulldorff, 1998). The GAM maps often give the appearance of excess clustering, with a high percentage of "false positive" circles (Fotheringham & Zhan, 1996). GAM maps for random point patterns have been generated, but it is difficult to compare these to actual GAM results. Still, GAM continues to be revised and improved, and it has paved the way for new exploratory spatial analysis methods linked to, or embedded in, GIS.

Spatial Scan Statistic

A method similar to GAM, but which takes into account the problem of multiple testing, is the spatial scan statistic (Kulldorff, 1997). Like GAM, the method utilizes a field approach and searches over a regular grid using circles of different sizes. For each circle, the method computes the likelihood that the risk of disease is elevated inside the circle compared to outside the circle. Alternative statistical models, including Poisson and Bernoulli distributions and Monte Carlo simulation, can be used in assessing significance. The circle with the highest likelihood value is the circle that has the highest probability of containing a disease cluster. Clustering in other circles can be tested by comparison with the maximum likelihood value. Software for the spatial scan statistic is available from the National Cancer Institute (Kulldorff, Rand, Gherman, Williams, & DiFrancesco, 1998).

Kulldorff, Feuer, Miller, and Freedman (1997) used the spatial scan statistic to test for clustering of breast cancer mortality in the northeast United States. They found one statistically significant cluster extending from the New York metropolitan area through parts of New Jersey to Philadelphia. Long Island is included in the region, lending support to the reported cluster of breast cancer there.

Rushton and Lolonis's Method

Rushton and Lolonis's (1996) method is a field-based method that incorporates innovative procedures for visualizing and analyzing cluster significance. Like kernel estimation, it uses a window of constant size to scan the study area for clusters; like GAM and the spatial scan statistic, it provides information about the likelihood that a cluster might have occurred by chance. The method uses Monte Carlo procedures to simulate possible spatial patterns of health events within a geographically fixed risk population—in effect, it simulates alternative maps of health events. Assuming that disease risk is constant, or that it can be estimated based on known risk factors, the simulations provide a null hypothesis distribution of possible health outcomes in different parts of the study area for comparison with actual patterns. Clusters are places where the actual number of health events is significantly larger than that found in the corresponding null hypothesis distribution.

Rushton and Lolonis's (1996) method typically utilizes point location data for both individuals at risk and cases of disease to generate simulated patterns of health events. Together, these cases and noncases form the total risk population. If the incidence of ill health was the same everywhere, or if it was simply based on known risk factors, then each of these individuals would face a predictable risk of ill health. Based on this assumption, the method simulates alternative spatial patterns of health events to provide a benchmark for comparison. For each individual at risk, the method randomly generates an outcome (event/nonevent) based on the known incidence rate for the study area. This process is repeated for each individual at risk, creating a simulated pattern of health events within the risk population. The number of events in the simulated pattern need not equal the number of events in the actual data set, though the overall risk is constant.

Rushton and Lolonis (1996) recommend generating several thousand of these simulated patterns. As with other field methods, a regular grid of points is superimposed on the study area each time a simulated pattern is generated. Overlapping circular zones are created around each grid point (Figure 5.11). Within each of these circular zones an incidence rate is computed for each simulated pattern. The full set of 1,000 or more simulated rates serves as a benchmark distribution for that circular zone. The zone's actual rate is compared to its simulated rates, and the percentage of simulated rates that are less than the actual rate provides a measure of significance. A high percentage means that in that zone the vast majority of simulated rates fall below the actual rate, indicating that the actual rate is unusually high. The percentages can be displayed on an isarithmic map to show areas with significantly high rates.

This method consists of an interplay of GIS operations and statisti-

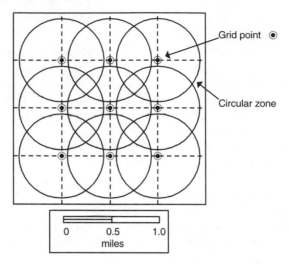

FIGURE 5.11. Overlapping circular zones generated around grid points in the Rushton and Lolonis method of analyzing clusters. From Rushton and Lolonis (1996). Copyright 1996 by John Wiley & Sons, Ltd. Reproduced by permission.

cal simulation procedures. The GIS functions are relatively straightforward: first, create grid points and circles, and second, count the numbers of cases and noncases within each circle. After that it is necessary to generate the simulated, random patterns of health events. Using a random number generator, the analyst generates a simulated outcome (either event or no event) for each individual at risk. Then the system is used to compute the numbers of simulated events and nonevents within each circle to derive a simulated rate. This is repeated thousands of times to determine the benchmark distributions for comparison with actual rates. Most existing GIS cannot perform statistical simulations, so it is necessary to use statistical programs or to write specialized software for this purpose.

Rushton and Lolonis (1996) used this method to analyze spatial clustering of birth defects in Des Moines, Iowa. Local health officials were concerned about poor infant health indicators in the city and wanted to be able to identify neighborhoods where birth defect rates were significantly high. From birth records, the researchers knew the residential locations of all births in the city—the risk population—as well as the locations of infants born with birth defects—the health event. One thousand simulated patterns of birth defects were generated. Figure 5.12 shows areas where the actual birth defect rate exceeded 95% of the simulated rates. The map depicts an elongated cluster of high rates in the east central portion of the city.

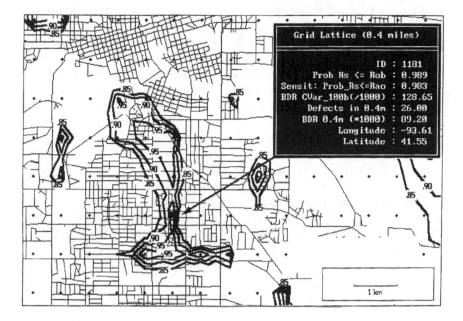

FIGURE 5.12. Areas with statistically significant high birth defect rates in Des Moines, Iowa, based on the Rushton and Lolonis method. From Rushton and Lolonis (1996). Copyright 1996 by John Wiley & Sons, Ltd. Reproduced by permission.

An Object Approach to Clustering: Besag and Newell's Method

Unlike the previous methods, which search for clusters across the entire study area, Besag and Newell (1991) devised a spatial clustering method that only searches for clusters around cases. Their method adopts an "object" approach, treating health events as objects, instead of the "field" approach of the previous methods. Besag and Newell's logical premise is that *clustering can only exist in places where cases exist*, so instead of searching over the entire study region, we need only search around cases. This greatly reduces the amount of spatial search and computation required and provides a finite limit to the number of significant clusters that can be detected.

Assume that we have point data for cases but area data for risk population. The actual locations of health events are known, while data on risk population is available for areas such as counties, census tracts, or blocks. Let k be the minimum number of cases needed to constitute a disease cluster. Besag and Newell's method tests for clustering around a case i by analyzing the number of nearest neighbor areas (M_i) needed to accumulate the k cases closest to i. In other words, if we rank cases according to their distance from i and identify the k nearest cases, M_i identifies the geographical areas that contain those k cases (Figure 5.13). Defining x_j as the number of cases in area j and p_j as its risk population, then the total number of cases in M_i is $X_j = \Sigma x_j$ and the total risk population is $P_i = \Sigma p_j$. To test for clustering around i, we analyze whether the total number of cases in M_i is large relative to total risk population. Once again the Poisson test is used to assess significance, with λ set at the incidence rate for the entire study area.

Besag and Newell's method involves a sequence of operations that can be implemented in GIS. At each case location, we first compute distances to all other cases and rank the distances to determine the k nearest. Point-in-polygon operations identify the areas in which the k nearest cases are located to identify the set M_i for case i. We then sum cases and risk population across those areas and calculate the statistical test to determine if the number of cases is significantly high relative to the risk population. If prevalence is high, one can draw a circle encompassing that cluster and display the cluster on a map. As in the GAM, clusters often appear as overlapping concentrations of circles.

A critical issue in Besag and Newell's (1991) method is the choice of k,

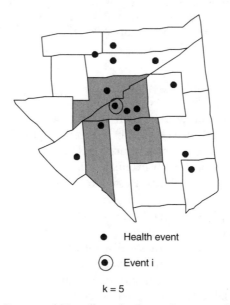

●   Health event

⊙   Event i

k = 5

FIGURE 5.13. The Besag and Newell method searches around each health event i to find the k nearest health events. The areas containing those events are shaded. The risk population within the shaded areas is the denominator for the Poisson test.

the cluster size parameter. The value of k must be large enough to identify real clusters of cases, not just isolated groupings. But it must be small enough to permit the identification of distinct clusters within a region. Values of between 2 and 5 are common, representing clusters of 3 to 6 cases including the centroid case. Besag and Newell recommend trying several k values and analyzing the sensitivity of the results to the choice of k.

A modified version of Besag and Newell's method was used to search for spatial clustering of breast cancer cases among long-term residents of West Islip, New York (Timander & McLafferty, 1998). West Islip is a middle-income community of approximately 40,000 people located on Long Island. As in many communities on Long Island, residents of West Islip were worried about high rates of breast cancer and possible links to environmental factors: hazardous waste sites, contaminants in the water supply, and electromagnetic fields. Taking the matter into their own hands, they conducted a survey of local residents to find out about breast cancer prevalence and risk factors (Grimson, 1999).

The survey data were entered into a GIS, geocoded, and displayed on a community map. To see if cases were clustered within West Islip, a modified version of Besag and Newell's (1991) clustering method was used and implemented in a GIS. Because breast cancer takes many years to develop, the research focused on long-term residents, survey respondents who had lived at their current addresses for more than 25 years. These people would be most affected by hazards in the local environment near their homes. The GIS analysis showed no strong evidence of spatial clustering of breast cancer in West Islip. Four significant overlapping clusters were uncovered in the south central portion of the town (Figure 5.14), but the clusters disappeared when known risk factors for breast cancer, like family history and age at first pregnancy, were controlled.

Compared to the GAM, Besag and Newell's (1991) procedure provides a clearer description of cluster locations. Because the method only checks for clusters around cases, it is more conservative in detecting clusters and is less likely to identify false positives (Fotheringham & Zhan, 1996). By limiting the search process, it is also less computationally intensive than GAM and thus represents an efficient option for cluster detection.

USES OF SPATIAL CLUSTERING METHODS

Spatial clustering methods are exploratory tools that help researchers and policymakers make sense of complex geographic patterns. Knowing whether or not clusters exist and where they are located provides an important foundation for health research and policy formulation. State health

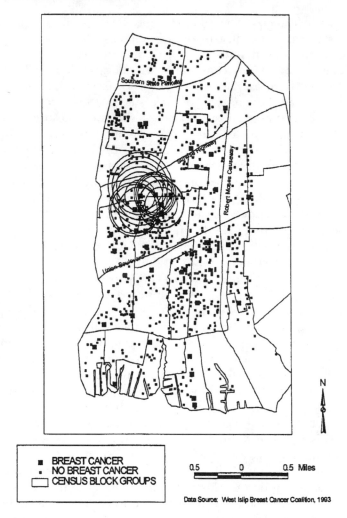

FIGURE 5.14. Spatial clusters of breast cancer in West Islip, New York, based on a modified Besag and Newell method, for $k = 4$, 5, and 6. There were four significant circles in the set of circles for which $k = 4$; there were six significant circles each in the sets of circles for which $k = 5$ and $k = 6$. Reprinted from Timander and McLafferty (1988), with permission from Elsevier Science.

departments receive literally thousands of requests for spatial cluster investigations from individuals and community groups every year (Greenberg & Wartenberg, 1991). The methods discussed here can be used to confirm or deny the existence of suspected clusters in an efficient and effective manner.

Responding to community concerns, however, only deals with a fraction of potential clusters and is likely to miss clusters in communities that lack political and economic clout. To overcome this bias, cluster detection needs to be incorporated in ongoing public health surveillance efforts (Rushton, 1998). With GIS, health departments can monitor health records as they come in, using spatial clustering methods to search for unusual patterns. Of course, once a cluster is identified, only detailed epidemiological investigation can determine if the cluster is a "random" event or if it is linked to some environmental, occupational, or social cause. A small number of clusters will occur by chance, even if health risks are not elevated. Therefore, it is essential that statistically significant clusters be examined in more detail. Spatial cluster analysis is not an end in and of itself; it is a screening tool that assists in guiding public health surveillance efforts.

Incorporating spatial clustering methods in GIS also makes it possible to conduct exploratory analyses to help in identifying the causes and correlates of health problems. Overlaying cluster maps with other spatial databases, including environmental, social, transportation, and facilities data, can provide clues about the causes of disease, while identifying variations in health linked to differences in physical and social environments. These map overlays have always been important hypothesis-generating tools in public health research and policymaking (Croner, Pickle, Wolf, & White, 1992). Now they can be done efficiently and effectively, in an automated GIS environment. These overlay procedures are discussed in more detail in the chapters that follow.

CHALLENGES

Much progress has been made in designing algorithms for spatial clustering analysis, but many challenges remain. One challenge comes from the interrelated problems of disease latency and migration bias. *Latency* refers to the length of time between exposure to a disease-causing agent and the appearance of symptoms. While some health problems develop quickly, others (e.g., many cancers) take months or years to develop. *Migration bias* refers to the effects of migration on the results of a clustering analysis. Most cluster methods only work with single addresses at single points in time. Yet people in the United States move frequently, and they face different environments at each place of residence. A person's current address may have little connection to his or her environmental exposures over the life span. Migration effects are most relevant for diseases such as many cancers, heart disease, and multiple sclerosis, those with long latency periods that result from environmental, social, behavioral, and genetic factors interacting over long periods of time.

How can these problems be addressed? One approach is to focus on long-term residents or people who have spent most of their lives in the local area, as was done in the West Islip breast cancer study. Another approach is to collect and utilize information on migration histories. We need to devise methods that assess clustering through space and time based on individuals' life paths. This second approach presents its own challenges, though, because we no longer are dealing with a geographically defined population. The "population" encompasses people at different locations, at different points in time.

Confounding factors, known risk factors, also present challenges in spatial clustering analysis. For many health problems, some fraction of cases can be explained by known risk factors. These include basic demographic factors like age, as well as behavioral and genetic factors, such as smoking and family history. It is critically important to control for these factors in analyzing spatial clustering. Methods are currently being developed to incorporate confounding factors directly in clustering analyses. These methods often involve using statistical methods to control for known risk factors and then analyzing "unexplained" clustering (Kingham, Gatrell, & Rowlingson, 1995). Alternatively, one can identify cohorts of similar individuals and examine spatial clustering of disease within those cohorts. Finally, cluster analysis can be embedded in case–control designs or integrated with traditional age–sex standardization procedures (Rushton, Krishnamurthy, Krishnamurti, Lolonis, & Song, 1996).

The theoretical basis of clustering methods is also important. Most methods make naive assumptions about the environmental or social processes that generate observed patterns. Clusters of motor vehicle accidents will be arrayed in a linear pattern constrained by the road network. Clusters that are environmental in origin may follow contamination footprints or plumes of air pollution. Communicable disease clusters are shaped by human interactions that are unlikely to fit simple geometric forms. These types of GIS-based health analyses are discussed in Chapters 6 through 8.

Finally, most spatial cluster methods are not available in commercial GIS. Typically the analyst must use specialized programs and import/export data and results to a GIS. Fortunately, computer programs to perform many of the clustering methods described here are available commercially or as shareware. It is also possible to write macros in some GIS systems to implement clustering procedures, but this requires programming skills, and many GIS still do not incorporate the advanced statistical functions that form the foundation of clustering methods. This situation is changing rapidly, however. Many GIS are developing closer and more seamless links with powerful statistical packages. The marriage of statistical and geographical power will greatly enhance our ability to use a diverse set of clustering methods and explore the sensitivity of results to changes in parameter values.

CONCLUSION

This chapter has discussed a representative set of methods for analyzing spatial clustering of health events using area or point data. Many other methods exist, and we encourage readers to look beyond this chapter to find the method that best fits their data and clustering problem. Good general references include Marshall (1991), Kulldorff (1998), and Gatrell and Bailey (1996). What does the future hold? Given the rapid advances in GIS and computer technology and the growing spatial analysis capabilities of GIS, it is likely that desktop GIS will soon be able to perform spatial clustering tests. This will give public health departments an expanded and enhanced set of tools for performing one of their most basic surveillance tasks: the search for clusters of health problems.

CHAPTER 6

Analyzing Environmental Hazards

Environmental health, "the prevention and control of health problems related to the environment" (Thacker, Stroup, Parrish, & Anderson, 1996, p. 633), is an important function of health departments at the local, state, and federal levels. Environmental health problems involve agents that produce adverse health outcomes in humans. These *agents* can be physical (ultraviolet radiation), chemical (lead), or biological (cryptosporidium) in nature. Human populations encounter these agents by breathing, eating and drinking, or coming into physical contact with agents present in the atmosphere, the food and water supply, and the natural and built environments. GIS modeling of health problems involving biological agents is discussed in Chapters 7 and 8. This chapter focuses primarily on *toxicants*, natural or synthetic chemicals that produce adverse health outcomes.

The process by which an agent in the environment produces an adverse health outcome in a person can be modeled as a hazard–exposure–outcome process (Figure 6.1). Information systems for monitoring environmental health problems viewed in this way require longitudinal data on the amount, nature, and sources of environmental hazards; the environmental quality in the places where people live and conduct their daily activities; the presence of the agents in human populations; and the adverse health outcomes that can be linked to exposure. In cases where these data exist to support hazard surveillance for a particular agent, exposure and outcome data will rarely be available from the same single data source. Instead, data must be drawn from multiple sources and integrated in the surveillance system. Although not always explicit, time and space are the basis for data integration in a way that logically models haz-

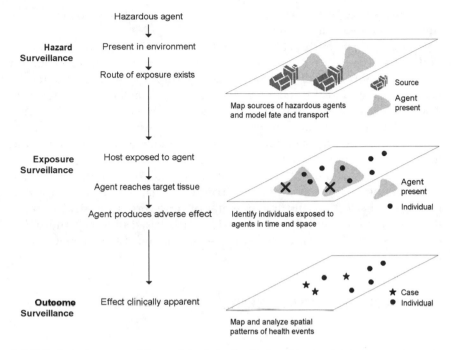

Hazard Surveillance

Hazardous agent
↓
Present in environment
↓
Route of exposure exists

Map sources of hazardous agents and model fate and transport

Source
Agent present

Exposure Surveillance

Host exposed to agent
↓
Agent reaches target tissue
↓
Agent produces adverse effect

Identify individuals exposed to agents in time and space

Agent present
Individual

Outcome Surveillance

Effect clinically apparent

Map and analyze spatial patterns of health events

Case
Individual

FIGURE 6.1. A geographic model of the hazard–exposure–outcome process.

ard–exposure–outcome processes. Integration of geographic data drawn from many sources is one of the main uses of GIS.

This chapter discusses GIS applications in environmental health. GIS have been used to display sources of environmental contaminants of concern for human health and to model the zones of contamination around these sources. Geographic variations in environmental quality measured at monitoring stations have also been modeled using GIS. The geographical distributions of populations at risk and spatial patterns of health outcomes, reviewed in Chapter 4, have also been reported and analyzed using GIS technology.

These applications suggest that complete environmental health surveillance systems are in place for only a few of the thousands of potentially hazardous agents. We have not identified all hazardous agents with demonstrated links to specific diseases, let alone described their presence in the environment in relation to susceptible populations. Somewhat more complete data are available on health outcomes, and these have been used to conduct epidemiological investigations to identify potential hazardous agents. This means that, for particular environmental health problems, surveillance systems will differentially emphasize hazard, exposure, or outcome surveillance.

The first part of this chapter briefly considers how an agent is identified as hazardous based on risk assessment and subsequently becomes a focus for reporting and regulation. The geography of hazard or potential hazard sources and the role of GIS in hazard surveillance are discussed. The following sections in the chapter address some of the most challenging aspects of environmental health surveillance using GIS: modeling exposure of susceptible populations to environmental contaminants and linking health outcome data to exposure.

The final sections of the chapter consider the role of GIS in risk management and issues in mapping environmental hazards. *Risk management* involves the selection and implementation of appropriate strategies for the regulation or control of identified hazards based on social and political factors (Ruckleshaus, 1983). Risk assessment and risk management are complementary.

HOW ENVIRONMENTAL AGENTS ARE IDENTIFIED AS HAZARDS

Before the source locations of hazards and the associated contamination fields can be modeled in a GIS, hazardous agents must be identified. Human experience has been an important source of awareness of the harmful effects of many toxicants. Our recognition of lead, mercury, and other chemicals as hazards to human health is centuries-old. The establishment of quantitative standards for risk, however, is largely a development of the last 100 years. In part, this reflects the growth and geographical dispersion of chemical production on an industrial scale (Cutter, 1993). In addition to naturally occurring chemicals, approximately 4,000 synthetic chemical substances are in commercial use worldwide, accounting for more than 99% of the total volume of synthetics (Moochhala, Shahi, & Cote, 1997). To cite just one example, more than 600 generic pesticides are commercially available. With the production, storage, transportation, use, and disposal of all these chemicals have come increased risks to workers, other susceptible populations, and the environment.

Quantitative risk assessment is the process of characterizing the health effects expected from exposure to an agent, estimating the probability of occurrence of health effects, estimating the number of occurrences in a population, and recommending acceptable concentrations of the agent in air, water, or food (Hallenbeck, 1993). In the United States, the development of quantitative standards for risk grew out of the Pure Food Act of 1906 (Hattis, 1996). Subsequent federal legislation has been the major impetus for conducting risk assessments. The statutes and their amendments do not generally define "acceptable risk"; the responsibility for determining acceptable risk is left to the various federal regulatory agencies implementing the legislation.

Three basic categories of scientific information are used in quantitative risk assessment: toxicological studies, controlled clinical studies, and epidemiological studies (Moochhala, Shahi, & Cote, 1997). Each of these approaches has advantages and disadvantages. GIS can perhaps provide the greatest support to quantitative risk assessment through epidemiological studies. Toxicological and controlled clinical studies are conducted in laboratory or clinical settings.

Toxicological studies have been a major and controversial source of information for risk assessment. *Toxicology* is an experimental science that studies the effects of toxic substances in selected animals or cells. Toxicological studies provide the greatest degree of control over populations exposed, exposure conditions, and measured effects. They are most often used to evaluate agents for which epidemiological studies would be premature because of the lags between exposure and outcome and for which controlled clinical studies would be unethical. Aside from the growing public debate over the ethical treatment of animals in human health research (Rowan, 1997; Barnard & Kaufman, 1997; Botting & Morrison, 1997), the major scientific limitation of toxicology studies is uncertainty in extrapolating the exposure–outcome relationships observed in animals to humans.

Controlled clinical studies, like toxicological investigations, provide the opportunity to control and quantify exposure but focus directly on the effects of agents on the health of human subjects instead of animals. The U.S. National Ambient Air Quality Standards for ozone and sulphur dioxide (SO_2) were developed in part based on controlled clinical studies of changes in airway resistance of asthma sufferers who were exposed while exercising (McDonnell et al., 1991). These effects would be difficult to detect in an epidemiological investigation of the general population. The major limitation of controlled clinical studies in producing data for risk assessment is that, for ethical reasons, research must be limited to exposures producing nothing worse than short-term health effects that are reversible. The number of human subjects is generally very small in these studies because of the costs of the research. Some susceptible individuals would never be considered appropriate human subjects for clinical studies because of the potential for harm.

An interesting issue in controlled clinical studies is the extent to which the human subjects are homogeneous with respect to housing and other aspects of environmental quality. A search of the literature suggests that the residential locations of participants in controlled clinical studies is rarely considered explicitly as part of the study sample design. As noted in the Introduction, a random selection of all people will not be a random selection of all places unless the population from which the sample is drawn is uniformly distributed (Goodchild, 1984). If there are important geographical differences in exposure, these could be explicitly considered in a spatially stratified sampling scheme for participants in controlled clinical studies.

The method of hazard identification where GIS can make the strongest contribution is environmental epidemiology. *Environmental epidemiology* research attempts to associate adverse health outcomes with environmental exposures. The main advantage of these studies is that they measure health effects in people based on actual exposure conditions. Epidemiological studies are particularly useful in situations where exposure concentrations are relatively high during the time period of investigation (e.g., exposure to benzene in workplaces) or when exposed populations are very large (e.g., large urban populations exposed to air pollution).

There are also limitations to epidemiological studies for risk assessment. Frequently, high-quality hazard information may not be available to assess exposure, as in the case of indoor air quality or water quality at the tap. Also, effects in worker populations may be unsuitable for estimating health effects in the total population because occupational exposures generally involve smaller populations at a limited number of sources and higher doses. Finally, from a public health perspective, it is most desirable to identify hazards *before* exposure has produced adverse human health effects. Epidemiological investigations, relying as they do on the lagged association between adverse outcomes and exposures, are not protective of human health because the adverse impacts have already been manifested.

Epidemiological investigations are designed to find out whether or not a statistically significant adverse health outcome is observed in an exposed group. Very large sample sizes are necessary to detect small increases in disease incidence with exposure. Characterizing exposure involves locating sources of potential toxicants; analyzing the transport and ultimate fate of toxicants released from these sources; collecting and analyzing samples that offer a measure of the environmental quality at various locations from air, water, and soil; describing the locations and demographic characteristics of exposed and susceptible populations; and modeling the conditions of human exposure. GIS can be useful in many of these analyses.

GIS ANALYSIS OF SOURCE LOCATIONS OF ENVIRONMENTAL HAZARDS

One way of classifying hazard sources is based on the geography of the discharge process. *Point source* pollution occurs when contaminants are discharged into the environment at a single discharge point, for example, a smokestack or a sewer (Puckett, 1994). Many of the air and water pollution control measures adopted in the early 1970s were directed at point sources because of the volume of pollutants they discharged and the relative ease of identifying them in the landscape. More recently, pollution control efforts have broadened to include nonpoint sources. *Nonpoint sources* contribute pollutants to the air, water, or soil at numerous and widespread locations rather than at a few localized discharge points. Motor vehicle emissions are a nonpoint source of air pollution. Commercial fertilizer and animal manure are important nonpoint sources of nitrogen, which affects water quality.

Some challenges in using GIS to represent the distribution of point and nonpoint pollution sources include quality of positional information, completeness of data, and acquisition of data from different regulatory agencies or other data sources. These factors can make compilation of source data difficult.

Databases of Known Point Sources

The Toxics Release Inventory

One of the most important sources of information on environmental release of toxic substances in the United States from point sources is the *Toxics Release Inventory* (TRI) developed by the Environmental Protection Agency (EPA) in 1986 as part of the Superfund reauthorization. Approximately 30 states and cities had already enacted some form of pollution disclosure law by this time (Hearne, 1996). After Congress passed Section 313 of the Emergency Planning and Community Right-to-Know (EPCRA) law, U.S. manufacturers were required to report to the EPA on an annual basis the amounts of toxic chemicals they release into the environment or ship off-site as waste (Doa, 1992). An important component of the law was creation of an unrestricted online reporting system. The Pollution Prevention Act of 1991 broadened the TRI to include reports on source reduction, recycling, and treatment. The law covers all manufacturing facilities in all U.S. states and jurisdictions employing the equivalent of 10 full-time employees in industries in *Standard Industrial Classification* (SIC) codes 20 through 39 that produce, import, or process 25,000 pounds or more of any of the 600 individual chemicals and 28 chemical categories on the TRI list of toxic chemicals or that use in any other manner 10,000 pounds or more of a TRI chemical during the reporting year (Environmental Protection Agency, 2000). The EPA requires manufacturers to submit complete TRI data forms for *each* chemical covered by the TRI if they meet the requirements. For example, a facility required to report on three TRI chemicals would submit three separate forms. The first year for which TRI data are available is calendar year 1987.

An important category of reporting information for the purposes of GIS analysis is facility information (Figure 6.2). This category includes lat/lon coordinates that identify where the release occurred. A variety of methods could be used to generate these coordinates: address matching, GPS, digitizing, cadastral survey, to name a few. When data produced by these relatively accurate methods are not available, the EPA provides instructions for determining coordinates from USGS topographic maps (Environmental Protection Agency, 2000). Since the positional data in the TRI comes from multiple sources, positional accuracy is highly variable. For large-scale mapping and analysis, locational information should be checked and verified or corrected to ensure that positional accuracy is within tolerable limits (Burke, 1993).

The geographic information in the TRI has provided a basis for describing geographic patterns of TRI facilities and releases (Stockwell et al., 1993). Considering the use of TRI data in an environmental hazard surveillance system, however, it is worth pointing out that TRI reporting requirements cover only a selected set of industries that release toxicants in their current operations. TRI data cannot be regarded as providing a complete spatial and temporal picture of environmental contamination.

Other Point Source Databases

To create a comprehensive picture of sources of environmental contamination in a particular region, public health analysts have to draw on multiple sources of information. Many state environmental protection agencies have compiled databases of sources of environmental contamination. In Connecticut, for example, the Department of Environmental Protection maintains a Point Source Inventory. The Point Source Inventory includes all sources in the state capable of emitting more than 5 tons per year of any one of a specified set of pollutants including carbon monoxide (CO), volatile organic compounds, lead, and particulates. Most of the sources are combustion sources, but these are sometimes operated by facilities like hospitals or schools that public health analysts might not readily think of as sources of environmental contaminants.

The Point Source Inventory includes state plane coordinate locations for each stack and a base elevation for the stack. This makes it possible to integrate data from the Point Source Inventory with other GIS databases maintained by the Connecticut Department of Environmental Protection. Mapping the locations of point sources reveals how widely distributed they are across the state (Figure 6.3). State environmental regulation and permitting statutes are an important place to identify the kinds of sources that are regulated in a state and that might be identified in a database compiled by a state regulatory agency.

SECTION 4. FACILITY IDENTIFICATION								
4.1	Facility or Establishment Name			TRI Facility ID Number		Facility or Establishment Name or Mailing Address(if different from street address)		
	Street			Mailing Address				
	City/County/State/Zip Code			City/County/State/Zip Code				
4.2	This report contains information for: (Important: check a or b; check c if applicable)	a. ☐	An entire facility	b. ☐	Part of a facility	c. ☐	A Federal facility	
4.3	Technical Contact Name					Telephone Number (include area code)		
4.4	Public Contact Name					Telephone Number (include area code)		
4.5	SIC Code (s) (4 digits)	a.	Primary	b.	c.	d.	e.	f.
4.6	Latitude	Degrees	Minutes	Seconds	Longitude	Degrees	Minutes	Seconds
4.7	Dun & Bradstreet Number(s) (9 digits)	**4.8**	EPA Identification Number (RCRA I.D. No.) (12 characters)	**4.9**	Facility NPDES Permit Number(s) (9 characters)	**4.10**	Underground Injection Well Code (UIC) I.D. Number(s) (12 digits)	
a.		a.		a.		a.		
b.		b.		b.		b.		

FIGURE 6.2. Reporting of facility information for the Toxics Release Inventory.

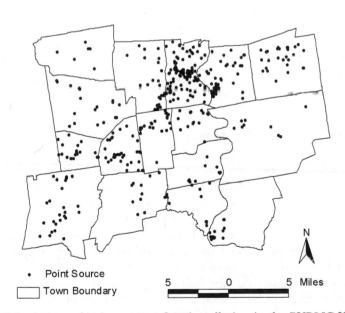

• Point Source
☐ Town Boundary

5　　　0　　　5　Miles

N

FIGURE 6.3. A map of point sources for air pollution in the PUBLIC HEALTH GIS study area. Data provided by the Connecticut Department of Environmental Protection.

Using GIS to Develop Databases of Potential Point Sources

In some cases, regulatory agencies find it difficult to identify all of the entities that may release toxicants and be subject to some kind of permitting or enforcement action. In these cases, GIS analysis has been used as a screening tool to identify the locations of industries that might be discharging wastes. An analysis taking this approach was conducted in seven counties in Pennsylvania to identify industries in the region likely to have shallow injection wells based on their SIC codes from the Dun and Bradstreet Baseline database (Davis & Flores, 1992). A GIS database of the locations of 14 types of industrial facilities was created based on the lat/lon reported in the Dun and Bradstreet database. This database, like the TRI, contains a variable describing how the coordinates of the facilities were determined. A GIS database of principal sewer systems was also created from maps of sewered and unsewered areas provided by local officials in the counties.

The analysts were interested in identifying facilities in unsewered areas because these facilities would likely be using injection wells to dispose of their liquid wastes. The cartographic overlay function of the GIS was used to overlay the two coverages. "In this way, the facilities outside sewered areas were easily identified" (Davis & Flores, 1992, p. 117). Using the GIS functions that enable selection of objects by feature attribute, companies that had yearly sales figures of more than $1,000,000 were selected and mapped separately because it was assumed that they generated higher levels of waste. A second group of companies having 20 or more employees was also selected because their septic systems required permitting.

Modeling Nonpoint Sources

GIS has also been useful in modeling the locations of nonpoint pollution sources. Septic system discharge in soils unsuitable for waste purification has been identified as an important source of groundwater pollution (Bicki & Brown, 1991). In Pennsylvania, where soil wetness, shallow bedrock, slow percolation, and steep slopes limit septic system performance, a GIS analysis was performed to model nitrogen loadings from septic systems on a statewide basis (Nizeyimana et al., 1996). It would be difficult to pinpoint the locations of more than one million septic systems on a statewide basis. The 1990 Census of Population and Housing, however, reports the number of housing units on septic tanks or cesspools by census tract. These data were used with data on the number of persons and housing units to estimate the amount of nitrogen produced in each tract. The census tract data were integrated with a database of watersheds in the state. Figure 6.4

shows the density of persons using septic systems per hectare by watershed in the state.

The Changing Geography of Hazards

Because modern industrial and agricultural activities involve assembly of raw materials from many sources and distribution of finished products and waste materials to many locations, hazard geography is not static. More than 1 billion tons of hazardous materials are transported in the United States annually across all modes (Lepofsky, Abkowitz, & Cheng, 1993). These shipments occur in all regions of the country. The Hazardous Materials Transportation Uniform Safety Act of 1990 provided a legislative basis for regulating these shipments.

In California, the Highway Patrol developed a GIS to support risk assessment and risk management of hazardous materials shipments (Lepofsky et al., 1993). Particular attention was paid to poisonous gases. The geographic database included a digitized network of all interstates, most federal and state highways, and selected county and local roads ex-

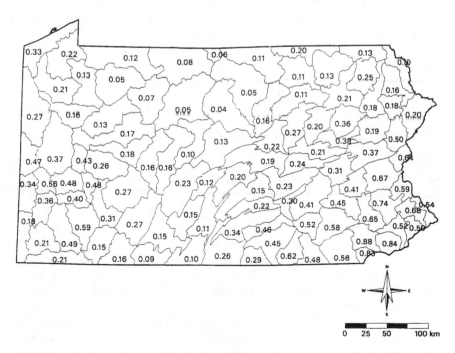

FIGURE 6.4. An estimate of persons using septic systems per hectare by watershed area in Pennsylvania. From Nizeyimana et al. (1996). Copyright 1996 by the *Journal of Environmental Quality*. Reprinted by permission.

tracted from the National Highway Planning Network and augmented to include all highways in the state and some additional county and local roads. In some cases, location data can be obtained in real time from vehicles fitted with monitoring devices.

As the economics of production change, producers of goods and services change their locations. Local land use and zoning controls provide some basis for evaluating potential impacts from new activities making use of toxic substances or generating them during the production process. It may be more difficult to detect historical patterns of contamination, particularly when land use change has occurred. Nevertheless, it is possible to reconstruct past community landscapes. Old telephone directories, Sanborn fire insurance maps (Geography and Map Division, Library of Congress, 1981; Keister, 1993), reports and case studies of contamination events (Colten, 1991), and other archival materials can be used to reconstruct the locations of tanneries, paint manufacturers, metal processors, and other businesses that might have polluted the environment or even the geographical patterns of past contamination events.

Computer models have also been developed to estimate quantities of hazardous wastes generated at industrial facilities based on their number of employees and the products they manufacture (Ashact, Ltd. & Dagh Watson, Spa., 1989). The locations of the industrial facilities can then be determined from directories, remote sensing data, or field surveys. This approach is potentially useful in environmental health analyses conducted in situations where facilities are not required to disclose hazardous material inventories (Lowry, Miller, & Hepner, 1995).

Integrating Databases Describing Sources of Contaminants

GIS applications have used TRI data in conjunction with other source data to describe the sources of environmental contaminants more completely. As part of a project to monitor environmental conditions within the Greenpoint/Williamsburg section of Brooklyn, New York, data on the locations of approximately 20 TRI sites were integrated with data on the locations of other potential sources of environmental contaminants (Osleeb & Kahn, 1999). These included a sewage treatment plant and incinerator, a low-level radioactive waste repository, more than 200 hazardous-materials processors, a major expressway, and a large number of chemical and petroleum bulk storage tanks.

As these applications show, GIS have been used to describe the sources of environmental contaminants. But even when these databases are relatively complete, the location of pollution sources only partially describes the geography of environmental hazards. Contamination zones around these sources also need to be evaluated.

MODELING FATE AND TRANSPORT AND ENVIRONMENTAL QUALITY IN A GIS

Fate and Transport Modeling

After the locations of sources of toxicants have been identified and analyzed, it is necessary to understand how these agents affect environmental quality *in situ* and elsewhere. *Fate and transport models* are used to investigate what happens to agents that are released into the environment. These models require geographic and physical descriptions of the source and information on the rate of release into the atmosphere, the hydrosphere (surface water and groundwater), and the lithosphere (land). Given the location of the source, the meteorology of the receiving air (including rainfall patterns), the hydrology and hydrogeology of the receiving water features, and the physical and geologic characteristics of the receiving land can be evaluated.

Models that attempt to describe the areas ultimately impacted by discharges into the air, water, or soil generally consist of two major components: a chemical dispersion model and a GIS database (Chakraborty & Armstrong, 1995). Given information about the types of chemical released and local environmental conditions (Figure 6.5), the chemical dispersion model provides the dispersal "footprint." The plume footprint can then be incorporated into a GIS database by locating the source of the release as the origin of the footprint and computing the planar coordinates of the footprint polygon. By overlaying the plume footprint with census data, the characteristics of the population within the footprint area of risk or exposure can be modeled.

A variety of dispersion models are available. Some of these are relatively simple, while others are complex three-dimensional models capturing vertical as well as horizontal spread (Brutsaert, 1982). Composite plume models are developed from a set of dispersion footprints generated for the same source but incorporating different air temperatures, relative humidities, cloud covers, and wind speeds and directions, reflecting variability in climatic conditions. If the locations of releases are known, composite plume models can be developed around each origin. By identifying the locations of 45 intersections in Des Moines, Iowa, with the highest numbers of truck accidents and then developing composite plume models for each intersection based on long-term average monthly climate data, Chakraborty and Armstrong (1995) were able to identify residential populations most at risk for exposure to gases released following a collision.

Fate and transport modeling is also an important technique for investigating water quality degradation. Solute transport models incorporating GIS for spatial data compilation, analysis, and visualization have been developed at a variety of spatial scales from the individual farm to the multistate region (Wagenet & Hutson, 1996). In a study of a relatively

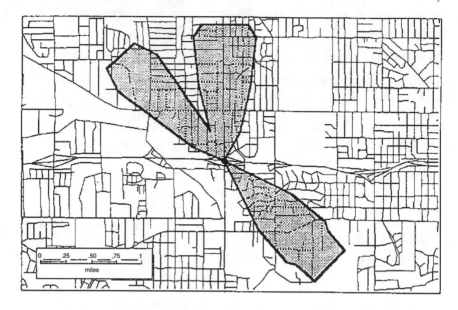

FIGURE 6.5. A composite of 12 monthly dispersion footprints generated for the same accident location in Des Moines, Iowa, reflects seasonal variations in prevailing wind direction. Reprinted from Chakraborty and Armstrong (1995), with permission from Elsevier Science.

small geographical area (7 kilometers × 10 kilometers in upstate New York), a GIS was used to overlay slope, land use, and soils databases to produce a composite identifying those soils found in agricultural areas with slopes less than 10%. The hydraulic properties of the soils were used to identify main hydraulic groups. Pesticide data for four chemicals along with pesticide application rates and typical corn planting dates and growth patterns were obtained for the region. In this application, the GIS was particularly useful for preprocessing input data for the solute transport model from a variety of sources and for postprocessing the results of the various simulations and generating maps.

Assessments of environmental conditions resulting from fate and transport modeling can be confirmed or contradicted by field measurements. In addition to describing the sources of environmental contaminants and their fields of impact, measuring environmental quality is an important component of environmental health analysis.

Environmental Quality

The cumulative effects of physical processes and human activities in the environment manifest themselves in environmental quality. While the sources of environmental contaminants and their dispersion patterns have generally been modeled as object data (points and areas), environmental quality is a field variable, as defined in Chapter 2. Dimensions of environmental quality—atmospheric conditions, water quality, soils—are continuous and can be observed everywhere. These phenomena are usually measured based on a partitioning of the surface that creates a spatial framework for locating monitoring stations. Given the spatial distribution of monitoring sites and the observations recorded at them, the spatial distribution of environmental quality is modeled as a mathematical function. The resulting distribution is often mapped as an isoline map.

Sampling Networks for Measuring Environmental Quality

An important issue in describing environmental quality, and ultimately its association with patterns of human health and disease, is the design of the sampling network. In a study of outdoor air pollution and asthma in Brooklyn and Queens, New York, there were too few air monitoring stations for measuring inhalable particulate matter and ozone and the stations were too clustered in the western portion of the study area to interpolate air quality adequately (Weisner, 1994). Designing a monitoring network involves defining the number, locations, sample pattern, and sample frequency of sampling sites (Olea, 1984). How many sampling sites are necessary to determine and map some dimension of environmental quality in a region is both a statistical question and a spatial question. Statistical analyses have generally focused on detecting statistically significant variations in environmental quality, that is, evaluating the statistical accuracy of the estimations. Some evidence suggests that more frequent sampling does not necessarily greatly increase the power of the statistical tests or the precision in the estimates (Hsueh & Rajagopal, 1988). The quality of environmental data for both statistical purposes and for mapping are also greatly affected by the spatial sampling strategies used to set up the monitoring network (Luzzader-Beach, 1995).

Because one of the most critical factors in monitoring environmental quality is the availability of data that can support comparisons across locations through time, environmental analysts recommend using spatial–statistical methods in the design of sampling networks (Nelson & Ward, 1981; Beach, 1987). Three main approaches to designing monitoring networks for groundwater quality have been described in the literature (Loaiciga, 1989): optimization, simulation, and variance reduction. *Optimization models* seek to optimize some function, for example, variance of estimation error, subject to resource and unbiasedness constraints (Hsueh & Rajagopal, 1988; Loaiciga, 1989). *Simulation models* involve repeated generation of synthetic plumes to describe temporal and spatial variation in the variable of interest. The *variance reduction model* is an interactive approach first applied to measuring water tables or elevations (Rouhani, 1985). From a set of known sampling locations, the sampling site that contributes most to reducing variance of estimation error for the variable of interest is selected. Additional sites are added to the network one at a time until the variance cannot be reduced further or the gain in accuracy is outweighed by other factors such as the cost of adding the site. This approach is related to *kriging*, discussed in greater depth in Chapter 7.

The variance reduction approach has been extended "to demonstrate how sample density affects the spatial and statistical representation of a unitless groundwater quality variable in a hypothetical basin" (Luzzader-Beach, 1995, p. 384). The hypothetical basin was designed to approximate in size and dimensions a basin that might be found in northern California and exhibited three groundwater quality patterns of different geographical extent (one large and two small areas). A rectangular grid was overlayed on the hypothetical water quality map and a model well from which water samples could be taken was located at each intersection in the grid.

Sections of the grid were grouped into hypothetical "townships" to facilitate a spatially stratified random sampling scheme for 22 sample densities ranging from 100% of the hypothetical wells down to 5% of the hypothetical wells. In addition, a sample was drawn at 2.8% coverage to simulate a policy recommended by the California Department of Water Resources Task Force to sample one well per township. For each level of sampling density, the pattern of water quality resulting from the sampled wells was mapped by kriging.

The results of the analysis supported the point that relatively few sample sites are required to accurately represent an environmental feature like ambient groundwater quality in a hypothetical basin. A standard of one well per township, however, was inadequate to capture variation in groundwater quality. The smaller, more localized groundwater patterns were harder to detect as sampling density decreased (Figure 6.6), and a density of five wells per township appeared to be the threshold density for ensuring adequate sampling. Once appropriate sampling networks are in place for individual components of environmental quality, it is also possible to develop composite indices of environmental quality at particular locations.

Integrated Index of Environmental Quality

In the same way that GIS have been used to developed composite databases of the sources of environmental contaminants (Osleeb & Kahn, 1999), systems have also been developed to integrate data measuring individual components of environmental quality. One integrated index of this type was developed in the Netherlands specifically to support land use zoning that was sensitive to environmental issues (Sol, Lammers, Aiking, De

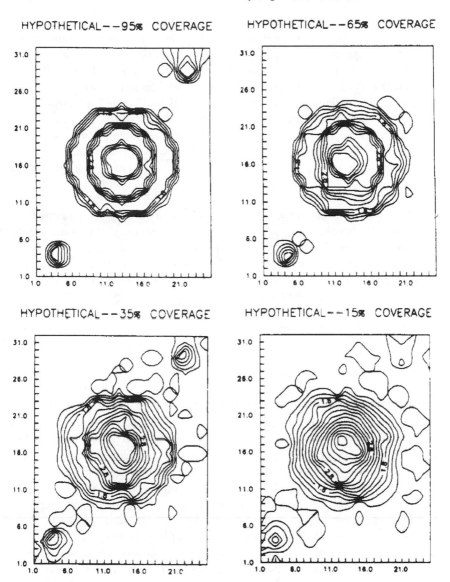

FIGURE 6.6. Contour maps of groundwater quality based on diminishing sample sizes (expressed as the percent of available sample wells in a hypothetical basin) show different patterns of groundwater quality. From Luzzader-Beach (1995). Copyright 1995 by Springer-Verlag. Reprinted by permission.

Boer, & Feenstra, 1995). High values of the index at a location would be used to support planning restrictions on housing units, for example, while low values might indicate areas where no restrictions on residential development would be needed. The construction of an integrated index of environmental quality involves five basic steps: (1) identification of polluting agents, (2) assessment of the magnitude of health effects, (3) summation to combine the effects of different agents producing comparable health effects by the same mechanism, (4) valuation of combined health effects to express them as dimensionless units on an arbitrary numerical scale, and (5) aggregation to combine the values associated with the identified agents. Individual and composite index scores can be mapped using a GIS, as in the Netherlands study.

An important advantage of this approach is its integrative aspect. In the context of a regulatory system where individual pollutants are monitored and compared to a corresponding regulatory standard, the integrated index is important for identifying areas where environmental quality is unacceptable even though individual pollutants do not exceed their standards. A major difficulty of this approach, aside from the uncertainty of risk in the assessment process, is the difficulty of finding suitable methods for valuation of health effects.

GIS AND EXPOSURE MODELING

Toxicants in the environment can affect a person's health only if the person is exposed. *Exposure* may consist of a single occurrence, be repeated, or be long term and continuous. The *effective exposure time* is the minimum time interval required from exposure to produce a health effect. With exposure to some toxicants, the effect may be almost immediate; with other substances, effects may not be induced for years. The *latent period* is the time interval from first exposure to observed health effect. The latent period is a function of many factors, including the dose and dose rate; characteristics of the person like age, sex, and length of time exposed; and the frequency and nature of health observations. *Threshold toxicants* are substances that are known or believed to cause adverse health effects above a specified dose or dose rate. *Nonthreshold toxicants* are known or believed to cause adverse health effects at any dose. In order for adverse health effects to be detected, studies must follow subjects for longer than the minimum latent period. Studies that do not follow individuals over the lifetime most likely underestimate true risk.

The Agency for Toxic Substances and Disease Registry has developed an exposure history form for use by medical practitioners because many environmental diseases have nonspecific symptoms (Frank, 1992). The form suggests some of the complexities in developing valid exposure histories for a person. In addition to recording basic demographic information such as age and sex, the exposure history form explores the substances someone has come into contact with, but does not attempt to quantify the level of exposure. The form also asks for an occupational history and a history of the residential environment.

The basic demographic characteristics are an indicator that individuals vary in susceptibility to toxic substances. Questions that probe occupational environment, residential environment, and recreational activities remind us that the home location is not the only place where individuals are exposed to toxicants because the home is only one node in a person's activity space (described in the Introduction). Questions detailing employment history highlight the importance of assessing exposures throughout the lifetime.

Ideally, the environmental health analyst has quantitative data on characteristics of the exposed population, including numbers by age and sex, and on the route and duration of exposure along with the concentration of the contaminant. In most epidemiological investigations, however, exposure data are "problematic" (Hallenbeck, 1993). Often, no exposure data are available for the locations and time periods of interest or data are of limited validity and reliability due to measurement problems.

GIS analyses can contribute to epidemiological studies by modeling the geographical distributions of contamination zones composited across a range of contaminants and overlay these with distributions of locations where susceptible populations live, work, attend school, and engage in other activities (Lowry et al., 1995; Chakraborty & Armstrong, 1995). The automated environment of the GIS also enables the analyst to evaluate the sensitivity of the exposure estimates.

GIS applications in environmental health, emphasizing colocation in time and space of susceptible populations and facilities that release harmful substances, have been open to criticism for apparently substituting proximity to hazardous facilities for quantitative data on actual exposure at the individual level. Systems like LandView III, a joint project of the U.S. Bureau of the Census and the EPA, enabling users to draw a circle around a user-selected point and generate a demographic and environmental profile of the area within the circle, may be useful for environmental risk management, but they fail to exploit the full capabilities of GIS for more accurate modeling of spatial processes in the hazard–exposure–outcome cycle. If, for example, we knew the location of a contaminated public drinking water well, we would not want to assess the exposed population based on a circular buffer around the well location. Water from the well is not equally likely to travel in every direction around the well, as the circle implies, because the water is delivered through a distribution network (Aye & Archambault, 1997). GIS can model that distribution network to produce a more accurate representation of the areas served whose water might be contaminated (Figure 6.7).

Estimating Populations in Hazard Zones

A controversial area of environmental health analysis has been the investigation of possible links between electromagnetic fields (EMFs) and a variety of human health problems. EMFs arise from the operation of electrical generators, distributors, and appliances, and are omnipresent in post-industrial societies. Epidemiological research has focused attention on the EMFs associated with electrical power systems, including generating stations, high-voltage transmission lines, and distribution lines.

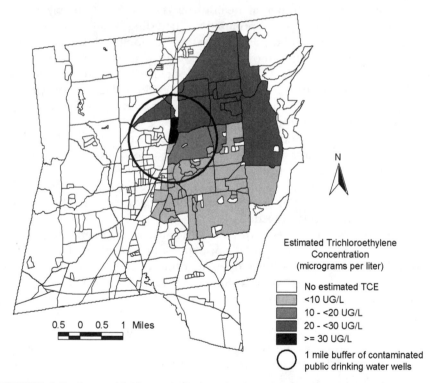

Estimated Trichloroethylene
Concentration
(micrograms per liter)

☐ No estimated TCE
▨ <10 UG/L
▨ 10 - <20 UG/L
▨ 20 - <30 UG/L
■ >= 30 UG/L
◯ 1 mile buffer of contaminated
public drinking water wells

0.5   0   0.5   1   Miles

FIGURE 6.7. Census block areas that received contaminated drinking water from wells adjacent to a National Priority List hazardous waste site. A hydrological analysis of the water supply system estimated that areas northeast of the contaminated wells received the highest exposures. The geographical pattern of water contamination impact was influenced by water usage, competing sources of water, and hydrologic pressures in the water distribution system, and not simply by distance from the contaminated wells. From Aye and Archambault (1997). Adapted by permission.

To map and analyze EMFs associated with high-voltage transmission lines in Hartford County, Connecticut (Cromley & Joy, 1995), a GIS database of transmission lines located in the study area (Figure 6.8) was created by digitizing maps of line location and type obtained from the utility and registering the digitized lines to a less complete but more spatially accurate database of transmission lines compiled by the Connecticut Department of Environmental Protection. The FIELDS program, a software system available from Southern California Edison Company, was used to calculate the EMF field around each transmission line segment in the study area. The FIELDS program requires input on phase coordinates (horizontal and vertical), number of subconductors per bundle, conductor diameter, bundle diameter, line kilovolts, phase current in amps for the relevant time period, phase angle in degrees, ground wire coordinates (horizontal and vertical), ground wire diameter, ground wire current amps, and ground wire phase angle. These data were also obtained from the utility. Variables used to calculate the exposure fields were based on what a line was rated to carry during the winter and summer months. Ac-

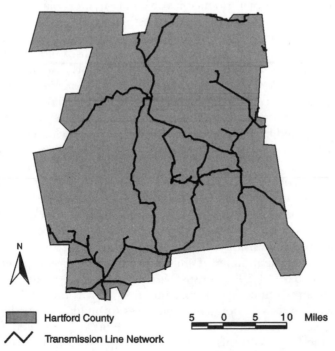

N

| | Hartford County | | 5 | 0 | 5 | 10 | Miles |
| | Transmission Line Network | | | | | | |

FIGURE 6.8. Electrical transmission lines in Hartford County. From Joy (1994). Copyright 1994 by K. P. Joy. Adapted by permission of the author.

tual readings are taken along line segments every 15 seconds by the utility, but these data would be too voluminous to process.

Based on the results of the analysis for each line segment, the center of each line segment right-of-way as represented in the GIS was buffered to the distance calculated for an exposure field in excess of 2 milligauss. This buffered area minus the line segment right-of-way—where no development can exist—represented the area of 2 milligauss or greater exposure. This data layer represented the area where homes or schools might be exposed to EMFs at the specified level of interest.

To find out how many children in the study area might live or attend school within this zone, two analyses were performed. To estimate the number of children attending school within this zone, a simple point-in-polygon overlay was performed to identify schools located within the zone of interest. School lat/lon data were obtained from a gazetteer and converted to the Connecticut State Plane Coordinate System. Information on 1990 school enrollment was collected from the Connecticut Department of Education and individual schools.

Estimating the number of children residing within this zone was more difficult because data on numbers of children were available only for areas (census blocks) and not points (individual schools). The estimate of children exposed by residence involved areal interpolation. *Areal interpolation* refers to a set of techniques to estimate the distribution of a phenomenon (in this case children under 18 years of age) across one set of spatial units called *source units* (in this case 1990 census blocks) in terms of a second set of spatial units called *target units* (in this case the 2-milligauss exposure zones). A common approach to areal interpolation is the area-weighting method, relying on the concept of map overlay (Lam, 1983). In this approach, the variable "number of children under 18 in the census block" is weighted by the proportion of the census block's area that lies in the target EMF zone. The resulting number of children is then assigned to the EMF zone as part of that unit's population (Figure 6.9).

Areal interpolation can be enhanced by incorporating ancillary data (Flowerdew & Green, 1989). For example, if we know based on the distribution of streets or houses that no one actually lives in a certain part of the census block, we can derive a better estimate of the population residing in the area of overlap.

To estimate the number of children under 18 exposed based on residence, a database of 1990 census blocks was digitized using coincident features from Connecticut Department of Environmental Protection road, stream, and town boundary databases to build a census block database of greater positional accuracy than could be compiled from the TIGER/Line files. With this database, it was possible to identify by polygon overlay all of the 1990 census blocks in each study area town within 1 mile of a transmission line. Clearly, some areas in a town are not close to transmission lines, but it may also be that no one actually lives in those ar-

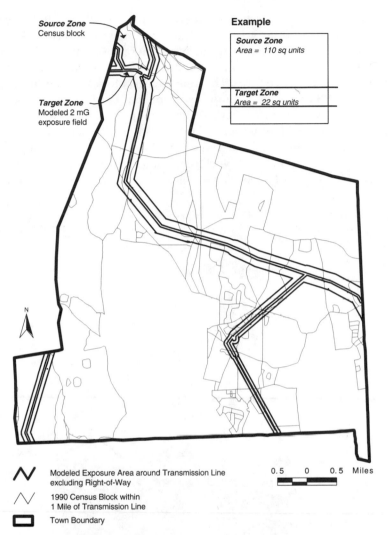

FIGURE 6.9. Areal interpolation by the area-weighting method to determine population within a risk area. In the example, 20% of the population in the source zone would be estimated to be within the target zone because the target zone covers 22/110, or 20% of the source zone. The map shows the complex arrangement of 1990 census blocks as source zones with target zones determined by modeling the 2-milligauss exposure field around transmission lines excluding the power line right-of-way where no development can occur. From Joy (1994). Copyright 1994 by K. P. Joy. Adapted by permission of the author.

eas. To develop a better picture of where people actually reside in the census blocks, a 300′ buffer was created around the street network—excluding major highways—to represent the area where residential development is most likely to occur based on residential setback and lot configurations in the study area (Figure 6.10). The 1990 census block population for children under 18 was assigned uniformly to this buffered street area and this area was overlayed with the database containing the 2-milligauss exposure fields. The estimated number of children exposed was calculated by multiplying the total number of children in the block by the percentage of the buffered street region in that block that coincided with an exposure field (Figure 6.11). Approximately 2% of children under age 18 were estimated

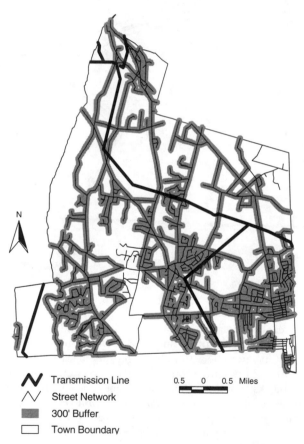

N

/\/	Transmission Line
/\/	Street Network
▨	300' Buffer
☐	Town Boundary

0.5   0   0.5 Miles

FIGURE 6.10. The buffered street network is a form of ancillary data that can be used to localize population within a source zone like a census block to improve estimates based on areal interpolation. From Joy (1994). Copyright 1994 by K. P. Joy. Adapted by permission of the author.

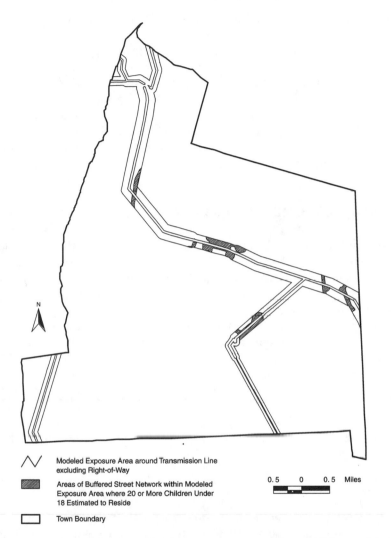

FIGURE 6.11. Areas within a modeled exposure zone where children might live based on position of the street network in relation to the exposure zone and the child population of the census block where the street segment is located. From Joy (1994). Copyright 1994 by K. P. Joy. Adapted by permission of the author.

to be exposed to transmission line EMFs based on this analysis, which also revealed the neighborhoods where that exposure was likely to occur.

Another approach to simulate the location and characteristics of the general population that might be exposed to an environmental hazard involves linking aggregate data on age, sex, and race/ethnicity for census block groups to residential addresses in a study area (Knapp, Archambault, & Aye, 1998). The 1990 census block group totals for each block group are converted into a table containing a record for each individual. The age, sex, or race/ethnicity characteristics of these "individuals" sum to the block group totals. A residential address obtained from an electronic telephone number database is randomly assigned to each individual in the table. This makes it possible to assess the characteristics of populations as well as cases affected by environmental contamination events. The next step in such an analysis, after exposure areas have been identified, is outcome surveillance.

GIS AND OUTCOME SURVEILLANCE

Physical and chemical agents like those studied in the earlier examples in this chapter may produce several different kinds of adverse health and environmental effects (Hallenbeck, 1993; Stockwell et al., 1993). First, cancer is an effect due to toxic mechanisms operating in nonreproductive cells. Developmental effects, like death of the fetus; structural abnormalities, like cleft palate, that are observable at birth; or postnatal functional disabilities of the central nervous, respiratory, and intestinal systems can also result from toxic mechanisms operating in nonreproductive cells. When DNA-interactive mechanisms operate in reproductive cells, hereditary effects can occur. Finally, organ and tissue effects, like damage to the liver, kidneys, or lungs or to nerve tissue, are due to nongenotoxic mechanisms operating in nonreproductive cells. The following sections offer examples of how GIS techniques have been used to investigate these various health outcomes.

Cancer

A GIS developed to model household magnetic fields from power lines found a significant association with childhood leukemia in Los Angeles County after analyzing both exposure measurements based on wire codes and 24-hour measurements of the magnetic fields taken in the bedrooms of cases and controls (Bowman, 2000). To develop the wire code model for magnetic fields associated with electric transmission and distribution systems, magnetic field measurements were fitted by nonlinear regression to a function of wire configuration attributes (Bowman, Thomas, Jiang, Jiang, & Peters, 1999). These measurements were 24-hour bedroom measurements taken at 288 homes. Case–control data on childhood leukemia in Los Angeles County were reanalyzed to investigate associations between observed magnetic fields and the predicted magnetic fields and childhood leukemia (Thomas, Bowman, Jiang, Jiang, & Peters, 1999). Although the measured fields were not associated with childhood leukemia, the risks were significant for predicted magnetic fields above 1.25 milligauss and a significant dose–response effect was noted.

Using GIS to display the spatial structure of the transmission system and its wire code characteristics appeared to assess the leukemia risk associated with a child's long-term residential magnetic field exposure better than 24-hour measurements. The GIS approach enabled assessment of exposure with more subjects and more previous residences because it did not entail obtaining measurements in the field at hundreds of homes. This increased the power of the analysis. Also, 24-hour EMF measurements are strongly affected by short-term fluctuations in usage that do not yield a reliable picture of long-term exposure. The GIS model also creates a tool for retrospective studies of exposure because it only requires data on the wire code configuration and the locations of residences. Also, the model can be used to investigate possible links between other cancers, like breast cancer, and EMFs.

Reproductive Outcomes

Reproductive outcomes are believed to be sensitive to many environmental influences (Stallones, Nuckols, & Berry, 1992). A hospital-based case–control study of stillbirths in a community in central Texas investigated the effects of chronic inhalation of low levels of arsenic (Ihrig, Shalat, & Baynes, 1998). A plant in the community producing arsenic-based agricultural products had been in operation for more than 60 years. Arsenic exposure levels were estimated from airborne emission estimates by using an atmospheric dispersion model linked to a GIS. Exposure was then assessed based on the residential address of the mother at the time of delivery. Exposure was included as a categorical variable in a conditional logistic regression model. An exposure-and-race/ethnicity interaction variable was also included to reflect the fact that members of particular groups within the population may be concentrated in certain residential neighborhoods. The prevalence of stillbirth was significantly higher among Hispanics living in high exposure areas.

Elevated Blood Lead Levels

Data on health problems like cancer or birth defects can be obtained from tumor registries or vital statistics registration systems, as discussed in Chapter 3. Data on other health effects, like elevated blood lead levels, are often collected as part of screening programs. *Screening* is "the presumptive identification of unrecognized disease or defect by the application of tests, examinations, or other procedures . . . [that] can be applied rapidly and usually cheaply" (Eylenbosch & Noah, 1988, p. 279). Unlike vital statistics databases or tumor registries, which are relatively complete, screening databases can be highly biased in representing the geographical distribution of a health problem, particularly if screening is not mandatory. Figure 6.12 reveals how misleading maps of the distribution of health problems can be if spatial biases in screening are not explicitly described.

For some health problems, like lead poisoning, links to a toxicant have been established, and environmental risk factors have been identified based on our understanding of the distribution of the toxicant and how people come into contact with it in their daily lives. For these problems, GIS analysis has been used to map known risk factors and health outcomes to support the design of public health intervention strategies. In New Jersey, analysts mapped data related to several known risk factors for lead poisoning (Guthe, Tucker, & Murphy, 1992).

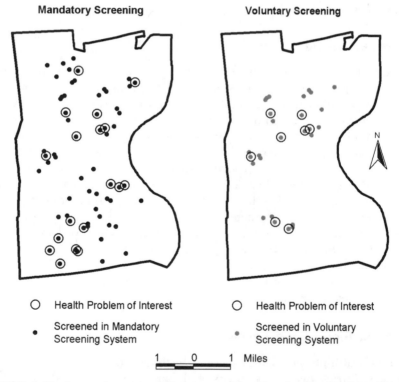

Mandatory Screening   **Voluntary Screening**

○ Health Problem of Interest   ○ Health Problem of Interest

• Screened in Mandatory   • Screened in Voluntary
   Screening System   Screening System

1   0   1   Miles

FIGURE 6.12. A mandatory screening system identifies the distribution of health problems of interest within the screened population. If the screening system is voluntary, fewer people may be screened and the distribution of identified health problems of interest may be biased. In the example above, an apparent concentration of cases in the north end of town is probably a result of more people having been screened there. Cases in the south end of town were not detected because the voluntary system was less effective in screening people in that section of town.

Data from the TRI on industrial sites emitting lead and from a state database of hazardous waste site locations were obtained. Traffic volume estimates from the New Jersey Department of Transportation were used to identify segments in the road network with high traffic volumes. EPA lead emission factors were then applied to estimate lead emissions from vehicles. In addition, data identifying census tracts exceeding threshold levels for number of structures built before 1940 and number of children under 5 years of age were compiled to depict exposure to lead paint in residences. The GIS was used to integrate these data and display the risk factors in relation to the distribution of children with high blood lead levels.

Overall, the results of the analysis showed a spatial correlation among sources of lead, susceptible populations, and health outcomes in the study area. In addition to identifying neighborhoods where numerous sources of lead and high blood lead levels were observed, the analysis highlighted other regions within the study area where frequencies of elevated blood lead levels were higher or lower than expected based on the sources of lead present. These results suggested limitations in the screening data and in the lead source databases. The spatial patterns observed aided the New Jersey Department of Health in developing soil sampling and lead exposure research and in community outreach efforts to prevent lead exposure.

GIS AND ENVIRONMENTAL RISK MANAGEMENT

GIS can make contributions to risk assessment, primarily by supporting better modeling of geographical distributions of hazards, susceptible populations, exposures, and health outcomes. GIS also has a role to play in *environmental risk assessment*, a social and political process that involves the selection and implementation of strategies for the regulation or control of identified hazards. Once priorities have been set for regulation or control of particular hazards, GIS can be used to identify the locations of entities producing toxicants for targeting intervention activities.

During the late 1980s, comparative risk assessment as an approach to prioritizing environmental management efforts of environmental management emerged (Finkel & Golding, 1994). The "risk-based" paradigm is concerned with evaluating whether the relative efforts—regulation, allocation of resources for monitoring and mitigation—devoted to reducing risks are in reasonable proportion to the seriousness of the risks being compared. The opportunities for integrating risk assessment models into GIS are being explored. A highway transportation risk assessment software system uses a GIS to allow analysts to select highway or rail routes interactively and obtain a route-specific risk assessment for shipment of radioactive materials (Moore, Sandquist, & Slaughter, 1994).

The EPA's interest in comparative risk assessment provoked a debate raising methodological, procedural, and implementation concerns about adopting comparative risk assessment as the basis for environmental protection resource allocation, and a fundamental objection to "ranking" instead of "addressing" environmental problems (O'Brien, 1994). Although GIS can aid the process of quantitative risk assessment through epidemiological investigation and can be used to support targeting geographical areas for protection (Habicht, 1994), the role of GIS in *risk management* is not inextricably tied to the risk-based paradigm. GIS can be used to depict the geographical structure of an environmental problem of interest, for example, delineating watershed and wellhead protection areas (Chernin, 1993; Rifai, Hendricks, Kilborn, & Bedient, 1993; Hammen & Gerla, 1994), regardless of the problem's rank in a list of environmental problems prioritized by risk.

ISSUES IN ENVIRONMENTAL HAZARD MAPPING

GIS are making it easier for environmental analysts to produce hazards maps demonstrating sensitivity of hazard patterns to changes in modeling criteria (Tim, 1995). However, "GIS-generated maps may be viewed by users as having greater reliability than is warranted" (Wagenet & Hutson, 1996). Depending on the modeling criteria, vulnerability and hazard maps produced from the same data may appear very different. It is important to define and understand exactly the databases that a particular map displays.

Because maps are often interpreted as precise portrayals of reality rather than an analyst's view of data, efforts to map hazards, environmental quality, and community vulnerability should be undertaken with particular care. Many residents of environmentally degraded areas do not need analyses and maps to describe the hazards in their communities or the adverse psychological and financial impacts that may exacerbate both the direct health effects of exposure to contaminants and the incidence of stress-related diseases. Community groups with vested political and economic interests will not always welcome these maps, even when the data are complete and accurate, the analyses are conceptually sound, and the results are robust.

The momentum for disclosure of information on environmental hazards like the disclosure regulations put into place through the Emergency Planning and Community Right-to-Know Act continues to build. The Safe Drinking Water Act signed in 1996 expanded consumers' "right to know" and established a National Contaminants Occurrence Database, enhanced surveillance of waterborne diseases, and set up a loan fund to improve water treatment infrastructure to protect public drinking water sources. In this context, it is important to recognize the role GIS can play not just in mapping environmental health problems, but in managing and making accessible to the public the large, spatially referenced databases of environmental information that citizens have the right to know.

CONCLUSION

The decline in incidence of infectious disease in the United States in the 1950s and 1960s shifted the focus of public health and medical research efforts to diseases like heart disease, cancer, asthma, and other chronic health problems that were increasing in incidence. Many researchers have investigated environmental risk factors as explanations for these observed health outcomes. This research is now being supported by the use of GIS to model complex hazard–exposure–outcome processes in time and space.

An interesting development in our understanding of chronic disease is a growing body of research suggesting that some health problems like arteriosclerosis may be partly the result of infectious agents (Ewald & Cochran, 1999). This introduces a new level of information that may need to be considered to understand how environmental conditions, human behavior, and infectious agents work together to cause disease and how we can design public health interventions to reduce the occurrence of disease. The role of GIS in analyzing infectious disease is considered in Chapters 7 and 8.

CHAPTER 7

Analyzing the Risk and Spread of Infectious Diseases

The resurgence of infectious diseases, some new and unfamiliar, others with a long history in human populations, has been identified as a global threat to human health at the end of a century of scientific and medical advances that had seemingly conquered infection as a cause of death (Working Group on Emerging and Re-emerging Infectious Diseases, 1995). In addition to the immediate public health need for improved infectious disease surveillance and response, the renewed concern for infectious disease has been accompanied by a reevaluation of contemporary risk factor epidemiology (Susser & Susser, 1996a, 1996b; Pearce, 1996). In studying rising chronic disease mortality in the period after World War II, researchers developed and refined methods like those discussed in Chapters 4 and 6 for identifying individual risk factors. Although the risk factor approach recognizes that many public health problems are multicausal, critics argue that focusing even on multiple individual risk factors has disconnected epidemiology "from an examination of the broader historical and social forces that help to shape disease patterns in populations" (Nasca, 1997) and from the "way in which people interpret their health-related behavior" (Lawson & Floyd, 1996).

Factors cited as contributing to the reemergence of infectious disease include land use change affecting vector and host habitats and human interaction with vector and host populations, urbanization, transportation technology affecting migration and population mobility, and changes in the ways water and food are delivered (Working Group on Emerging and

Re-emerging Infectious Diseases, 1995; Walker et al., 1996). Many of these factors have an important geographical dimension.

The biological basis of infectious diseases is crucial for understanding where and why the diseases occur. Infectious diseases are caused by living microorganisms, the disease *agents* or *pathogens*. They spread among human or animal *hosts*, either by direct transmission or via a *vector* that transmits the disease from host to host. Thus, the occurrence and spread of infectious disease depend on hosts' exposure and susceptibility to pathogens and interactions among hosts, agents, and vectors.

Chapters 7 and 8 explore how GIS have been used in the study of emerging and reemerging infectious diseases, particularly those transmitted directly from person to person (Chapter 7) and those transmitted by vector (Chapter 8). For many infectious diseases, unlike cancers, birth defects, and other health problems associated with exposure to toxicants, etiology is known and the diseases spread via contact among hosts or their exposures to vectors. These differences in disease process give rise to different modeling approaches.

This chapter examines the use of GIS in analyzing infectious diseases that spread directly from person to person. These "nonvectored" diseases include some of the most significant public health concerns in the United States: HIV/AIDS, tuberculosis, measles, influenza, and gonorrhea, among others. Their uneven geographical distributions reflect the social and environmental conditions that affect risk and susceptibility and the social interactions and behaviors that facilitate transmission. A distinctive feature of these diseases is that they spread over time from person to person and from place to place, often in epidemic and pandemic forms.

Nonvectored diseases spread through a variety of different means. Many, like HIV/AIDS, syphilis, and impetigo, spread directly through skin or sexual contact. Others can exist in the environment, persisting in air, water, soil, or food. These diseases spread via our most basic, everyday behaviors: eating, drinking, breathing, and working. Airborne transmission occurs when pathogens spread from host to host through the process of respiration, as occurs with influenza, tuberculosis, or the common cold. Other diseases, such as cryptosporidiosis and cholera, are transmitted through contaminated water or food. Some pathogens can persist in soil, giving rise to the transmission of diseases like tetanus.

The mode of transmission is a critical factor in any GIS assessment of nonvectored diseases. It influences the kinds of geographical questions asked about the disease, the types of analyses performed, and the types of data layers that need to be included in a GIS. In mapping and analyzing waterborne diseases, for example, the water distribution network, including reservoirs, mains, and private wells, is crucial. By comparison, airborne diseases emerge out of geographical patterns of human contact and interaction, which are linked to housing conditions, crowding, and personal contact in facilities such as schools, daycare centers, jails, and workplaces. Sexually transmitted diseases (STDs), on the other hand, reflect intimate relations that are embedded in broader concepts of identity, sexuality, and gender. With STDs, the relationships among people that channel disease spread are hidden from view, not clearly visible in the day-to-day movements of people that comprise traditional spatial patterns of human interaction.

Transmission of infectious diseases also depends on the host's *immunity*, the host's ability to resist the pathogenic effects of infection. Some immunity is acquired in response to repeated infection, as occurs with malaria, influenza, or the common cold. *Immunization* is a way of artificially inducing acquired immunity by injecting small doses of toxins in the host. *Innate immunity* refers to the body's ability to harness its own biological resources to ward off infection. Although immunity rests partly in biology—for example, the host's genetic makeup—it also has an important social basis. Nutrition and malnutrition, exposure to environmental contaminants, and past exposure to infections affect the immune response. These reflect people's access to nutritious food, their home and work environments, and the stresses and risks they face in their daily lives. Understanding how these social and geographical processes influence the immune response, the susceptibility to and risk of infection, and the severity of illness is crucial in explaining the geography of infectious diseases.

The spread of infectious diseases among hosts can be described in general terms using *epidemic models* (Thomas, 1992) that chart the extent of disease spread as a function of the sizes of susceptible and infected populations, the degree of mixing between them, and the transmission rate and incubation period for the disease. The simplest models assume a population consisting of three groups: susceptibles (S), infecteds (I), and recovereds (R), and even mixing of the S and I populations. According to these models, an epidemic begins slowly, but builds up as the number of infecteds increases (Figure 7.1). The peak transmission occurs when the S and I populations are approximately equal in size. After that, the epidemic diminishes as the number of susceptibles declines. More complex models have been developed; these have proven fairly accurate in charting the course of epidemics over time. However, many models are "single region" and thus ignore the geographical dimensions of disease spread (Cliff & Haggett, 1996; Thomas, 1992).

SPATIAL DIFFUSION

The geographical patterns of interaction between infected and susceptible hosts are crucial for understanding how and where infectious diseases spread. *Spatial diffusion* describes the movement of phenomena—people,

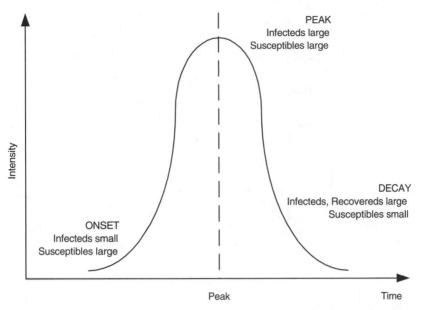

FIGURE 7.1. An epidemic curve, showing changes in susceptible and infected populations.

goods, ideas, innovations, and diseases—through space and time. Spatial diffusion of disease occurs when a disease is transmitted to new locations. Sometimes diseases follow a pattern of *contagious diffusion*, that is, they spread gradually outward from a point of origin to nearby locations (Cliff & Haggett, 1988). Contagious diffusion reflects the localized nature of human spatial interaction: people are more likely to interact with their neighbors than with those located farther away. Constraints on mobility related to age, low income, disability, or poor access to transportation may lead to highly localized patterns of spatial interaction. Diseases also spread contagiously between cities and surrounding suburbs, following commuting flows and social interactions. The prevalence of AIDS in suburban communities is strongly correlated with the volume of workers who commute to central cities (Figure 7.2). These connections among diverse communities are critically important for health policy: the health problems of central city and suburban areas are inextricably linked by flows of people and the interactions among them. Inner-city clusters of communicable disease can act as epidemic pumps that spread disease to suburban areas (Wallace & Wallace, 1998).

When we examine disease diffusion patterns, we find that diseases often "jump" from place to place, rather than following the gradual outward expansion of contagious diffusion. In *hierarchical diffusion*, diseases spread

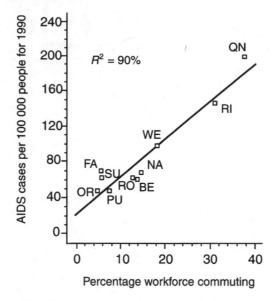

FIGURE 7.2. For 10 affluent counties in the New York metropolitan region, cumulative AIDS cases through 1990 per 1,000 people is highly correlated with the percentage of workforce commuting into Manhattan. Spatial diffusion of communicable diseases is often channeled through commuting flows. From Wallace and Wallace (1998). Copyright 1998 by Verso Books. Reprinted by permission.

via the urban hierarchy, starting in large cities and spreading over time to medium-sized cities, then to smaller cities and towns. The large populations, strong transportation connections, and movements of people among large cities channel hierarchical diffusion. Transmission occurs over long distances—for example, from New York City to Chicago and Los Angeles—propelled by the strong interactions among large urban populations. *Network diffusion* refers to the spread of disease through transportation or social networks. As with the other types of diffusion, network diffusion reflects the geographical and social structuring of human interactions.

Centuries ago, most diseases spread primarily through contagious diffusion; today, however, patterns of disease spread often show a mix of hierarchical, network, and contagious diffusion (Figure 7.3). Mixed patterns are clearly evident in the spread of HIV/AIDS, both in the United States and worldwide (Gould, 1995).

Efforts are underway to link epidemic models with spatial diffusion models to better depict the movement of infectious diseases through time and space (Cliff & Haggett, 1996). These efforts typically involve modeling disease spread within regions and modeling the flows of infected and

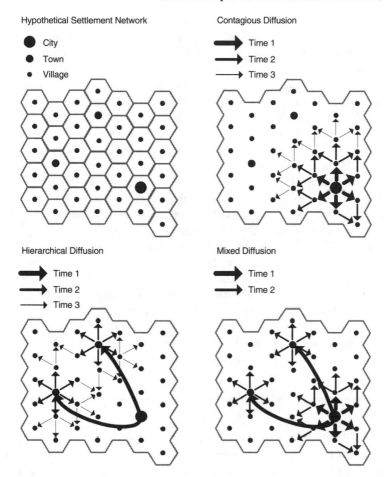

FIGURE 7.3. Spatial diffusion patterns.

susceptible populations among regions based on spatial interaction patterns. In the coming years, these efforts will rely more heavily on GIS both for modeling spatial interactions and patterns and for managing the large spatial data sets that underpin these models (Cliff & Haggett, 1996).

MAPPING CASE DISTRIBUTIONS

Where are infectious diseases most prevalent? Which populations and geographical areas are most in need of treatment and prevention programs? These questions motivate much geographical analysis of diseases that spread directly from person to person. These analyses require data on case locations that come from some type of surveillance system, a topic discussed in Chapter 3. But before mapping case distributions, we need to consider how cases in the database were identified. Changes in case definition over time can affect the stage during an illness when disease is diagnosed and the number of individuals eligible for a diagnosis. The definition for AIDS originally developed in 1982 was revised in 1985 and again in 1987 (Chang, Katz, & Hernandez, 1992). The 1992 definition, which became effective in January 1993, significantly increased the number of AIDS cases reported as was expected (Centers for Disease Control and Prevention, 1993a, 1993b, 1993c). The new definition brought in many women with AIDS who had been excluded under earlier definitions that failed to include "women's diseases," like pelvic inflammatory disease, as opportunistic infections. A revised surveillance case definition for HIV became effective in January 2000 (Centers for Disease Control and Prevention, 1999a). These changes underline the need to make case definition explicit in GIS databases and metadata.

Researchers have used several of the methods discussed in Chapter 5 to pinpoint spatial clusters of infectious diseases and plan public health interventions. This type of research is illustrated in a recent study of pertussis. Pertussis (whooping cough) is a serious contagious disease that spreads rapidly from person to person via airborne transmission. An effective vaccine, administered during childhood, can prevent the spread of infection. Concern about the presence and persistence of whooping cough in Denver during the early 1990s led to an analysis of the spatial clustering of cases using GIS (Siegel et al., 1997). Pertussis cases were first identified through a retrospective surveillance system and then geocoded using an address-matching procedure. The incidence of pertussis by census tract was computed by overlaying the geocoded cases on a tract map, and summing cases by tract (Figure 7.4). A nonlinear smoothing method was used to estimate the age-standardized incidence rate for each tract. The map of smoothed rates revealed clustering of high pertussis tracts in areas of high poverty, suggesting the need for more effective immunization programs and improved health care access in those areas.

The real value of mapping emerges when maps are linked to disease control and prevention efforts. Increasingly, public health professionals are using GIS to develop more effective immunization programs. During a measles epidemic in Auckland, New Zealand, public health analysts displayed measles surveillance data on GIS maps in order to direct epidemic control efforts (Jones, Bloomfield, Rainger, & Taylor, 1998). Intensive vaccination campaigns were targeted to neighborhoods where the incidence of measles was highest. In the final phase of the epidemic, mobile vaccinators were sent to streets where new cases of measles were occurring. In this example, geocoded health surveillance data was critically important in developing an effective public health response.

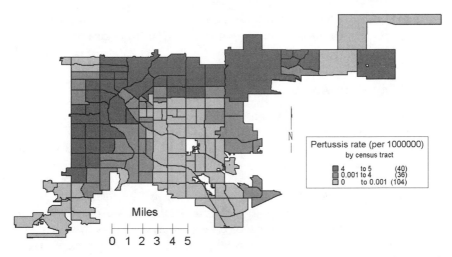

FIGURE 7.4. Smoothed age-adjusted pertussis rates, Denver County, 1986 through 1994. From Siegel et al. (1997). Copyright 1997 by American Public Health Association. Reprinted by permission.

Although most infectious disease surveillance data include the residential address as a geographical identifier, for some diseases transmission can occur outside the home. In many countries, the spread of HIV is linked to long-distance truck drivers and migrant workers who spend much time away from home (Gould, 1995). Their risks of acquiring and transmitting HIV extend over a far-flung network in which the home is just a single node. A recent study of syphilis in North Carolina found high rates clustered along the main interstate highway (Cook, Royce, Thomas, & Hanusa, 1999). For transmission processes like these, a map of case locations geocoded to residence, while depicting where infected people live, only partially represents the geography of disease risk.

In preparing maps of case locations, analysts must also be sensitive to reporting and sampling bias. Surveillance data come from physicians, laboratories, and health care facilities that, though mandated to report, may choose not to do so. Significant underreporting exists for diseases that carry social stigma, like STDs. The implications for mapping depend on the geographical distribution of reporting bias. If underreporting is uniform over space, then rates will be low across the board. However, research on STDs shows strong class differences in underreporting, since high-income people "are more likely to visit a private physician and private physicians are more likely than public clinics not to report an infection" (Thomas & Tucker, 1996, p. S139). This class-based disparity leads to lower rates of reporting in high-income areas and exaggerates the apparent degree of clustering in low-income areas. The result is an uneven geographical distribution of reporting bias and an uneven pattern of error in case maps.

Identifying Core Areas

A special application of infectious disease mapping is the analysis of core groups and core areas. Studies of STDs have drawn attention to the clustering of cases in "core" population groups. A *core group* is a "geographically and socially defined sexual network" (Thomas & Tucker, 1996, p. S134) within which the rate of infection is disproportionately high. As concentrated, high-risk populations, core groups have great importance in efforts to control and prevent STD infection (Yorke, Hethcote, & Nold, 1978). *Core areas*, the geographical analogues of core groups, are areas in which STD incidence and transmission are unusually high. For diseases like gonorrhea that have an effective cure, the high transmission density in core areas maintains infection and creates a reservoir for epidemic spread (Zenilman, Ellish, Fresia, & Glass, 1999). As with core groups, core areas are critically important for planning and targeting STD treatment and prevention efforts.

GIS can be used in identifying core areas and analyzing the patterns of disease transmission within core groups. This approach was employed in a GIS to analyze core areas for gonorrhea in Baltimore, a city with one of the highest incidence rates of STDs in the United States (Becker, Glass, Braithwaite, & Zenilman, 1998). The GIS worked with disease surveillance data for gonorrhea. Residential addresses of persons diagnosed with gonorrhea were geocoded and assigned to their corresponding census tract. Using 1990 census data to estimate denominator populations, incidence rates were computed by tract. The rates were arranged in rank order, and core areas were defined as the 13 tracts in the upper quartile of the distribution. Core areas contained 15.5% of gonorrhea cases and just 6.5% of population. Incidence rates in the core tracts were more than double the citywide rate.

Successful mapping of core areas requires an appropriate definition of core incidence. Some researchers have used counts of cases in identifying core areas (Rothenberg, 1983). When counts are used, the core areas that emerge may be areas with large populations but low disease rates. Using counts ensures that core areas contain a large proportion of cases. In the Baltimore study, which used rates instead of counts, focusing public health resources in core areas would reach just 15.5% of reported gonorrhea cases. Another problem with using rates in identifying core areas is the instability and unreliability of the rates for areas with small populations. Typically, the highest and lowest incidence rates are found in these areas. Thus, core areas defined based on rates will often include areas with low populations. To address this problem, methods like probability mapping and empirical Bayes smoothing, discussed in Chapter 5, should be used in identifying core areas. An even better approach is to work with point-based methods; however, point data are often unavailable for communicable diseases because of privacy concerns.

Defining the cut-off point for identifying core areas, based either on counts, rates, or smoothed rates, provides an opportunity for creatively combining mapping and descriptive statistics. In analyzing core areas for chlamydia and gonorrhea in Winnipeg, the distribution of ranked incidence rates by postal code was displayed alongside maps of core areas (Blanchard et al., 1998). Core areas were defined according to natural breaks in the distribution curves (Figure 7.5). A GIS might include a "sliding bar" that allows the analyst to move the cut-off point along the distribution curve while simultaneously displaying the associated map of core areas for each cut-off value.

Core areas are critical to disease transmission. Their high rates of transmission are thought to sustain diseases during nonepidemic periods and act as reservoirs for infection to areas outside (Rothenberg, 1983). Given detailed data, researchers can explore the geography of STD trans-

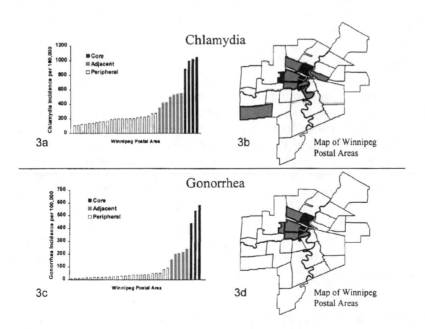

FIGURE 7.5. Mapping core areas of chlamydia and gonorrhea in Winnepeg based on natural breaks. From Blanchard et al. (1998). Copyright 1998 by American Public Health Association. Reprinted by permission.

mission patterns inside and outside of core areas to describe the densities, locations, and distances between sexual partners. Such issues were examined in a study of sexual partnerships in Baltimore (Zenilman et al., 1999). The research involved geocoding residential addresses of sexual partners, computing the Euclidean distance between partners, and comparing those distances with distances to randomly chosen residential locations. Residents of core areas lived much closer to their sexual partners than did persons living outside the core, and both distances were significantly less than random. Sexual partnerships were highly localized, especially in core areas, suggesting the potential benefits of geographically targeted prevention programs.

Identifying and mapping core areas raises several important broader issues. Displaying the areas on maps may unfairly stigmatize the residents of core areas and lead to place-based redlining and discrimination. The areas can become labeled as places where disease risk is high, and therefore to be avoided by businesses, service providers, and individuals. Part of the problem stems from defining places as in- or outside the core when in fact disease incidence is not so polarized. Typically the vast majority of cases are located outside core areas, and the vast majority of core area residents do not have the disease. In the Baltimore example, almost 85% of people with gonorrhea lived outside core neighborhoods, and well over 90% of core area residents did not have gonorrhea. These patterns are typical of STDs and should be emphasized when presenting maps of core areas.

Core area mapping projects also need to recognize the social and economic conditions that underpin high prevalence. The higher risk of disease in core areas is often rooted in patterns of social deprivation, including high unemployment, low incomes, deteriorated housing, and poor access to health care. The withdrawal of fire services, housing, and jobs from New York City's inner-city neighborhoods in the 1970s triggered the emergence of core areas that then became nodes for the outward spread of HIV/AIDS, tuberculosis, and other communicable diseases (Wallace & Wallace, 1999). As the work of Wallace and Wallace vividly portrays, core areas are not zones of "deviant" behavior, but rather products of a multitude of social and political inequalities and misguided social policies. From this perspective, developing effective intervention programs requires an understanding of the social and political ecology of core areas and how people's access to work, housing, and services in core communities structures their health.

MAPPING VARIABILITY IN DISEASE AGENTS

A critical feature of infectious diseases is that the agent is a living organism that evolves over time to enhance its reproductive success. A single agent can have a multiplicity of genetic forms that evolve in response to changes in the environment, hosts, and medical treatments (Ewald, 1994). The best-known example of this is the influenza virus whose rapid mutation leads to the emergence of new epidemic strains on an almost yearly basis. The agents for tuberculosis, malaria, staph, and strep have evolved new drug-resistant forms that are resistant to conventional treatments. Mapping the genetic diversity of infectious agents is an important and largely neglected application area for GIS. Scientists have long used mapping as a tool for understanding the emergence and evolution of pathogens over time (Myers, MacInnes, & Myers, 1993), but the applications are rather limited in scope and do not take full advantage of the analytical capabilities of GIS.

Where are new and resistant strains emerging and why are they emerging in those areas? Research by Bifani et al.(1999) combined DNA fingerprinting with GIS to examine the geographical distribution of tuberculosis strains in the New York metropolitan region. While no spatial clustering of new strains was observed outside New York City, maps revealed the emergence of new strains in New Jersey. Such large-scale mapping of genetic variability will become increasingly common as DNA fingerprinting and GIS technologies become more available and accessible.

The reasons why new strains emerge can also be explored through GIS. One study (Chen et al., 1998) analyzed whether drug-resistant streptococcal pneumonia was more likely to emerge among persons of high socioeconomic status because of their greater access to antibiotic treatments. Cases of resistant and nonresistant S. *pneumoniae* were geocoded to census tracts, and the median household income level of the tract was used to approximate socioeconomic status. Results showed a positive association between median income and the proportion of drug-resistant S. *pneumoniae* by tract. Though ecological in nature, the findings suggest the links between income, access to drug treatments, and the emergence of drug resistance.

ANALYZING TEMPORAL AND GEOGRAPHIC TRENDS IN DISEASE OUTBREAKS

An important issue in monitoring communicable diseases and planning interventions is to understand the patterns of spread through space and time. A public health department might want to know when the peak outbreaks of disease typically occur and how those peaks move from place to place. Many communicable diseases like influenza and the common cold show distinct seasonal patterns of occurrence. For these types of diseases, the patterns of spread reflect when and where the disease was introduced, weather conditions, and the interactions and movements of infected and susceptible populations.

One way to visualize temporal and spatial trends is to prepare a map showing for each location the date (month or week) of peak disease incidence -- that is, the week or month when the largest number of cases occurred. The timing of peak activity for rotavirus infection in the United States was mapped in this way (Torok et al., 1997). Rotavirus is a major cause of gastroenteritis among infants and children. In the United States, the timing of peak rotavirus infection shows strong seasonal and geographical trends, with epidemics beginning in the Southwest in the fall and spreading north and east. To display these trends, data from the National Respiratory and Enteric Virus Surveillance system gathered from 69 laboratories in 42 states were analyzed. The weeks of the year were represented by numbers (1 to 52), and for each laboratory the week of peak infection was recorded.

To create a clear and effective map of the geographical distribution of peak times, the geostatistical procedure kriging was used (Figure 7.6). The earliest peaks occur in the southwest United States in the late fall, and the peaks spread north and west through the winter months. In the eastern and northern United States, the epidemic reaches its maximum in late spring (Bosley, 1997).

Kriging

Kriging is a method used to represent measurements taken at a discrete set of control points as a continuous surface. In the rotavirus example, the

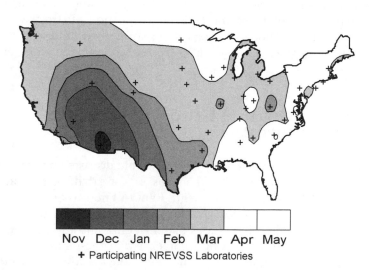

FIGURE 7.6. A kriged map of temporal peaks in rotavirus infection in the United States. From Bosley (1997).

control points are the 69 surveillance laboratories and the measurement for each laboratory is the week (1–52) of peak rotavirus incidence. To generate the representation of the epidemic as a continuous surface, a grid is overlayed on the control points, just as in kernel smoothing, which was discussed in Chapter 5. Values—in this case, the estimated week of peak incidence—are estimated at each grid point based on the distances to control points. What distinguishes kriging from other spatial interpolation methods is that it considers not only the distances to control points, but also the spatial autocorrelation of measurements among control points. *Spatial autocorrelation* refers to the similarity or association of values over space as measured in statistics like the G^* statistic discussed in Chapter 5.

To measure spatial autocorrelation, kriging uses the measure of *semivariance* (variance divided by 2). If Y_i is the measurement at control point i, d_{ij} is the distance between control points i and j, and h denotes a distance among control points, then the semivariance at distance h is:

$$\frac{\sum_{d_{ij} \leq h}(y_i - y_j)^2}{2n(h)}$$

where $n(h)$ is the number of pairs of control points that are distance h apart. The semivariance thus measures the variance of values for control points separated by distance h. A small semivariance indicates that measurements at distance h are similar to each other, whereas a large semivariance indicates a large disparity in measured values. As h varies, different values for the semivariance will be obtained. The *semivariogram* is a graph that shows the values of semivariance at different values of h (Figure 7.7). In general, the semivariance increases with increasing h, reflecting spatial dependence in the phenomena being investigated. Nearby control points will tend to have similar values, and thus a small semivariance, whereas distant locations tend to have less similar values and thus a larger variance.

In kriging, the semivariogram is used to generate a set of spatial weights or $\lambda_i(s)$ for each control point i and grid point s. Computing these weights involves matrix algebra (Isaaks & Srivastava, 1989). Once the weights have been computed, we estimate the value $Y(s)$ at grid point s as a weighted linear combination of the values at various control points (Figure 7.8). The estimated value at grid point s is:

$$Y(s) = \sum \lambda_i(s) \times Y_i$$

Computing these estimated values for all grid points s produces a fine mesh of values that appear as a continuous surface when mapped, as in Figure 7.9.

Kriging is a well-developed methodology that is widely used in the

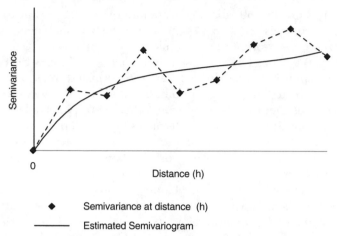

FIGURE 7.7. The semivariogram describes the relationship between semivariance and distance. It is estimated as a curvilinear function that best fits the actual semivariance values.

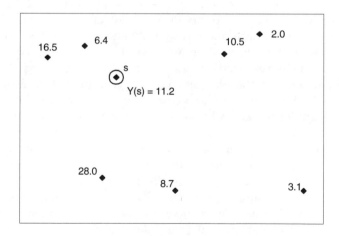

• Control point

$Y(s) = (\textbf{0.17} \times 16.5) + (\textbf{0.32} \times 6.4) + (\textbf{0.13} \times 28.0) + (\textbf{0.08} \times 8.7) +$
$(\textbf{0.15} \times 10.5) + (\textbf{0.06} \times 2.0) + (\textbf{0.09} \times 3.1) = 11.2$

FIGURE 7.8. A schematic example of using kriging to estimate the value at a particular place(s) based on known values at control points. The known values are multiplied by their respective kriging weights (λ), which come from the semivariogram. Kriging weights are shown in bold.

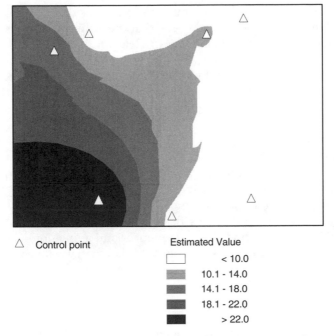

FIGURE 7.9. The results of a kriging analysis displayed as a continuous map.

earth sciences and geography. Although complex, it is generally considered the best method for creating a continuous surface map of estimated values from measurements taken at discrete control points. For communicable diseases, these measurements can show the time of peak incidence, as in the rotavirus example, or they may simply represent the level of disease incidence or prevalence at discrete locations. Kriging has been used for exploring other types of health problem like lead poisoning (Griffith, Doyle, Wheeler, & Johnson, 1998).

The main advantages of kriging are the following:

- Unlike many other interpolation methods, the estimated values can fall outside the range of the known data values.
- Kriging gives a standard error (kriging variance) for the estimated grid point values, making it possible to compute confidence intervals around the predictions.
- Kriging incorporates and indeed models the spatial dependence in the data.

Despite these advantages, kriging, like all statistical methods, requires caution in its application. The accuracy of kriging estimates depends heavily on the accuracy of the semivariogram that generates them. Before embarking on kriging, it is important to check that the semivariogram is properly specified and fits well the data being modeled. Still, kriging has great potential as a tool for visualizing health information, not only for communicable diseases, but for many health conditions that vary over space. It is also a valuable tool for estimating the incidence, prevalence, or timing of health conditions at locations outside the bounds of traditional surveillance systems.

Maps showing the timing of epidemic peaks capture only a limited aspect of disease diffusion. A more complete picture would reveal the movement of disease through both time and space in a dynamic sequence of images. Unfortunately, most current GIS systems are not well suited to tracing changes over space and time (Langran, 1992). Time adds a "third dimension" that does not always fit comfortably in the two-dimensional world of GIS. Two methods—map sequences and animation—can be used in conjunction with GIS to analyze and display spatial patterns of disease diffusion.

Map Sequences

Map sequences—or lag maps—have been widely used in studying the spread of infectious disease. A *map sequence* is a series of maps, displayed side by side, that show the disease distribution at different points in time. Each map represents a cross section, or slice, through time of the geographical pattern of disease. In their research on the diffusion of measles, Cliff and Haggett (1988) created map sequences of measles in Iceland during various epidemic periods (Figure 7.10). Patterns of contagious and hierarchical diffusion were clearly evident. Contagious diffusion dominated the map sequences for early epidemics when transportation connections were limited. In contrast, map sequences for the 1940s showed increasing evidence of hierarchical spread, reflecting higher rates of mobility and transportation access.

Map sequences can be created for almost any type of spatial health information that varies over time. The maps can display case locations, incidence rates, or rates of change over time. Ancillary features like transportation routes or commuting flows can be added to show the connections between transportation improvements and the spread of disease.

One of the main advantages of map sequences is the ease of comparing geographical patterns at various points in time. All maps are on the same page, allowing the viewer to shift from one map to the other while searching for similarities and differences and to focus easily on time periods that hold special interest. At the same time, it is often difficult to make sense of time trends in map sequences depending on the difficulty of comparing maps as the viewer shifts from one image to another. De-

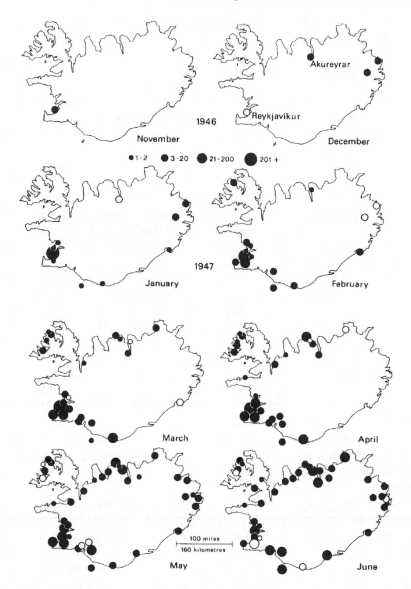

FIGURE 7.10. A map sequence of measles cases in Iceland by month from November 1946 through June 1947. From Cliff and Haggett (1988). Copyright 1988 by Blackwell Publishers Ltd. Reprinted by permission.

spite these shortcomings, map sequences offer a useful method for analyzing disease diffusion.

Animated Maps

Animated maps are "maps characterized by continuous or dynamic change"
(Slocum, 1999, p. 222). The maps are displayed dynamically, in sequence,
forming a constantly changing image or *animation*. The field of animation
has advanced rapidly in recent years, stimulated by developments in computer hardware and graphics software. These advances are fueling changes
in mapmaking as cartographers gain access to one of the first effective
tools for representing continuous change through space and time.

There are only a few examples of animated mapping of infectious diseases. One of the best is the work on HIV/AIDS, which began with Peter
Gould's animated maps of AIDS in Pennsylvania and now includes an animated sequence that shows the diffusion of AIDS in the United States
from 1983 to 1997 (Centers for Disease Control and Prevention, 1999b).
Created at the Centers for Disease Control, the latter shows dot density
maps of AIDS by year. The dots are yellow on a black background, and
the map "lights up" over time as the bright dots fill in the dark U.S. background. The animated maps are a vivid reminder of how AIDS emerged
just 2 decades ago and now affects the entire United States.

Designing map animations involves several considerations beyond
the traditional visual variables of static mapping, including duration, rate
of change, and order (DiBiasi, MacEachren, Krygier, & Reeves, 1992. *Duration* refers to the length of time each map is in view (Slocum, 1999). A
short duration means that each image disappears quickly, producing a
smooth but constantly changing animation. Lengthening the duration
gives the viewer more time to study each map, but the animation appears
choppy.

Rate of change describes the smoothness or variability of the animated
map sequence. It is computed as the amount of change between maps divided by the duration. If the positions or attributes of features on the map
change substantially during the animation, the animation has a high rate
of change. One can reduce rate of change by increasing the duration of
each map and thus smoothing the transition from map to map. Similarly,
reducing the amount of change between maps gives a lower rate of
change and a smoother animation. One way to accomplish this is by using
overlapping time intervals for the maps rather than discrete intervals. For
example, the first map might show disease incidence for weeks 1–4, the
second for weeks 2–6, the third for weeks 4–8, and so on. The 2-week
overlap means that some of the data on one map also appears on the next
map in the animated sequence.

Order defines the sequence of maps in the animation. Map animations typically rely on chronological order, a sensible choice for representing change over time. Slocum (1999) reports that using criteria other than time for ordering maps makes animations difficult to interpret. The viewer has to pay close attention to decipher the timing and sequencing of events.

Other visual variables mentioned in Chapter 2 and 4, such as hue, size, shape, and so on, can also be used effectively in map animation. Contrasting colors, changes in symbol size, and flashing symbols attract the eye to important data events.

Animation is an effective way of displaying the spread of infectious diseases through time and space. The smoothly changing patterns of contagious and hierarchical diffusion and the intensity of epidemic spread are all apparent on map animations. As in the AIDS example, animated maps reveal the expanding contours of disease emergence and the rapidity of spread. Animations, however, are primarily visual tools. They clearly show regular patterns, but if events move or vary in intensity unpredictably over time, the animation will be difficult to comprehend. Viewers also have trouble analyzing information on animated maps. The images move by quickly and are difficult to compare. Although one can often stop the animation to focus on a particularly interesting map, the contrast with other maps may not be apparent. For these reasons, animation will most likely remain a tool for visualization and display, not a method for spatial analysis.

PRIVACY AND CONFIDENTIALITY

Mapping communicable diseases at detailed geographic scales raises significant concerns about privacy and confidentiality. Just as maps of core areas can be used to stigmatize places, maps of case locations reveal personal information that can be used to stigmatize or discriminate against infected people. People's access to insurance or to health care and medical treatment may be denied because of geographical location. Curry (1999) calls this the "power of the visual," the violation of privacy for individuals or groups that results from creating maps of social and spatial information.

Even if health information is not displayed on a map, the spatial data management capabilities of GIS raise additional privacy concerns. These include the rapid growth of unregulated and potentially inaccurate spatial data, and the ability to create large dossiers on individuals by linking bits of information about people and places (Curry, 1998). GIS is central to these activities because it can be used to join data from different sources based on a common geographical location.

How can the needs of researchers and policymakers for geographically detailed health information be reconciled with the important right to privacy? In preparing maps, analysts can use several strategies to avoid the most obvious privacy violations. One is to aggregate health data to larger spatial units. Several of the studies mentioned earlier in this chapter began with residential addresses, but grouped the data by census tract for analysis and mapping (Becker et al., 1998). The address information is essentially discarded after assigning the cases to tracts. This is not a perfect solution because some of the tracts have such small populations that their tract totals might reveal personal information. To address this problem, we can omit tracts with small populations from analysis and mapping. In the Baltimore study, only tracts with more than 30 cases of gonorrhea were included in the GIS analysis (Becker et al., 1998).

Alternatively, one can retain the address information but only display it on small-scale maps, as was done in the study of sexual parternerships in Baltimore (Zenilman et al., 1999). Although each dot on the map represented a residential address, it would be extremely difficult to trace the addresses from the map because of the lack of detail on the Baltimore base map. This option, then, involves specifying a maximum scale for mapping.

It is also possible to develop "geographical masks" that preserve the security of individual health records while retaining enough location information to make it possible to answer questions that can only be answered with some knowledge of the geography of health events. Both the validity of these masks and their relative security have been examined (Armstrong, Rushton, & Zimmerman, 1999). Additional research is needed to investigate the impacts of geographical masking on the power of statistical tests for clustering or correlation.

None of these strategies deals with the issues of stigmatization, data linkage, and profiling, issues that are social and political in nature and not easily amenable to technical solutions. Addressing these issues will require multifaceted and multidisciplinary approaches (Curry, 1999) that are sensitive to the needs and concerns of individuals and communities and that emerge out of a legal, ethical, and political framework that is open and participatory.

Maintaining privacy and confidentiality is one of the most significant challenges in health mapping, especially for nonvectored infectious diseases, but also for a wide array of health issues including mental health and cancer. There are no easy solutions. Any attempt to address privacy and confidentiality involves balancing the competing interests of individuals and groups defined by class, ethnicity, race, or place, with the interests of protecting public health and providing high-quality data for public health research. While GIS researchers can offer general recommendations about aggregation and map scale, "solutions" will evolve in the political, legal, and social arenas.

CONCLUSION

Infectious diseases that spread directly from person to person are significant health concerns nationally and globally. Caused by living organisms that change in response to our efforts to control them, such diseases present a continually shifting challenge to public health. GIS mapping and analysis have an important role in depicting the large disparities among communities in infectious disease burden, in understanding how such diseases emerge and evolve, and in charting the dynamics of epidemics through space and time.

CHAPTER 8

Exploring the Ecology of Vector-Borne Disease

Vector-borne infectious disease involves a causative *agent*—usually some type of microorganism—that is the direct cause of the disease in the *host*. The *vector* is a living organism—usually an insect—involved in the transmission of the disease. For some vector-borne diseases, the transmission cycle also involves an *intermediate host* organism in which the agent develops or multiplies and a *reservoir* population of organisms that, in addition to human hosts, maintain the agent. GIS applications in the study of vector-borne disease attempt to model some aspect of how people live with animals and vectors in a particular ecological system.

New technologies in production and transportation and human population pressure are transforming ecological systems, even at the global scale. These transformations involve changes in land use, vegetation cover, species and species locations, and climate. Many of these factors have been suggested as explanations for the resurgence of infectious disease. "Ecoepidemology" is emerging in response to a perceived need to broaden the scope of assessment of the impacts of environmental change (Hales, Weinstein, & Woodward, 1997, p. 191). This approach entails a shift in emphasis from the study of direct, or toxicological, mechanisms to the study of indirect, or ecological, mechanisms and a shift from the individual to the region. Chapter 8 provides examples of GIS analyses of the distribution of vector and host populations, the land use and activity patterns that bring people into areas where vectors and hosts are present, and the resulting patterns of disease.

CASE DEFINITION FOR VECTOR-BORNE DISEASE

Like the infectious diseases discussed in Chapter 7, vector-borne diseases are often complex and difficult to diagnose. Lyme disease, the most common tick-borne disease in the United States, illustrates this problem. Lyme disease is a multistage multisystem disease caused in North America by *Borrelia burgdorferi*, a spirochete transmitted from mammal to mammal by ticks of the genus *Ixodes*. Humans "are inadvertent hosts of the spirochete" (Walker et al., 1996, p. 463). Early Lyme disease is often indicated by erythema migrans, a characteristic skin rash appearing around the site of the tick bite after a week. Late stage disease affecting the musculoskeletal and neurological systems can be more difficult to diagnose, particularly if there is no history of erythema migrans in a person who lives in or has visited an area where Lyme disease is *endemic*, or permanently present, and depends on laboratory confirmation. State criteria for defining a Lyme disease case vary (Vogt, 1992).

In 1990, the Center for Disease Control (CDC) and the Council of State and Territorial Epidemiologists made Lyme disease nationally notifiable and developed a national case definition (Centers for Disease Control and Prevention, 1997a). The complexity of the case definition reflects the difficulty of diagnosing cases of many vector-borne infectious diseases. A case of Lyme disease is confirmed if the person has the skin lesion erythema migrans or if at least one late manifestation of disease is present and the case is laboratory-confirmed. Erythema migrans must be diagnosed by a physician, and laboratory confirmation is recommended for persons with no known exposure. Exposure is defined as having been in a county where Lyme disease is endemic within 30 days before the onset of erythema migrans. The Lyme disease case definition contains a geographic standard for determining whether disease is endemic to a county: if at least two confirmed cases have been previously acquired or established populations of a known tick vector are infected with *B. burgdorferi*. The development of a standard is important in the design and implementation of a national reporting system so that the time and expense of reporting will result in consistent information on valid cases. The standard has, however, been problematic in some regions like the southeastern United States where erythema migrans and other Lyme disease symptoms have been observed in patients who live in areas where there is no documentation of transmission of *B. burgdorferi* to humans. Also, a "count by county" standard is not uniform across the country because counties vary considerably in land area, habitat area, and population size. The county of San Bernardino, California, for example, is larger in area than the state of Connecticut (about four times as large, or 20,064 square miles compared to 4,872) and Connecticut has eight counties.

TEMPORAL AND SPATIAL INTEGRATION OF SURVEILLANCE DATA

Case data from a surveillance system can be geocoded using the methods described in Chapter 3. One of the most important functions of a GIS is data integration. In the case of infectious disease epidemiology, GIS can be used effectively to integrate data temporally and spatially.

Temporal patterns are of particular concern with emerging and reemerging infectious diseases. In the case of Lyme disease, *B. burgdorferi* has been detected in mice specimens from the 1890s, but the lack of specimens has made the question of the origins of the disease in North America speculative (Ginsberg, 1993). The principal vectors differ in the different North American foci. In the northeastern focus, it is likely that the increase in ticks is explained either by diffusion from a few coastal islands in New England or by increase and local spread of a widely distributed but previously rare tick population.

The distribution of vector-borne infectious diseases is often assessed using case reports, in part because good baseline data on the distribution of vectors is often unavailable. Lyme disease case data reported for different surveillance periods in a region of Connecticut where the disease is hyperendemic illustrate the spread of the disease (Figure 8.1). Given the relatively recent recognition of Lyme disease, however, some of the increase is probably due to increased public and provider awareness and changing reporting requirements (Dennis, 1991; Ginsberg, 1993), although Connecticut has used a consistent case definition throughout. The apparent rapid spread of an infectious disease may be partly an artifact of changes in case definition or reporting.

Spatial integration of data is also an important GIS function in the study of infectious disease. Health problems like Lyme disease have been fairly intensively studied, but many other emerging diseases are less well understood. Human granulocytic ehrlichiosis (HGE) is a potentially life-threatening bacterial disease characterized by undifferentiated flu-like symptoms (Walker et al., 1996). HGE is not a notifiable disease, but the CDC has developed a national case definition (Centers for Disease Control and Prevention, 1997a).

An early focus of the disease in North America was Wisconsin and Minnesota, but cases have since been recognized in the northeastern United States and California, places that also have high incidence rates for Lyme disease. HGE in the northeastern United States is believed to be transmitted by the same tick that transmits *B. burgdorferi* to humans, either by a single tick or by different individual ticks (Reed, Mitchell, Persing, Kolbert, & Cameron, 1995). About 9% of patients with HGE also acquire concurrent Lyme disease or babesiosis and about 9% of Lyme disease patients also acquire HGE, although the incidence rate for HGE is much

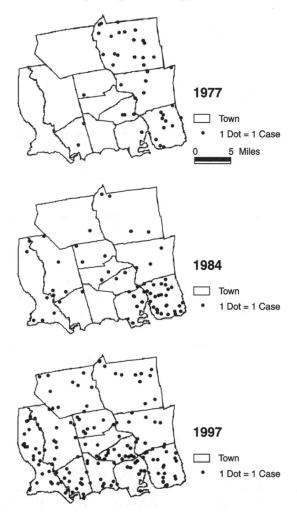

FIGURE 8.1. Dot density maps of Lyme disease cases by town illustrate the spread of the disease in a region in southern Connecticut where Lyme disease is hyperendemic. The data for 1977 were reported in Steere, Broderick, and Malawista (1978), used by permission. The data for 1984 and 1997 were provided by the Epidemiology Section, Connecticut Department of Public Health.

lower. GIS analysis has been used to compare the distributions of HGE and Lyme disease cases in a region in Connecticut where Lyme disease is hyperendemic by mapping case locations for each disease and indicating cases where an individual acquired Lyme disease and HGE. Coinfection is important because it may affect immunosuppressive response in the host, leading to more severe disease (Bakken et al., 1994). Because the diseases are believed to be transmitted by the same tick, interventions to control tick populations would obviously have implications for both diseases.

IDENTIFYING AREAS OF HIGH AND LOW INCIDENCE

In addition to describing temporal and spatial patterns in disaggregate case data from a surveillance system, GIS analysis can be used to identify areas of high and low incidence. Sometimes, as described in Chapter 5, the detection of disease clusters is part of an epidemiological research project to identify the cause or causes of a disease. For some emerging infectious diseases, temporal and spatial concentration of health problems with rapid onset may have been the clue that the disease was infectious or vector-borne in the first place. For infectious diseases of known etiology, the identification of areas of high and low incidence is relevant to the design of intervention strategies because high-incidence areas may indicate places where many people are being exposed to the disease agent, particularly if the time between exposure and onset is short. Areas of low incidence are either places where the agent–vector–host cycle is not established, or where people are not present, or both.

Surveillance systems usually report residential address. Distribution by residential location is almost always relevant for medical services planning, but the residence may not be the relevant location for identifying disease clusters. Questions about the relevant locations to map and the impacts of aggregating cases or populations at risk to geographical areas have been raised for decades (Maxcy, 1926). Spot maps of typhus cases in cities in the southeastern United States showed no particular concentration by residential neighborhood other than a tendency toward localization in the central portions of the cities (Figure 8.2). Spot maps by place of employment, however, revealed focal centers. Because exposure to Lyme disease in Connecticut is believed to occur primarily peridomestically, looking at residential locations makes sense. In other regions of the country where exposure may be more likely in recreational settings, the residential distribution of cases may not be useful in identifying areas where people are at risk for acquiring the disease.

Hantavirus pulmonary syndrome is another disease where place of exposure is not always known. Hantavirus pulmonary syndrome is a severe illness affecting the cardiovascular system and resulting in death in slightly less than half the cases (Centers for Disease Control and Prevention, 1998). The most frequently seen agent of the four different hantaviruses in North America is Sin Nombre virus, transmitted to humans from the deer mouse *Peromyscus maniculatus* by direct contact with infected mice, their droppings, or their nests, or by inhalation of virus particles from mouse excrement. Residence in a dwelling with substantial ro-

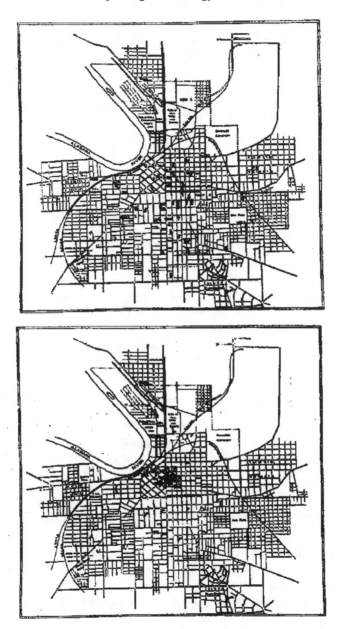

FIGURE 8.2. The top map of cases of mild typhus in Montgomery, Alabama, 1922-1925, according to residence shows no clustering. The bottom map of cases according to place of employment shows a concentration of cases near the center of the city. From Maxcy (1926).

dent infestations has been identified as an important source of exposure. Geocoding residential addresses from the surveillance records would therefore be a reasonable starting point for investigating where populations are at risk.

The distribution of cases shows the spatial pattern of the numerator. This distribution needs to be viewed in the context of the distribution of the denominator population. One approach for accomplishing this is to calculate rates for predetermined geographical areas, like census tracts. Some drawbacks to this approach are that the geographical areas often arbitrarily partition the numerator and the denominator: places with low rates may have large numbers of cases, places with high rates may have small numbers of cases, and some places may have no cases because no one lives there. As in documenting core areas for communicable disease transmission, GIS analysis enables us to look at the joint distributions of cases and population so that we can better classify areas.

Spatial databases can be used in GIS to show various representations of population distribution (Figure 8.3): the choropleth map of population counts by census tract, the land-use/land-cover representation derived from remote sensing data that shows areas of residential development of different density, and the street network representation that shows where structures are likely to be located. The land-use/land-cover representation depicts the settings of residential areas—for example, adjacent to commercial strips or surrounded by forested zones. The street network view helps the public health analyst better interpret the meaning of no cases or few cases reported from an area by providing a picture of whether or not residential or high-density residential development exists in the area.

There are a number of important considerations in identifying areas of high incidence. Although we will not observe a case in a place where there is no residence, it is not always true that disease patterns "follow" the distribution of residences. If it were, there would be no geographical variations in disease unexplained by the geographical distribution in population. The same case distributions can be embedded in different underlying population distributions (Figure 8.4), highlighting the need to view the joint distribution of numerator and denominator before calculating rates for areas that might arbitrarily partition the numerator and denominator or performing a clustering analysis with an arbitrary distance criterion. Maxcy (1926) recognized this problem in his study of typhus: "The question arises whether this apparent concentration is merely the result of a greater density of population in that part of the city. . . . The division of the city is peculiarly unfavorable for the purposes in mind [rate calculation], inasmuch as the wards are arranged radially in such manner that all except one include portions of the central part of the city."

A 1992 case–control study of Lyme disease in southeastern Connecti-

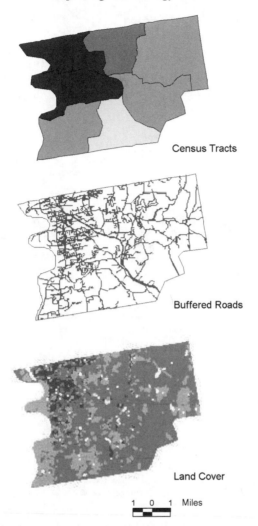

Census Tracts

Buffered Roads

Land Cover

1 0 1 Miles

FIGURE 8.3. Spatial databases in a GIS provide different kinds of information about the distribution of population within a PUBLIC HEALTH GIS study area town.

cut found that the only variable significantly associated with Lyme disease incidence was self-reported residence in a "village" or higher density residential setting. In the study area, these settings do not correspond to census or other political administrative units for reporting aggregate population. The hypothesis was tested using GIS (Cromley, Cartter, Mrozinski, & Ertel, 1998). Rather than calculating rates for administrative

POPULATION DISTRIBUTION   ○ 1 Person   CASE
                                                 DISTRIBUTION

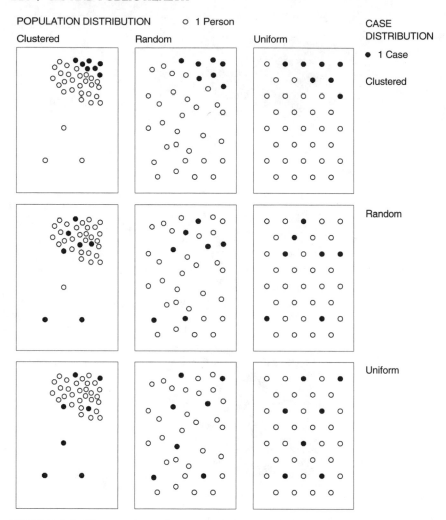

FIGURE 8.4. The number of cases and the population size is the same in each study area shown above, but similar case distributions can be embedded in different underlying population distributions.

units, the analysts calculated rates for regions defined by residential density. Geocoded cases acquired by active surveillance were classified as being located inside or outside of a village setting. "Village setting" was operationalized as any area of contiguous medium- or high-density residential development that was at least 30 acres in size. The study area population residing inside and outside villages was also estimated. The analysis confirmed a lower relative risk for people living in villages. Settlement density has also been identified as a risk factor for vector-borne disease in tropical settings (Laveissiere & Meda, 1999). Evaluating the environmental characteristics of locations where cases are observed and then comparing them with the characteristics of places where people live or engage in activities but do not acquire the disease can offer additional insights into the disease process.

EVALUATING THE ENVIRONMENTAL CHARACTERISTICS OF CASE LOCATIONS

A number of GIS applications have evaluated the local and neighborhood environmental characteristics of case locations, generally through point-in-polygon analysis, discussed in Chapter 4. Through this type of analysis, it is possible to take a point in one data layer and compare its location to a set of areas in another data layer to determine which area the point lies within (Figure 8.5). Once this determination is made, the attributes of the area can be associated with the point. Points can then be selected based on the attributes of the areas they lie within. Also, once the polygon in which the point lies is determined, the characteristics of adjacent areas can be evaluated and associated with the point (Figure 8.6).

In this way, the local and neighborhood characteristics of places with a high frequency of cases can be assessed. Once the characteristics of areas where many cases are observed have been determined, it is possible to develop maps showing regions with similar environmental conditions regardless of disease incidence. Maps of this type can be important for suggesting areas where disease may be underreported, where disease incidence may increase if people move in and local environmental conditions remain unchanged, or where disease may spread or emerge in the future.

In the analysis of Lyme disease, case databases have been integrated with other GIS data layers describing environmental characteristics like elevation, vegetation, and soils that may influence tick distribution. The relations between 127 environmental variables and Lyme disease incidence were explored in Baltimore County, Maryland (Glass et al., 1992). Empirical data on tick density and tick infection rates were not included. These data are difficult to collect for large geographical areas. Based on an overlay analysis of the distribution of cases and controls to determine the environmental characteristics of their residential locations, several environmental variables were found to be associated with increased risk, including location in one of two watersheds, on loamy soils, and in forested areas. Residence in highly developed areas was associated with a decreased risk. Only 14% of the land area in the county had environmental characteristics associated with increased risk for Lyme disease; approximately 8% of the county's population resided in these high-risk areas.

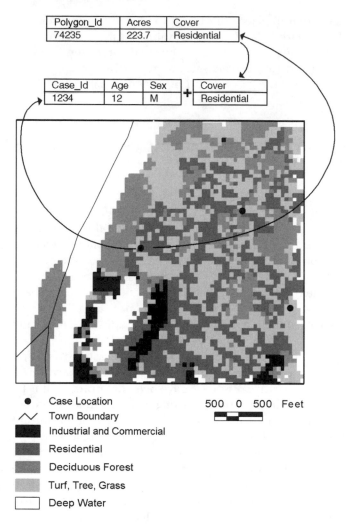

FIGURE 8.5. A point-in-polygon analysis identifies the land cover of the polygon where the case is located and assigns that land cover type as an attribute of the case through a spatial join procedure.

A similar conceptual approach was used to investigate the epidemiology of rodent bite and the distribution of the rat population in New York City (Childs et al., 1998). Rat bite fever, unlike Lyme disease, is a relatively rare but potentially fatal infection. Few epidemiological studies of rat bite have been conducted. Moreover, there have been very few attempts to describe the distribution of rat or mouse populations in urban centers by direct field observation. In the New York study, a GIS was developed to de-

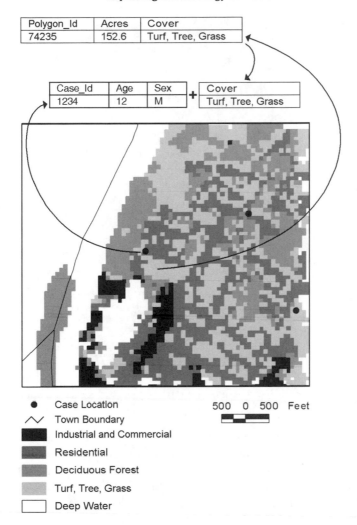

Polygon_Id	Acres	Cover
74235	152.6	Turf, Tree, Grass

Case_Id	Age	Sex		Cover
1234	12	M	+	Turf, Tree, Grass

●   Case Location
⋀⋁ Town Boundary
    Industrial and Commercial
    Residential
    Deciduous Forest
    Turf, Tree, Grass
    Deep Water

500   0   500   Feet

FIGURE 8.6. The land cover of the adjacent polygon is assigned as an attribute of the case.

termine the city block where the bite occurred and the environmental and social characteristics of the blocks (Figure 8.7). A set of control blocks where no bite had been reported was selected for comparison.

GIS analysis was used to produce maps of the distribution of blocks with different probabilities for rodent bite in each of the five boroughs. The predictive power of the maps was evaluated by comparing reports of rodent bite from a later year with the maps and by environmental sampling of randomly selected blocks in Manhattan and Brooklyn for evi-

Bite Characteristics	Census Block Characteristics				
Bite ID	+	Block ID	Total Pop	Pop Density	% Black	% Hispanic
118		202	1259	135866.4	45.0	74.0

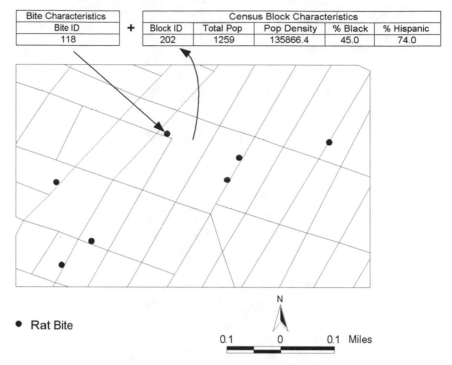

• Rat Bite

N

0.1   0   0.1   Miles

FIGURE 8.7. A point-in-polygon analysis to identify the local census block characteristics of a rat bite case and assign them as attributes of a case through a spatial join procedure.

dence of rat infestation. Blocks where rodent bites occurred tended to be closer to subways, railroads, and parks. These places are potential sources of exposed ground, providing rats with burrow sites and sites where human refuse accumulates where rats might forage.

ANALYZING THE GEOGRAPHICAL DISTRIBUTIONS OF VECTOR AND HOST POPULATIONS

Vector and host surveillance and analysis of the ecology of infectious diseases in animal populations are essential components of public health programs to address infectious disease. For some diseases, like rabies, the number of human cases is too low to provide a picture of where people may be at risk of coming into contact with the disease. Even for infectious diseases like Lyme disease with fairly high incidence rates, studying the ecology of the disease is important because there are often important regional variations in the disease cycle. GIS applications in infectious disease epidemiology illustrate these themes.

Rabies: Few Human Cases but a Widespread Problem

Rabies is a *zoonotic* disease caused by an RNA virus (Krebs, Wilson, & Childs, 1995). Animal hosts maintain and transmit the disease to humans, usually by bites, although nonbite exposures have been documented. Human infections are not important in maintaining the virus because humans do not contribute to the transmission cycle. Mammalian carnivores are the essential hosts, primarily dogs in the developing world and wildlife in developed countries where rabies in domesticated dogs has been brought under control through vaccination programs. In the United States, wildlife have been the principal reservoir since the 1960s (Krebs, Strine, & Childs, 1993). In humans, the virus affects the central nervous system and results in death unless effective postexposure treatment is provided.

Human rabies cases are rare. In 1997, only four cases were documented in the United States (Centers for Disease Control and Prevention, 1998). Bats are recognized as an important wildlife reservoir for variants of the rabies virus that are transmitted to humans, accounting for 58% of cases diagnosed in the United States from 1980 to 1998. Bat bites are of particular concern because injury from a bat bite is often more limited than injury from the bite of a terrestrial carnivore like a raccoon and people may not be aware that they have been bitten. Because "all bites by carnivores (especially raccoons, skunks, and foxes) and bats must be considered possible exposures" (Krebs et al., 1995, p. 689), understanding the geographical patterns of places where human contact with these animals has occurred is important. GIS can be used to portray these patterns.

Bretsky (1995) used GIS to map the spread of rabies in Connecticut from 1991 through 1994. Connecticut's experience during this time was part of the most intense outbreak of wildlife rabies ever to occur in the United States (Rupprecht, Smith, Fekadu, & Childs, 1995). From the time the index case was reported in West Virginia in 1977, it took approximately 14 years for the first case to arrive in the town of Ridgefield, Connecticut, on the New York border. Over the next 4 years, the disease spread throughout the state from southwest to northeast (Figure 8.8) and a second wave was reemerging in the southwestern part of the state. The initial epizootic wave had advanced approximately 30 kilometers per year (Wilson et al., 1997).

Lyme Disease: Regional Variations in the Transmission Cycle

Many vector-borne infectious diseases involve the same agent but different vectors and hosts in different regions. In the Northeast, the principal Lyme disease vector is *Ixodes scapularis* and the disease reservoir is the white-footed mouse. In California, the principal Lyme disease vector is *I. pacificus*, the western black-legged tick. The identification of the dusky-footed woodrat as a Lyme disease reservoir in California revealed a pattern

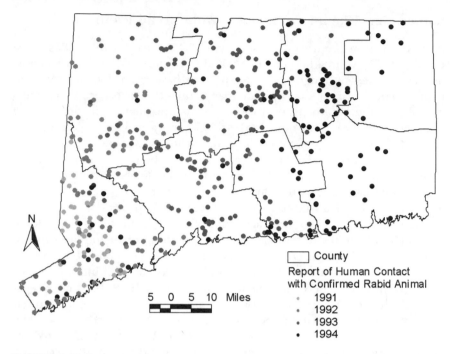

FIGURE 8.8. Reports of human contact with confirmed rabid animals during the 1991–1994 epizootic in Connecticut. From Connecticut Department of Environmental Protection.

of Lyme disease transmission very different from the cycle in the northeastern United States. In California, the pattern has two cycles involving two different ticks (Brown & Lane, 1992). *I. neotomae*, with higher observed infection rates, was identified as responsible for maintaining the disease in the woodrat population but not involved in the human disease because it does not bite humans. *I. pacificus* ticks were infected at lower rates, not enough to maintain endemic disease, but enough to transmit the disease to humans. The detection of infected woodrats and *I. pacificus* ticks in the mountains near Los Angeles suggests a Lyme disease cycle maintained in wildlife in a main recreational area for one of the largest metropolitan areas in the country.

Ecological studies are also valuable because they may give insight into factors that affect temporal cycles in infectious disease risk. Acorns from oak trees are an important source of food for the white-footed mouse *Peromyscus leucopus* that is the principal reservoir in the Lyme disease cycle in the northeastern United States (Jones, Ostfeld, Richard, Schauber, & Wolff, 1998). A large autumn crop of acorns also draws the white-tailed deer into oak forests. Large crops are not produced every autumn, however. Instead, large crops are produced every 2 to 5 years, with few or no acorns produced during the intervening years. Experimental addition of acorns resulted in increased density of mice and of ticks. These experiments suggest that it "may be feasible to predict the risk of contracting Lyme disease from infected nymphal ticks in oak forests on the basis of masting events, with the risk being greater 2 years after an abundant acorn crop" (Jones et al., 1998, p. 1025).

Issues in Vector/Host Surveillance and Risk Assessment

Monitoring infectious disease patterns through vector/host surveillance is not without difficulties. A number of GIS applications dealing with Lyme disease have used data from host animals to investigate vector distribution. For example, studies have attempted to model the distribution of infected deer ticks by collecting ticks from deer killed by hunters and hunter-reported location of kill (Kitron, Jones, Bouseman, Nelson, & Baumgartner, 1992; Amerasinghe et al., 1992; Glass, Amerasinghe, Morgan, & Scott, 1994). These studies are obviously limited by spatial biases in where deer are killed.

The emergence of vector-borne diseases has been associated with renewed efforts to monitor vector distribution directly and to analyze vector infection rates. As with other infectious disease surveillance programs, support for vector surveillance eroded during the 1970s and 1980s when vector-borne infectious disease was not at the forefront of public health concern. Vector surveillance is time-consuming and expensive, and good baseline data sets are often not available. Many tick collection studies undertaken in response to the emergence of Lyme disease were based on the first reported collection from the site where the study took place (Ginsberg, 1993).

Because of the difficulties of producing a map of infected vectors (or even vectors or hosts), GIS applications have also been developed to model habitat (Beck, Lobitz, & Wood, 2000). Research on Lyme disease has attempted to model habitat by using remote sensing data. This approach was used in Rhode Island to develop a scheme for surveying tick populations on a statewide basis (Nicholson & Mather, 1996). A GIS analysis partitioned the state into 42 zones 10 kilometers square. Road, land use, vegetation, and hydrography data were included. Forested habitats were identified as areas where more than 50% of the cover was tree canopy. Land-use/land-cover data are derived from remote sensing data. Eighty tick collection sites of approximately 4 hectares were selected based on location in the state, type and amount of forested habitat, and road accessibility. Each large zone had from one to three tick sampling sites located within it. After 18 samples were taken from each site, mean tick density and mean infection rate were calculated. An entomologic risk index was computed as the product of tick abundance and the local infection rate.

Modeling environmental risk based on habitat alone without follow-up data on the distribution of human cases and vectors is problematic. To test the adequacy of these indices, the geographical distribution of risk areas needs to be compared either to the distribution of vectors and hosts or to the distribution of human cases, and preferably both (Mather, Nicholson, Donnelly, & Matyas, 1996; Nicholson & Mather, 1996). In the Rhode Island research, a strong positive correlation was observed between the entomologic risk index and human cases.

Environmental data from remote sensing and GIS analysis have also been used to predict host infection status for the Sin Nombre virus (Boone et al., 2000). Vegetation type and density, elevation, slope, and hydrology were characterized for 144 field observation sites in the Walker River basin along the Nevada–California border. Deer mice were trapped at field sites and blood samples were taken to determine current or past infection with the virus. Field sites were classified as positive or negative based on the infection status of the mice captured. Discriminant analysis was then used to examine relationships between the environmental variables characterizing each site and the site's infection status. Combinations of environmental variables were found that could correctly predict the infection status of deer mice with 80% accuracy.

Using GIS to model habitat can make an important contribution to understanding vector-borne disease. Habitats are significantly affected by land use change. Residential development or other land use change in an area alters the environment in ways that will either increase or decrease exposure.

GLOBAL CHANGE AFFECTING VECTOR DISTRIBUTION

Global change in technology and global climate change are two factors cited in the spread of vector-borne disease. GIS are being used to establish proactive surveillance, prevention, and control programs and to study patterns of global climate change and their possible impacts on vector-borne disease.

West Nile Virus

During the summer and fall of 1999, an outbreak of West Nile encephalitis occurred in New York. This was the first evidence of the virus in the Western Hemisphere. West Nile fever is a mosquito-borne flavivirus infection endemic in Africa and Asia (Tsai, Popovici, Cernescu, Campbell, & Nedelcu, 1998). Outbreaks occurred in southern France in the early 1960s and in Romania in 1996 (Lundstrom, 1999). The outbreak in Romania resulted in a high fatality/case ratio (Tsai et al., 1998). Mosquitoes in the home and, for apartment dwellers, flooded basements, in addition to spending time outdoors, were confirmed as risk factors in two case–control studies conducted in Romania (Han et al., 1999).

In New York, 56 cases including seven deaths had occurred by late fall. One of the fatal cases was an international case involving a Canadian citizen who had visited New York late in the summer and had onset of encephalitis several weeks later. The outbreak of West Nile virus was accompanied by intense research efforts to determine the particular strain involved (Jia et al., 1999; Lanciotti et al., 1999; Anderson et al., 1999).

To limit the impact of the virus in the United States, the CDC and the U.S. Department of Agriculture cosponsored a meeting in November 1999 to develop programs to monitor virus activity and to prevent future outbreaks of disease (Centers for Disease Control and Prevention, 2000). The New York outbreak had resulted in extensive mortality in crows. Because of bird migration patterns, CDC efforts included surveillance of areas from Louisiana and Alabama along the Gulf Coast to Massachusetts and Maine. The surveillance guidelines called for active bird surveillance in both wild and sentinel populations, active mosquito surveillance to monitor virus activity and to identify potential vectors, active veterinary surveillance—particularly for horses (Nolen, 2000), and enhanced passive human surveillance for reporting viral encephalitis. The guidelines also described the minimal laboratory diagnostic support required and emphasized mosquito control methods for preventing further outbreaks of the disease.

In New York and neighboring states, the local response has involved using GIS technology, particularly in bird surveillance. The geocoded locations of dead wildlife in Rockland County, New York, were plotted with test results for West Nile virus (Figure I.4). Evidence that the virus remained in bird populations over the winter reinforced the importance of preparations for the following spring and summer.

The West Nile outbreak in the United States illustrates the impact that transportation and trade have on patterns of infectious disease. Global trade and changes in transportation technology have made it possible for translocation of species and for individuals to contract a disease in one place and be in another country by the time symptoms appear. At the same time, changes in climate and weather patterns associated with human activity may be altering the range of vectors.

Global Climate Change

In addition to biological and ecological determinants of vector-borne disease, climate factors are influencing the worldwide spread of infectious diseases. Global infection rates for vector-borne diseases like viral encephalitis, dengue, and malaria are increasing. These diseases are among those most sensitive to climate change. Climatologists have identified an upward trend in global temperatures that could lead to a rise of $2\,^{\circ}$C by the end of the 21st century (Patz, Epstein, Burke, & Balbus, 1996). For vector-borne disease, climate change is expected to directly affect disease transmission by affecting the vector's geographic range, increasing rates of reproduction, affecting biting behavior, and shortening incubation periods of the pathogen. Warming is also expected to affect ocean surface temperatures and raise sea levels, creating a scenario for higher incidence of water-borne diseases like cholera and contamination of fish. These hypothesized effects have been widely discussed. There is a growing body of literature testing hypotheses of the connections between climate and infectious disease using climate change models, remote sensing data, and GIS.

Climate Modeling and Disease Distribution

Remote sensing and spatial interpolation of climate data have been investigated as complementary approaches to predict spatial variations in monthly climate. In a study of patterns for continental Africa in 1990, information from the *Advanced Very High Resolution Radiometer* (AVHRR) of the National Oceanic and Atmospheric Administration's satellite was used to model land surface temperature and moisture (Hay & Lennon, 1999). Then, data on the duration of cold clouds were derived from the *High Resolution Radiometer* (HRR) on the European Meteorological Satellite platform as a remote sensing measure of rainfall. Finally, temperature, atmospheric moisture, and rainfall surfaces were estimated by spatial interpolation from measurements taken at World Meteorological Organization stations in Africa. The station data were used to test the accuracy of the climate patterns produced from the remote sensing data or by spatial interpolation. No clear conclusions were reported, but this and other research shows considerable potential for using a variety of methods to develop better techniques for epidemiological research (Cresswell, Morse, Thomson, & Connor, 1999), particularly in areas where temperature data are required but conventional climate monitoring stations are inadequate.

Transmission and Biting

The dynamics of vector-borne disease transmission associated with specific climate events like the El Niño southern oscillation (ENSO) have also been investigated using climate modeling techniques. The ENSO of 1991–1992 has been suggested as a major climate factor in the southwestern United States, creating favorable conditions for an increase in the rodent population, leading to the outbreak of hantavirus pulmonary syndrome. Springtime precipitation in 1992 and 1993 at 28 sites with confirmed human cases of hantavirus pulmonary syndrome and 170 control sites was estimated and compared to precipitation during the previous 6 years (Glass et al., 2000). Elevation and Landsat Thematic Mapper data collected the year before the outbreak were also used to estimate disease risk. An association between elevation and satellite data and hantavirus pulmonary syndrome risk the following year was shown.

Correlations between annual averages of the ENSO index, local temperature, and dengue fever were calculated for 14 island nations across the South Pacific (Hales, Weinstein, Souares, & Woodward, 1999). Positive correlations of the index and dengue fever were found in 10 countries. The study concluded that climate changes associated with El Niño could enhance transmission on the larger and more populated islands where the disease is endemic, while propagation from the larger to the smaller islands, which appeared to be independent of climate variations, was probably a function of population density and travel patterns.

Many vector-borne disease processes show seasonal variation along with large within-year variation of incidence. Variability in weather patterns has been investigated for possible associations with variability in the entomological parameters like biting rates. A soil moisture model of surface water availability combined with land cover and soil features improved prediction of biting rates for two Anopheles mosquitoes associated with malaria outbreaks in an endemic region of Kenya (Patz et al., 1998). Modeling soil moisture and lagged soil moisture substantially improved prediction of variability in bite rates over the predictions made from modeling rainfall alone.

Sea Surface Temperature

Outbreaks of cholera occur when *Vibrio cholerae*, the bacterium that causes the disease, is sufficiently present in drinking water to provide an infective dose if ingested. The connections between the pathogen and plankton, and between plankton and sea temperature, have been described by Colwell (1996). Water samples taken from research vessels have been an important means of assessing presence of the bacterium and factors like water temperature, nutrient concentration, and plankton that favor its reproduction. This type of data acquisition, like ground-based sampling for ticks or other vectors, is expensive, time-consuming, and yields data for only limited areas.

Remote sensing data for the Bay of Bengal were used to evaluate sea surface temperature and sea surface height and to compare these variables with cholera case data collected in Bangladesh from 1992 to 1995 (Lobitz et al., 2000). An annual cycle in sea surface temperature similar to the cycle evident in the cholera case data was detected. Sea surface height was also correlated with disease outbreaks, perhaps because rising water results in an incursion of plankton-rich water inland.

Climate Change in Perspective

The research on climate change and vector-borne disease does not suggest that increases in vector-borne disease risk can be attributed to climate trends alone. Although vector populations are sensitive to climate trends, there are multiple factors underlying the emergence and reemergence of vector-borne disease. Housing conditions, public health resources, and access to medical care are among the factors that are likely to influence emergence of vector-borne diseases even in areas where the potential for transmission may be increasing in response to climate change (Martens, 2000). Efforts to model climate change and disease emergence, some using GIS, seek to improve our understanding of complex vector-borne disease transmission cycles, to identify high-risk areas and assess their characteristics, and to develop effective control measures to protect communities.

ENVIRONMENTAL IMPACTS OF CONTROLLING VECTOR-BORNE DISEASE

Vector-borne infectious disease transmission depends on ecological systems that may be complex—involving more than one agent, vector, or host—and regionally variable. This complexity is reflected in efforts to control vector-borne disease. In some cases, efforts are made to prevent the introduction of disease into a new area by restricting migration and trade. In the case of West Nile virus, for example, international restrictions on the movement of horses were put into effect. Attempts to control a disease once it has become established in an area can conflict with efforts to protect the environment.

Failure to control disease can directly affect the health of wild animal populations. During the rabies epizootic in the 1980s and 1990s in the northeastern United States, for example, more than 20,000 rabies cases were reported in raccoons (Bretsky, 1995). For some diseases, like Lyme disease, direct effects of the disease in wildlife populations have not been reported, and animal populations are significantly impacted not by the disease itself, but by control measures that affect their habitat.

Six control methods for dealing with vector-borne infectious disease problems have been identified (Table 8.1). Only self-protection measures can be associated with minimal environmental impacts. Efforts to control vector-borne infectious disease by intervening in an ecological system are

TABLE 8.1. Intervention Options for Vector-Borne Disease Control and Potential Environmental Impacts

Control method	Environmental effects
Self-protection precautions	Negligible; possible health effects of vaccines, repellents on user
Habitat manipulation	Powerful effects in areas where habitat is disrupted (can be limited to areas with high human presence)
Manipulation of host populations	Powerful effects on host species and associates (efficacy not always established)
Biological control	Depends on species utilized (efficacy not always established)
Broadcast pesticide applications	Powerful effects on nontarget species in application areas
Targeted pesticide applications	Main effects confined to nest associates of targeted species (can be limited to areas with high human presence)

Note. Adapted from Ginsberg (1994, p. 347). Copyright 1994, reprinted by permission of Blackwell Science, Inc.

bound to have impacts on other aspects of the environment and may produce unintended, undesirable consequences.

Conflicts also arise when wildlife hosts seed epidemics of disease in domesticated animals like cattle that can then pose a threat to human health. An example is bovine tuberculosis (TB) in Great Britain. The likeliest source of infection of cattle is the badger, although this has not been fully proved (Krebs et al., 1998). Natural habitat for badgers is often found in or around cattle pasture areas. Different strategies ranging from severe culling to only partial removal of badgers have been implemented for the last 2 decades to control bovine TB. Because these strategies were implemented in succession rather than in parallel, it has been difficult to assess their relative effectiveness.

A major unanswered question in vector-borne disease control is how much reservoir or vector populations have to be reduced before there is an impact on human health. Total elimination is usually out of the question, but partial elimination may be ineffective because lowering vector abundance or agent prevalence may not produce equivalent declines in human exposure risk (Ginsberg, 1993) or may exacerbate the infectious disease problem by disrupting territorial systems and decreasing diversity

(Krebs et al., 1998). When ecosystem diversity decreases, the disease transmission cycle may actually become more efficient.

CONCLUSION

Emerging and reemerging vector-borne infectious diseases are challenges requiring new responses from public health and medical care systems. These diseases are often undiagnosed, untreated, and unreported, a situation of special concern because delays in diagnosis and treatment often result in severe chronic health problems or death. Ecological studies of agent–vector–host relationships and improved surveillance methods have been cited as important priorities for addressing these infectious disease problems.

The resurgence of interest in vector-borne disease no doubt reflects their emergence or reemergence in populations and areas of the world where it was believed these problems had been conquered. Vector-borne diseases have remained "common among populations lacking basic human rights such as control over their land, political rights and access to water and sanitation" (Winch, 1998, p. 47). The global distribution of many of the same diseases—cholera, malaria, encephalitis—that are now the subject of interest were studied in the late 1940s as part of a disease atlas project supervised by Dr. Jacques May under the auspices of the American Geographical Society (American Geographical Society, 1944).

GIS analysis is playing an important role in the renewal of efforts to view the problems of vector-borne disease at a variety of geographic scales, including the global scale. But, as many of these studies point out, the important issue from a human health perspective is how our improved understanding of the disease process leads to better prevention and intervention and improves access to health services.

CHAPTER 9

Analyzing Access
to Health Services

Fiscal and administrative pressures are transforming health care delivery in the United States. The growth of managed care, shifts in medical practice, and the ever-present pressure to contain health care costs are reshaping how health care is provided, where, and for whom. At the same time, more Americans lack health insurance, including 15% of all children (Gold, 1999), and the population is becoming more diverse in terms of class, culture, and ethnic background. These changes are having profound effects on access to health services. Some health care facilities are closing their doors, others are relocating or expanding, and most are offering different types of services in different settings. Moreover, despite the rhetoric of "choice," health care access is increasingly regulated by managed care providers and constrained by lack of insurance coverage. This chapter investigates the use of GIS to analyze access to health services in this dynamic context. We consider the role of GIS in providing and managing information about health service locations, the measurement of geographical access to services, and the analysis of changing service distribution patterns.

Health services are services whose aim is to improve health. Although we typically think of biomedical health service providers such as physicians and hospitals, a much broader array of activities such as education, water supply, mental health, and social services contribute to health and well-being. Health services are provided and organized in two basic ways. *Informal health care* is care provided by families and communities in a home or community setting (Moon & Gillespie, 1995). The vast majority of health care is provided informally. It is not monetized nor assigned a value through market mechanisms or budgeting processes. Women are critically important in providing informal health care, accounting for well over half the care provided at the global scale (Timyan, Griffey Brechin, Measham, & Ogunleye, 1993).

In contrast, *formal health care* is care provided by public, private, and voluntary organizations through providers such as hospitals or physicians. Formal care takes place in a variety of settings, including clinics, workplaces, schools, and, increasingly, in individuals' homes. This chapter focuses primarily on formal health services; however, there are important links between the two types of health care that can be examined geographically. Changes in the intensity and structures of formal health care affect the need for informal health services, and vice versa. For instance, reductions in the length of hospital stay are sending patients home earlier, shifting them from formal, hospital-based care to informal care provided in the home.

ACCESS

Access is a multidimensional concept that describes people's ability to use health services when and where they are needed (Aday & Anderson, 1981). It describes the relationship between attributes of service need and the characteristics of service delivery systems. Penchansky and Thomas (1981) identify five important dimensions of access. *Availability* defines the supply of services in relation to needs—are the capacity and types of services adequate to meet health care needs? *Accessibility* describes geographical barriers, including distance, transportation, travel time, and cost. It highlights the geographical location of services in relation to population in need. *Accommodation* identifies the degree to which services are organized to meet clients' needs, including hours of operation, application procedures, and waiting times. *Affordability* refers to the price of services in regard to people's ability to pay. Income levels and insurance coverage are critical aspects of affordability. Finally, *acceptability* describes clients' views of health services and how service providers interact with clients. Accessibility encompasses barriers linked to gender, culture, ethnicity, and sexual orientation that affect an individual's willingness to use particular health services and his or her sense of comfort and satisfaction in receiving services. Services are acceptable if clients are well treated and satisfied, if providers and clients communicate openly, and if providers are confident about the quality of care delivered.

Geographical Accessibility

GIS necessarily emphasize accessibility, the geographical dimension of access. People's access to health services is rooted in their daily activity patterns in time and space. The framework of time geography, discussed in the Introduction, offers important insights into individual health care decision making. With the home as a base, people move about in space to conduct various activities, including work, school, shopping, and the care of children or elderly dependents. These socially defined roles and responsibilities reflect the needs of the individual and the household and community of which she or he is a part. For many women, the "double day" of paid work outside the home and domestic work at home limits the time available for taking care of personal health care needs. Women with limited time, resources, and access to transportation may choose to neglect their own health care while prioritizing the needs of others around them (Young, 1999). These time–space constraints clearly have a central role in shaping access to health care.

After making a decision to utilize health care services when a perceived need exists, an individual must choose a health care provider. In making that choice, the person weighs the advantages and disadvantages of alternative providers who typically are located in or near his or her activity space. The alternative that best satisfies perceived health care needs, within the time–space constraints of daily life, is often chosen. When aggregated together, these individual choices form spatial patterns of health care utilization—the flows of people over space to health services.

A fundamental aspect of health care utilization patterns is *distance decay*, or the tendency for interaction with service facilities to decrease with increasing distance (Figure 9.1). For a wide range of services, including many types of health services, we find that utilization decreases as distance increases. Studies in a variety of contexts, for different types of health services, confirm the significant effect of distance on utilization and its persistence after controlling for age, illness, and other known risk factors (Joseph & Phillips, 1984; Shannon, Bashshur, & Metzner, 1969). Distance decay is a consequence of the added time, cost, and effort of traveling long distances. As an individual's costs increase, his or her ability and willingness to travel decrease. People's knowledge of and familiarity with service opportunities also decline with distance, exacerbating the pattern of distance decay.

The frictional effect of distance varies among health services. Studies reveal a pronounced decline in utilization with distance for hospital-based elective and psychiatric procedures, even after controlling for medical need. In contrast, acute emergency procedures show little or no distance decay (Haynes, Bentham, Lovett, & Gale, 1999; Joseph & Phillips, 1984; McGuirk & Porell, 1984). Similarly, Goodman, Fisher, Stuckel, and Chang (1997) found no decrease in utilization with increasing travel time for conditions in which there is strong medical consensus on the need for hospitalization, but significant decreases with distance for conditions where outpatient treatment is a reasonable alternative. Thus, the severity and urgency of the health episode and medical practice decisions about how and

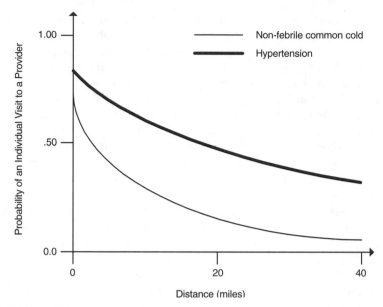

FIGURE 9.1. Distance decay in the utilization of health services. The frictional effect of distance varies among health services.

where such episodes should be treated all play a role in distance decay. The implications of such findings are unclear. Are rates of utilization excessive among those living near health facilities, or do those living far away forgo use of essential services? Do individuals distant from services rely more on informal care or formal home-based care? Regardless, geographical access has significant and varying effects on health care utilization patterns.

The role of geographical accessibility in service utilization also depends on population characteristics. People differ in their abilities to overcome distance and in how locational constraints affect their service use. Travel for health care is strongly affected by demographic and socioeconomic characteristics such as income, occupation, age, and gender. Research indicates that people whose mobility is limited by low incomes, age, or poor access to transportation are more sensitive to distance, and thus more likely to use the nearest health care provider (Bashshur, Shannon, & Metzner, 1971; Haynes & Bentham, 1982). A study in Savannah, Georgia, found that distance is a more important factor in health care–seeking behavior for inner-city residents than for those living in the suburbs or on the urban fringe (Gesler & Meade, 1988). Insurance coverage confounds these relationships. Uninsured patients may bypass nearby hospitals or physicians because the services are not affordable or do not accept people without insurance. Cultural differences come into play as well. For immigrant groups, language and cultural barriers inhibit utilization of health services, even when those services are geographically accessible (Dyck, 1990). Perceptions of place and location, and the meanings attached to them, vary through time and space (Kearns, 1993). Thus, the social and geographical dimensions of accessibility are closely intertwined.

. This brief discussion of accessibility highlights the interrelationships among the many dimensions of access to health care. Location and distance have significant effects on people's willingness and ability to use services, but these geographical effects vary in importance and meaning among places, populations, times, and individuals. In emphasizing spatial aspects of accessibility, GIS can easily hide or ignore its important social dimensions. This means that particular care needs to be taken in structuring GIS-based studies of access and interpreting the findings.

MAPPING SERVICE LOCATIONS

Preparing maps of health service locations is an important application area for GIS. Such maps can be used to display service location patterns, to provide information to residents about service locations and availability, and to visualize the spatial match between service needs and resources. Information about health services typically exists in tabular form, as lists of service providers and their addresses. Local, state, and federal agencies often maintain separate lists of their own services, as do private and voluntary organizations, leading to multiple lists that must be linked and collated for assessing service availability and accessibility. Using this tabular information to find out what types of services exist in an area, and where they are located, can be a difficult task.

Many health agencies now use GIS to manage spatial information about services. Addresses of health services are geocoded and then displayed on a map. Storing service data in a GIS can be beneficial for both service providers and the people who need services. Providers can quickly view their service portfolio to visualize areas of over- and undersupply. They can also query the GIS to examine types of services offered, utilization levels, staffing, and financial performance. For service clients, GIS offers a tool for identifying nearby service providers and finding out their attributes: services offered, hours of operation, and so on. Easy-to-use web-based systems are being developed to facilitate these querying and mapping functions.

Often health planners want to know not just about one type of service, but about an array of services that support health and well-being: education, childcare, jobs, mental health, substance abuse, and social welfare. To better integrate these services, Wolch (1996) calls for the creation of *service hubs*, a collection of small-scale health and social service agencies located in close proximity. The geographical concentration of interrelated agencies maximizes accessibility for service clients and promotes coordination among service providers. To analyze accessibility to service hubs and the full set of services that enhance health, one can overlay geocoded data for diverse services, displaying multiple layers of access to multiple service agencies. Morrison, Alexander, Fisk, and McGuire (1999) developed a GIS to allow welfare recipients to pinpoint the locations of essential health and social services, including job centers, childcare facilities, and primary health care centers. Bus routes were also displayed, along with the residential locations of employable welfare recipients.

MAPPING HEALTH NEEDS AND SERVICES

Service location information is particularly relevant when analyzed along with data on health care needs. Fundamentally, *need* describes the prevalence of health conditions that should be addressed by health care services. It can be measured and analyzed in many different ways. Typically, health planners use a combination of demographic, socioeconomic, and health outcome indicators, both quantitative and qualitative, in defining need. For example, in describing the need for prenatal care services, one would want to consider the number of pregnant women or the number of women in the childbearing age groups. In addition, because women who have high-risk pregnancies require more intensive and frequent prenatal services, indicators of pregnancy outcome or risk, such as low birthweight or maternal age, are also relevant. When examining need for particular health care services, characteristics of the service may be important, as services may be targeted to particular population groups or restricted to individuals who meet certain eligibility criteria. Need also has qualitative dimensions, as described by "perceived" need. When available, data from health surveys can be incorporated to capture individuals' views of their health care needs (Curtis & Woods, 1984).

In North Carolina, Hanchette (1998) used GIS to identify communities in need of universal lead screening. CDC guidelines recommended universal screening in areas where either a large fraction of young children had elevated blood lead or more than 27% of the housing stock was built before 1950. Using zip code areas as a base, data layers were created depicting the age of housing and the prevalence of elevated blood lead in earlier screening tests. Zip codes that met the CDC guidelines were selected by querying the data layers and then targeted for universal screening.

Are services located in areas of high need? Are some population groups or communities poorly served? Questions like these are central to health-planning activities in local health departments and many health care service organizations. They require an understanding of the geographical match between population health needs and appropriate service resources. It is increasingly common for health planners to use GIS to visualize and overlay the geographical distributions of health needs and service resources. In the area of dental public health, McSorley (1999) used GIS to identify communities where children's risk of dental caries was highest and where publicly funded dental services were most needed. Sociodemographic indicators such as the percentage of children below poverty and ethnic diversity of population served as indicators of need. Communities with optimally fluoridated municipal drinking water were excluded since fluoridation significantly reduces dental risk. By using Boolean operations to overlay maps of dental need with maps showing dental manpower shortage areas, the authors identified a set of high priority communities—those with both high need and a shortage of service providers (Figure 9.2).

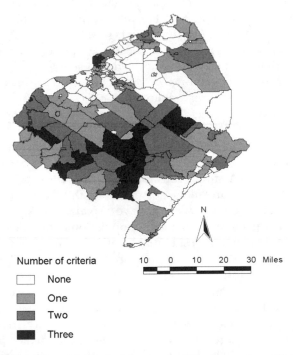

Number of criteria

☐ None

▨ One

▨ Two

■ Three

10 0 10 20 30 Miles

FIGURE 9.2. Identifying high-priority communities in southern New Jersey for a dental public health program. Criteria include: eligibility for fluoride program, race/ethnic diversity of population, and designation of the community as a dental health professional shortage area. The highest priority communities satisfy all three criteria. From McSorley (1999). Copyright 1999 by Kathryn McSorley. Adapted by author's permission.

Analyzing service needs in a GIS environment poses many challenges. For most health services the dimensions of need are not well defined; they may vary from person to person or by population group, and they may be challenging to measure. Combining and comparing indicators of need across individuals, groups, or areas are challenging tasks. Here the visualization and data-layering capabilities of GIS can be exploited to view and analyze different dimensions of need among different population groups.

ASSESSING POTENTIAL ACCESS TO HEALTH SERVICES

Which communities and populations have poor geographical access to health services? Since the early 1900s health planners in the United States have been concerned about this question, especially with regard to rural areas. Efforts have been made to identify communities with poor access (i.e., "shortage areas") and implement policies to improve service availability. These efforts focus on *potential accessibility*, the geographical match between people and essential health care services. At its core, the concept refers to the separation between services and population: How much distance, cost, time, and effort are involved in reaching service facilities? It may also incorporate *service capacity constraints*, restrictions on the numbers of people that can be served at each facility. There are many ways of characterizing potential access, and most can easily be implemented in GIS.

One of the simplest ways of measuring potential access is to calculate the average distance from the population in need of service to appropriate service providers. Assume that we have a data set containing the point locations of all service providers—for example, the locations of all hospitals in the state of Wyoming. We also have a spatial data set that describes the population in need of service. This population data set can either be a point data set that contains residential locations of people in need of service, or an area data set with counts of population by area. The latter must be converted to a point data set by finding the *centroid* of each populated area, as described in Chapter 5. To find average distance, we first identify the service provider closest to each population point/centroid, then calculate the distance to that service provider, and compute the average of those distances. The larger the average distance, the farther people must travel, on average, to their closest service facility, and the poorer the geographical accessibility.

In addition to determining average distance, examining the frequency distribution of distances can shed light on geographical access to services. Because people and health services typically cluster in urban areas, the frequency distribution of distances is often skewed, with a large proportion of the population close to services and a significant minority quite distant from services. Love and Lindquist (1995) created cumulative distributions to describe the geographical accessibility of aged population to hospital-based geriatric services in Illinois. The distributions show the proportion of aged population who reside within various distance bands of their closest service facility. Sixty percent of the aged population lived within 5.3 miles of a geriatric facility, and 80% lived within 16.3 miles. Geographical access problems were most acute in rural areas. Only 40% of the nonmetropolitan elderly lived within 20 miles of a geriatric facility, compared to over 90% for elderly living in metropolitan areas. Analyzing the distribution of distances can offer potent insights into the equality and inequality of geographical access among population groups.

Measuring Distance

Inherent in any assessment of geographical access is a measure of distance that represents the geographical separation, in distance, time, or cost, between people and services. There are many ways of measuring distance. For small-scale investigations, those at a national or regional scale, or when using unprojected coordinates such as lat/lon, distance is calculated along the curved surface of the earth. This is referred to as *spherical distance*, and it measures the distance along a great circle connecting two points. The spherical distance in kilometers between points i and j is:

$$d_{ij} = \arccos(z) \times 6371.11$$
$$z = \sin(Y_i) \sin(Y_j) + \cos(Y_i) \cos(Y_j) \cos(X_i - X_j)$$

where

$$Y = \text{latitude (in radians)}$$
$$X = \text{longitude (in radians)}$$

In analyzing geographical access to services in relatively small areas, such as cities, metropolitan areas, and small states, the earth's curvature does not present a major problem.

A more common measure of spatial separation is the Euclidean (straight-line) distance. If the coordinate locations of points A and B are (X_A, Y_A) and (X_B, Y_B), respectively, the Euclidean distance between A and B is:

$$\sqrt{(X_A - X_B)^2 + (Y_A - Y_B)^2}$$

Euclidean distances are appropriate if one is working with projected geographical coordinates, as in the state plane or universal transverse Mercator (UTM) coordinate systems; however, it is important to keep in mind that Euclidean distances do not take into account the curvature of the earth's surface. Most GIS use the Euclidean distance metric as the default in all distance calculations (i.e., in computing buffers and interpoint distances). In many situations, however, the Euclidean metric poorly represents travel patterns and travel potential.

One weakness of Euclidean distance is that it fails to take into account transportation routes and barriers to movement. Only rarely can people move from place to place along straight lines. In areas where the road network follows a grid pattern, one can approximate network distances by using the Manhattan metric to calculate distance. The *Manhattan metric* measures distance along the axes of a coordinate grid:

$$|X_A - X_B| + |Y_A - Y_B|$$

Since the distance measurements vary depending on the orientation of the grid, it is important that the grid be oriented along the main axes of the road network (Figure 9.3). Although Manhattan distances are not as accurate as distances measured along a transportation network, they can be computed very efficiently and work well as a surrogate for network distances in places where streets follow a grid pattern.

Most GIS include tools for calculating *network distances* that follow a street, bus, or rail network. Given a starting node and an ending node, the GIS will compute the length of the shortest path (see Chapter 10) along the transport network. This can be used as the network distance. Such distances offer a better approximation of the actual distances people must travel to obtain health services.

Although distance is a fundamental indicator of geographical access, travel time, cost, transportation access, and perceived distance are often much more relevant to health care utilization. Using GIS, one can estimate travel time along road networks, taking into account average speeds and speed limits on different classes of roads (Phibbs & Luft, 1995). To determine the travel time between two points, we identify the route connecting those points and sum the estimated travel times along each road segment in the route (Figure 9.4). Travel times provide a better indication of geographical barriers to health services than does travel distance, since by definition travel times incorporate access to transportation. In urban areas, a segment of the population often lacks access to cars, relying on public transportation, walking, and taxis to access health services. Often these are the most vulnerable, needy populations: people with low incomes, the aged, and some others. For these groups, travel times should be estimated based on the mode of transportation used. Travel times can be computed along public transportation routes for cases where people must change from one mode of transit to another. This is accomplished by weighting the various transit links based on the frequency of service,

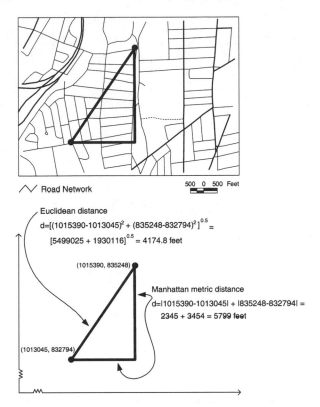

FIGURE 9.3. The calculation of Manhattan metric distance between an origin and a destination.

transfer times, and average speeds, providing a more realistic view of the travel burden for people whose mobility is limited by poor access to car transportation.

POTENTIAL ACCESSIBILITY MEASURES

Accessibility measures based on travel time, cost, or distance offer only a partial view of access to services. In reality, people trade off geographical and nongeographical factors in making decisions about health service use. The widely used gravity model and potential model offer a method for modeling these trade-offs in defining service access. The *gravity model* is based on an analogy with Newtonian physics in which the interaction between places is directly related to their relative sizes or attractiveness, and inversely proportional to the distance between them. People are willing to

ID	Name	Type	Length_ft	Travel Speed_mph	Travel Time_min
544	Country Club	Road	424.544	45	0.11
565	Country Club	Road	3094.514	45	0.78
580	Country Club	Road	830.618	45	0.21
584	Country Club	Road	519.34	45	0.13
557	Winding	Lane	443.895	25	0.20
611	Winding	Lane	1154.725	25	0.52
638	Stony	Way	519.055	25	0.21
655	Stony Corners	Cir	338.462	25	0.15
666	Stony Corners	Cir	399.896	25	0.18
695	Cotswold	Way	697.009	25	0.32
			8422.028		2.84

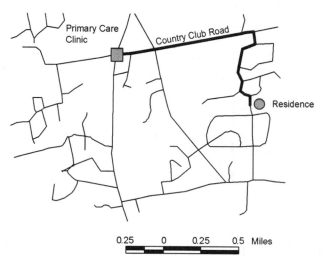

FIGURE 9.4. The measurement of travel time between an origin and a destination can be implemented in a GIS provided that data are available on the amount of time it takes to traverse a segment along the route of travel. For an automobile user traveling the speed limit, the 1.6-mile trip from the primary care clinic to the residence using the highlighted route would take about 3 minutes.

travel further to obtain better (more "attractive") health care services. Attractiveness depends on price, quality of services, accommodation, cultural appropriateness, and a host of service-related factors. Different population groups typically evaluate service attractiveness differently, depending on the service characteristics and qualities that are most relevant to their own needs. Gravity models belong to a more general class of *spatial interaction models,* tools for modeling interactions between places. We discuss the models later in this chapter as methods for predicting flows of people to health services.

The potential model uses gravity concepts to describe patterns of accessibility to services. Potential access is calculated for a particular individual or area, i, and it measures the area's overall accessibility to services. Defining A_j as the attractiveness of health service j, and d_{ij} as the distance (or travel time or cost) from i to j, we can compute the potential accessibility of individual or neighborhood i to health services as:

$$\sum_j A_j / d_{ij}^\beta$$

Higher values reflect higher levels of potential accessibility, which occurs when people live close to high-quality service facilities.

The distance exponent, β, describes the frictional effect of distance on service accessibility. When $\beta = 0$, distance has no impact on service utilization or access—access depends only on the attractiveness of service providers. Conversely, when β is large, distance has a strong frictional effect, and access depends only on the distance to service facilities. Large values clearly give more weight to nearby services in computing potential accessibility.

The above measure of potential accessibility does not incorporate differences in population or mobility across areas, but it can easily be modified to do so. Knox (1978) devised a measure of potential accessibility that takes into account the numbers of people living in various areas and the fractions of those people who have access to a car.

Estimating potential accessibility is greatly simplified in a GIS environment. Distances between people or communities and service facilities are easily computed, and service attractiveness data can be tied to geographic locations. For each person or community i, one can calculate the potential accessibility to health services using GIS spreadsheet operations (Geertman & Ritsema Van Eck, 1995).

Figure 9.5 shows a map of potential accessibility to hospitals in the study region. Accessibility values were calculated for census tracts, with several simplifying assumptions. First, straight-line, Euclidean distances from the centroid of the census tract to each hospital were used to represent geographical separation, and second, hospital size (number of beds) was employed as a surrogate for attractiveness. The differential shading of the census tracts reflects their varying levels of potential accessibility. Note the high levels of accessibility for census tracts located near the cluster of large hospitals in the center of the region.

Defining and measuring the attractiveness term is an important issue in applying potential models. "Attractiveness" is a multidimensional concept that describes the range and number of services offered, appropriateness, price, and quality of treatment. To define attractiveness, researchers have used service availability—number of physicians, number of hospital beds—as a surrogate measure (Morrill & Earickson, 1968), but clearly this is a limited tool. A better approach is to use a set of variables describing attributes of the health care provider and the range and quality of care de-

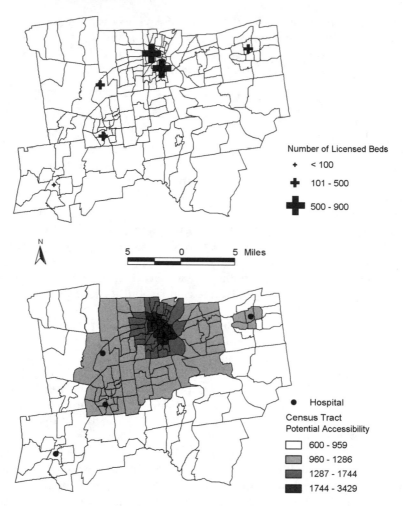

FIGURE 9.5. The top map shows the locations of community hospitals in the PUBLIC HEALTH GIS study region. The bottom map shows potential accessibility to hospitals in the region based on the number of licensed beds as a measure of hospital attractiveness and distance from hospital to census tract centroid. Census tracts in the center of the study region close to large hospitals have the highest potential accessibility. Census tracts close to small hospitals and census tracts located far from hospitals have lower potential accessibility.

livered. In a study of patient flows to hospitals, Folland (1983) utilized number of beds, price, accreditation, and the presence of specialized services as indicators of attractiveness. The potential model was expanded to include these diverse variables, each with a separate exponent that describes its effect on potential access.

The second issue concerns the distance exponent. In the classic gravity model, accessibility is directly proportional to attractiveness and inversely proportional to distance squared ($\beta = 2$)—a direct analogy with Newtonian physics. However, there is no reason to assume that these Newtonian exponents necessarily apply in modeling access to health care. Researchers have used multivariate statistical methods to find the distance exponent that best describes actual patterns of health service utilization (McGuirk & Porell, 1984). Using empirical data on patient travel to health services, one can calibrate a gravity model and determine the exponent that "best fits" actual travel patterns. In this case, "best fit" means that the predicted flows of patients from residential areas to health service facilities are as close to the actual flows as possible. Most studies have found distance exponent values ranging from 1.0 to 2.0 (Folland, 1983).

Assuming that the patterns of health service use are similar across areas, one can use a gravity model calibrated for one study area to predict potential accessibility in another study area. Knox (1978) did this in estimating intraurban patterns of potential accessibility to general practitioner services. The precise form of the distance function ($e^{-1.52d_{ij}}$) came from an earlier study of general practitioner use. The advantages of defining the exponent value based on actual patterns of service use are clear, but this method does have certain limitations. The effects of distance and attractiveness can vary over time and space, leading to errors in estimating potential accessibility. Similarly, the frictional effect of distance can differ substantially among population groups, reflecting differences in income, access to transportation, and sociocultural factors. Therefore, access changes as groups move in and out of areas and as their knowledge, preferences, and resources change.

Another serious problem is that the distance exponent depends in part on the spatial configuration of service opportunities (Haynes & Fotheringham, 1984). Research indicates that the distance exponent tends to be less negative for centrally located zones that are accessible to a large number of service facilities than for peripheral zones located distant from service opportunities. If this is the case, the distance exponent will not be transferable from one study area to another unless the two areas contain similar geographical arrangements of service opportunities and population groups—a highly unlikely situation. To address this problem, one can calculate potential accessibility over a range of exponent values and explore the stability of the observed accessibility patterns.

Visualizing Accessibility

Regardless of how it is measured, potential accessibility to health services is distributed unevenly over space. This reflects the way most health services are provided: at fixed sites, serving a dispersed population. Some individuals will always live closer to the service sites than others. GIS provides a tool for viewing geographical variation in accessibility and seeing if differences in accessibility stem from obvious gaps in service coverage or are structured along class, ethnic, or racial lines. Talen (1998) describes a GIS for "visualizing fairness" in service distribution patterns. The system incorporates a variety of accessibility measures, including average travel distance and population coverage. The GIS produces maps of accessibility that can be viewed individually and also related to maps that show the distributions of populations groups, housing values, and environmental features. Maps and statistics reveal the differential patterning of accessibility. Figure 9.6 presents an example of an "equity map" that describes patterns of accessibility to prenatal care services.

Accessibility and Activity Spaces

Accessibility can also be assessed in relation to *activity spaces*, the spaces that enclose daily travel patterns. As described in the Introduction, an in-

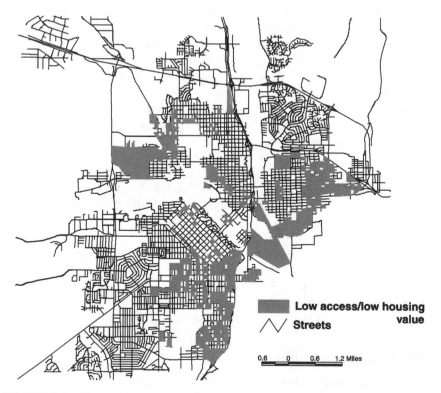

FIGURE 9.6. Census blocks in the central area of Pueblo, Colorado, with both low access to parks based on a gravity model and low housing value. From Talen (1998). Reprinted by permission of the *Journal of the American Planning Association.*

dividual's activity space consists of the set of locations that he or she visits regularly during everyday life: workplaces, schools, shopping centers, and the like. It is the space that an individual travels within on a daily or weekly basis (Cromley & Shannon, 1986). Health care services located in or near an individual's activity space are more accessible and conveniently reached than those located far away. Note that the activity spaces need not be regular in shape nor follow proscribed travel pathways. Using the concept of activity spaces, Cromley and Shannon (1986) analyzed accessibility to ambulatory medical services among elderly residents. Information was gathered on the locations of daily activities, and these were geocoded to create activity spaces. The authors grouped activity spaces that had similar geographical locations, producing "aggregate" activity spaces (Figure 9.7). Accessible service locations were sites that fell within the nested areas of these aggregate activity spaces. The advantage of such an approach is that accessibility is defined in relation to the routine patterns of everyday life, rather than in relation to some potentially arbitrary distance metric.

ANALYZING SERVICE UTILIZATION

GIS are also valuable tools for analyzing *revealed accessibility* to health care services, that is, patterns of health service utilization. Such patterns are the result of individual choices about when and where to use services, the geographical configuration of health care opportunities, and the mediating effects of medical referrals and regulations. This section examines GIS-based methods for investigating several key questions relating to utilization: What is the market area for a health care facility? How will changes in health care delivery—for instance, the closing of hospitals—affect market areas and utilization? Are services and procedures over- or underutilized in particular areas?

Identifying Service Areas

The *service area* or *catchment area* for a health care provider is the geographical area that contains the bulk of population served. For a health care provider, the service area ties the client population to a geographical area: a neighborhood, a community, or a set of communities. Some health facilities have *mandated service areas* in that they are required to serve the population living within a particular region, say, a county or set of zip codes. Public schools often have mandated catchment areas: all children who live within a given area are required to attend a particular school. Such mandated areas are less common in the case of health services in the United States, although some publicly provided services have mandated catchment areas. Furthermore, many managed care plans restrict health care choices

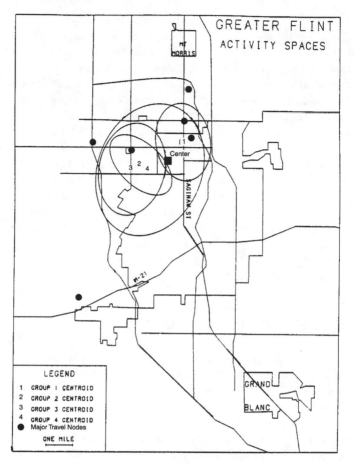

FIGURE 9.7. Groups of elderly residents of Flint, Michigan, were identified based on the set of neighborhood locations they regularly visited. The ellipses summarize dispersion and orientation of activity sites regularly visited around the centroids of sites visited by each group. Although residents lived in the same part of Flint, their travel and activity patterns differed. From Cromley and Shannon (1986). Reprinted with the permission of the Health Research and Educational Trust, copyright 1986.

to a given set of providers, resulting in mandated service areas for those who belong to a managed care plan.

More commonly, health care services have "natural" service areas that arise through individual choices and medical referral patterns. The service areas for different health care providers typically overlap, reflecting the diversity of health care needs and choices among people living in the same area. Patient origin information is essential for identifying "natural" service areas. The analyst geocodes the addresses of patients who use the health care facility and plots those address locations on a map (Parker & Campbell, 1998). The resulting geographical distribution of addresses defines the natural service area for the health care facility (Figure 9.8). The map of addresses may reveal "outlier" patients who reside very far from the service facility. To focus on the primary service area, we can plot the 80 or 90% of clients who live closest to the facility and identify the service area this way (Figure 9.8).

If client data are not available by residential address, only by area, the analyst can construct service area maps in several different ways. One is to rank the areas based on their respective shares of the health facility's clients and define the service area as those areas that make up a prespecified percentage of the facility's clients (Figure 9.9). Alternatively, the analyst can use a plurality rule that defines the service area as those areas in which a plurality of patients utilize the particular health care facility (Wennberg, 1998).

Understanding service areas is important for health care providers because it ties the client population to a particular area or set of communities. This area can be examined in its own right to see if all populations are being adequately served and to assess the diversity of population health needs. Analyzing the social and demographic characteristics of service areas may reveal populations with unmet needs. Providers who want to expand their client base can use the service area map to identify places and populations that are not being well served and to chart out areas for future expansion.

Spatial Interaction Models of Health Care Utilization

Although maps of service areas are useful descriptive tools, they do not address the determinants of service utilization patterns, and thus have limited value for forecasting and planning. What are the effects of distance, facility size, and service level on utilization? Spatial interaction models provide an essential tool for examining this question. *Spatial interaction models* describe and explain the movements or interactions between places as a function of distance and other factors. As noted earlier, spatial interaction models were first developed based on an analogy to Newtonian physics; however, they have been extended and enhanced greatly over the past decades. Today, there is a suite of methods that can be applied to a variety of health-planning problems (Lowe & Sen, 1996).

A particular form of spatial interaction model—the origin-constrained model—has been widely used in the United States for health care planning (Folland, 1983). This model assumes that the number of trips from an origin area—for example, a town, zip code, or census tract—is known and fixed. Interaction with health care facilities results from decisions in which

Hospital Service Area Based on Geocoded Patient
Residential Locations for All Patients

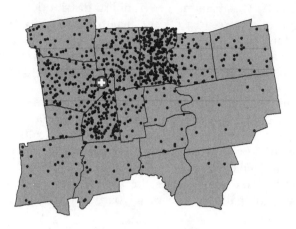

Hospital Service Area Based on Geocoded Patient
Residential Locations Excluding Outliers

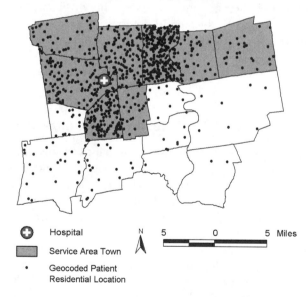

FIGURE 9.8. The primary service area of a health care facility identified by mapping patient residential locations in the PUBLIC HEALTH GIS study region. When the locations of all patients are considered, all towns in the study region would be included in the service area. When small numbers of patients in outlying communities are excluded, the primary service area includes fewer towns, but these towns account for approximately 90% of the total number of patients using the hospital.

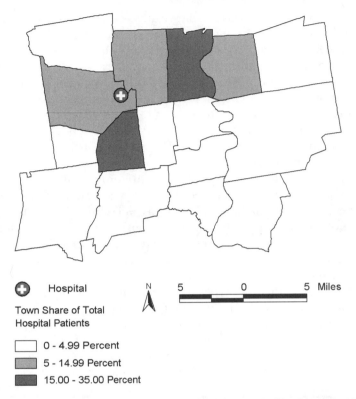

⊕ Hospital	

Town Share of Total
Hospital Patients

☐ 0 - 4.99 Percent

▨ 5 - 14.99 Percent

■ 15.00 - 35.00 Percent

N   5   0   5 Miles

FIGURE 9.9. The primary service area of a health care facility identified by mapping patient area of origin in the PUBLIC HEALTH GIS study region. In this case, 11 towns in the study region each accounted for less than 5% of the total number of patients served by the hospital. About half of the patients served by the hospital resided in one of two towns.

people compare available facilities and select the one that is best in terms of distance, quality, and other characteristics. The model expresses the allocation of those trips among health care facilities. For residents of area i, one can express the "utility" or value (U_{ij}) of health care facility j as a function of the distance or travel time to that facility (d_{ij}) and other attributes (k) of the facility that represent its attractiveness (A_{kj}):

$$U_{ij} = \prod_k (A_{kj}^{b_k}) / d_{ij}^{b_{k+1}}$$

The likelihood that an individual will utilize facility j (I_{ij}) depends on the utility of that facility compared to the total utility of all facilities that could have been chosen:

$$I_{ij} = U_{ij} / \sum_m U_{im}$$

The parameters b_k measure the relative effects of service attributes (A_{jk}) and distance on utilization decisions. As with the potential model discussed earlier, the larger the parameter value, the more weight given to that particular factor in hospital choice. Parameter values can be estimated empirically via multivariate statistical methods. Given data on flows of patients from origin areas to health care facilities, we find the parameter values that best describe these actual patient flows.

Folland (1983) calibrated a spatial interaction model to predict the flows of patients to hospitals in South Dakota. He concluded that distance was the single most important determinant of hospital utilization, accounting for roughly half the explained variation in utilization patterns when other factors were controlled. Hospital size, measured by the number of beds, was also highly significant, as were variables measuring the presence of specialized psychiatric and intensive care services. Thus, hospital choice in South Dakota represented a trade-off between the frictional effect of distance and the greater attractiveness of larger, more specialized hospitals.

There are several other types of spatial interaction models. The destination-constrained model assumes that the total capacity of each facility (i.e., the destination) is fixed, so each facility can only serve a predefined number of clients. Given this constraint, the model describes the flows of patients to facilities. These types of models have been widely used in Great Britain, where health care is centrally planned and financed, and planning authorities often dictate the capacities of health care facilities (Mayhew, Gibbard, & Hall, 1986).

The value of spatial interaction models for public health analysis lies in their ability to explain and predict health service utilization patterns. Researchers have used the models to estimate the changes in service areas that might occur when health facilities close, new facilities open, or with other policy changes. McLafferty (1988) developed a model to predict the changes in hospitalization and travel distance resulting from the closure of a public hospital in New York City. The model was estimated based on the flows of patients to hospitals before the hospital closed. Then, assuming that the model parameters remained constant, patients who attended the closed facility were reallocated among the remaining hospitals based on the model. Admissions at several nearby hospitals were predicted to increase as a result of the reallocation of patients. To check the validity of the procedure, the author examined patient flows after closure and found some predictive errors. Patients were more likely to shift into nearby hospitals than was predicted by the model, a reflection of the fact that the closed hospital was a small, community-based facility offering routine services for which there is a strong distance decay in utilization. These results highlight the importance of using spatial interaction models that are appropriate to the type of health service and population being studied.

Lowe and Sen (1996) examined a range of spatial interaction model applications in health care, including the impacts of hospital closure and universal health insurance on utilization and access. A key factor in their models was insurance match, or the willingness of a hospital to accept the patient's insurance. Health care choices were strongly conditioned by the availability and type of insurance. In exploring the impacts of universal health insurance, the authors assumed that insurance barriers would disappear and that hospital utilization would be based solely on distance and attractiveness. The gravity model predictions revealed a marked increase in geographical access to hospitals for residents of high-poverty zip codes following the adoption of universal insurance coverage.

These studies illustrate the wide range of spatial interaction model applications in the context of changing health care delivery systems. As health facilities open and close, and as managed care and other new forms of health care delivery affect affordability and access to care, the models offer a valuable forecasting tool. Using the models in a predictive context raises several important issues, however. Because geographical patterns of health care utilization vary for diverse population groups, for different types of health services, and in different places, it is crucial that the models be tailored to the particular study context (Handy & Niemeier, 1997). A spatial interaction model that describes hospital utilization patterns in Montana is inappropriate for describing hospital utilization in Chicago, and vice versa. In general, a model should fit as closely as possible the type of service, population, and geographical area in which it is applied.

The accuracy of spatial interaction models also depends on the level of aggregation of the data on which they are calibrated. Many gravity models used in health planning rely on patient origin data at the county or zip code level. In general, the models "fit the data quite well" (Lowe & Sen, 1996). Little is known, however, about the accuracy of such aggregate models in predicting changes in service utilization that result from policy changes or changes in service delivery. Models estimated from individual or small area data are generally thought to be more accurate for prediction since they describe better the forces that influence individual health care choices (Handy & Niemeier, 1997).

Small Area Variation in Health Care Utilization

A growing body of research demonstrates that rates of utilization for specific types of health services or medical-surgical procedures vary substantially from place to place in the United States (Wennberg, 1998). The authors of the *Dartmouth Atlas of Health Care, 1998* (Wennberg, 1998, p. 2) go so far as to say that "in health care, geography is destiny. The amount of health care consumed by Americans is highly dependent on where they live."

The Dartmouth project on small area variations uses GIS to create geographical areas for the comparison of utilization rates. Starting with Medicare data by zip code, the zip codes are grouped into hospital service areas, areas in which the Medicare population primarily uses a particular hospital. In turn, hospital service areas are aggregated into hospital referral regions, regions in which the bulk of population was referred to the given hospital for high-level surgical procedures like neurosurgery. The regions reflect actual patterns of hospital utilization (Figure 9.10), with adjustments to ensure contiguity and minimum population size. These regions form the base for statistical analysis and mapping of geographical variations in service utilization at the national scale.

Their mapping of health care utilization patterns of Medicare recipients reveals for some types of procedures two- or threefold variation in hospitalization rates among geographical areas, even after adjusting for age, gender, and race. The authors attribute much of the variation in hospitalization rates not to illness rates, but to hospital capacity, as the pressure to fill beds stimulates utilization. Practice variations, differences in medical decision making, are also thought to be important. The authors discount other possible explanatory factors such as variations in access and need. The research cited earlier clearly demonstrates that variations in utilization are affected by distance, even within a medical service area and within a population with few economic barriers to health care. Furthermore, how well do we understand the true geographical distribution of morbidity as a measure of need when most of our information about the health status of the population comes only from contact with the medical care system?

By focusing on Medicare recipients, the research considers a population that faces few economic barriers to accessing health care. Although the Medicare program removes most economic barriers to health care, social, cultural, and geographical barriers may limit utilization by Medicare recipients. These other types of barriers need to be carefully examined before drawing conclusions about "excessive" health care utilization among Medicare recipients.

For other population groups, economic, social, and geographical access barriers can lead to substantial differences in rates of health care utilization. These issues are examined in research on *ambulatory care sensitive conditions* (ACSC), medical conditions that generally can be treated successfully in an ambulatory care setting (Billings et al., 1993). Hospitalization should only be required in the case of severe illness or emergency. Although there is some disagreement on which conditions should be considered as ambulatory-care-sensitive, the list generally includes asthma, diabetes, and hypertension, among others. Small area variations in hospital use rates for these conditions reflect underlying differences in illness, poor access to primary care, or poor quality of preventive care. Individuals who have no health insurance or no regular source of primary care

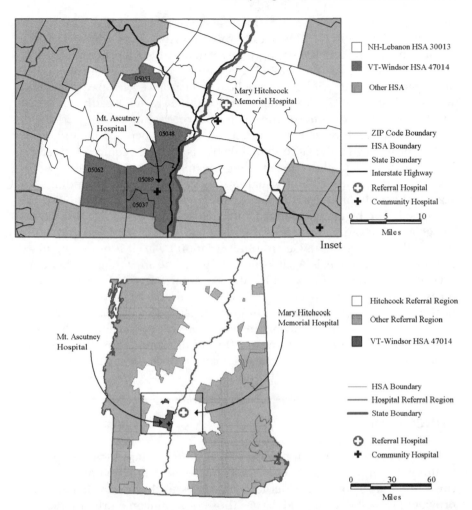

FIGURE 9.10. The inset shows a hospital service area (HSA) defined by patterns of utilization of Medicare enrollees by zip code area. Medicare enrollees in five zip code areas most often used the Mt. Ascutney Hospital in Windsor, Vermont. To preserve geographic contiguity in hospital service areas, zip code area 05053 was reassigned to a different hospital service area. The service areas of community hospitals like the Mt. Ascutney Hospital are nested within the larger service areas of referral hospitals like the Mary Hitchcock Memorial Hospital in Lebanon, New Hampshire, as shown in the main map. From Wennberg (1998). Copyright 1998 by American Hospital Publishing. Reprinted by permission.

do not get early, preventive treatment and are more likely to end up in the hospital acutely ill. Hospitalization rates for ACSC differ sharply among small areas and are strongly correlated with socioeconomic status. The risk of hospitalization for ACSC is much higher in low-income areas and among people who have no health insurance (Pappas, Hadden, Kozak, & Fisher, 1997). Hospitalization for these chronic health problems can be viewed as a failure of the medical care system.

As in research on practice variations, GIS can be used in studies of ACSC for managing the large spatial data sets that are required for examining small area variations, for creating meaningful geographical areas to analyze, and for display and visualization. The sensitivity of findings to scale and area boundaries (the modifiable area unit problem) can also be examined. The biggest challenge is interpretation, how to make sense of the geographic variations in health service use evident on the map (Goodman & Wennberg, 1999). Geographic variation by itself is not surprising; the essential question is what processes give rise to it. The ACSC and Medicare literatures offer sharply different interpretations of similar patterns, one emphasizing overreliance on hospitals caused by poor access to health care, and the other excess utilization caused by provider decisions. Research on individual behaviors in varying geographical and health care contexts is needed to sort out these different interpretations. With its emphasis on standardization, will managed care reduce these small area variations?

CONCLUSION

Differential access to health care has been an important theme in public health policy in the United States for many years. The access problems of rural residents who often travel long distances to the nearest health care provider are well documented, as are those of low-income urban residents whose choices are limited by time–space constraints, lack of insurance, and poor transportation access. The restructuring of health care will continue to alter these patterns, yet the implications are poorly understood. By documenting changes in service availability in their geographical and social contexts, and analyzing the differential impacts on population groups and places, GIS can play an important role in understanding evolving patterns of accessibility and their consequences.

CHAPTER 10

Locating Health Services

The geography of health services delivery is an essential component of GIS applications in public health. To the extent that our information about health problems is obtained through medical care contact, our understanding of the distribution of health problems is filtered by the geographical distribution of health services and geographical factors that affect their functioning and utilization (Shannon, 1980). In addition to documenting the geographical variations in access to health services described in Chapter 9, GIS analyses have addressed issues in health services planning. Concern for the organization of health services is a logical outgrowth of the study of health and disease. Describing patterns of environmental contamination or uncovering the causes of disease leads us to intervention and prevention. Activities designed to prevent or address health problems include education, enforcement, and environmental modification, in addition to medical care delivery. As long as our activities occur in time and space, knowing how patterns of health, disease, and health services characterize regions will be essential to our efforts to advance human health. Like the environmental systems through which human populations are exposed to disease, health service systems have important geographies that can be effectively modeled using GIS.

As discussed in Chapter 9, the location of health services is a key factor affecting accessibility to care. The way we choose to model the distribution of health services influences the identification of underserved areas. It also influences our decisions about where additional health professionals and facilities should be located.

This chapter considers the basic components and dimensions of health service delivery systems and how they can be modeled. Given a geographical distribution of people who need access to some type of health service and a set of objectives for providing that service, patterns of health service organization can be evaluated and managed. *Location-allocation models* have been developed and applied to the problems of health services delivery.This chapter reviews some basic models and their use in health services research. Issues in integrating these models into a GIS are also considered. GIS can become *spatial decision support systems* in the health services planning process, allowing decision makers to explore complex, multiobjective problems.

The development of GIS has coincided with important changes in health services delivery in the United States. Through the 1960s and 1970s, the federal government's role in health services delivery expanded dramatically even as many public health programs like infectious disease surveillance experienced funding cuts. Federal financial support for graduate medical education increased, and the federal government became a major purchaser of health services through Medicare and Medicaid (Kovner, 1990). The Health Care Planning and Development Act, passed in 1976, marked the culmination of almost 2 decades of federal support for health care planning by funding health system agencies across the United States. At the beginning of the 1980s, that federal support was eliminated and the federal focus on health services shifted from providing health care to cost containment, deregulation, and privatization.

At the beginning of the 21st century, major insurers and providers of medical care services in the private sector are using GIS technology for institutional health services planning (McManus, 1993; Kennedy, 1999), but these applications have not generally been described in the research literature. This is due, in part, to the fact that the locations of service centers, the structure of provider networks, and patient-origin patterns represent important business information that would be of value to competitors. At the same time, agencies in the public sector have recognized weaknesses in methods developed in the 1970s to identify underserved areas. Location modeling based in GIS can address some of these shortcomings.

HEALTH CARE SHORTAGE AREAS

During the period of expansion of the federal role in health services financing and delivery, two main systems were adopted by the federal government for identifying locations where barriers to obtaining primary health care exist (General Accounting Office, 1995). The system for designating Health Professional Shortage Areas (HPSAs) was first used in 1978 to direct placements of National Health Service Corps employees to counties or facilities with a critical shortage of physicians. By the mid-1990s, close to 30 other federal programs had adopted the HPSA approach. The Medically Underserved Areas (MUAs) system was developed in 1976 to identify areas eligible for federally funded community health centers; the Community Health Center program was the system's main user.

An evaluation of these approaches to identifying underserved areas conducted in 1995 concluded that these methods did not effectively identify areas with primary care shortages or target resources to benefit the underserved (General Accounting Office, 1995). Instead of identifying specific populations in need of care and the system resources available to meet that need, these approaches began with a place—a geographic area like a county or a specific facility like a prison—and characterized the place based on medical resource availability and population characteristics. The data used to describe the number of available physicians in a place were often neither timely nor accurate, especially when compared with information in health directories like those discussed in Chapter 3. As a result, analysts relying on these methods were not able to identify who was underserved and why.

GIS provide the means to capture and verify health service capacity in locally defined service areas using data that may not be available at the national level. GIS functions can be used to display the components of health service systems, to investigate the distributions of specific client populations affected by different barriers to care, and to incorporate location models that assess how well the distribution of services fits the distribution of populations in need.

COMPONENTS AND DIMENSIONS OF HEALTH SERVICE DELIVERY SYSTEMS

Technological advances in communication have made it possible to distribute information about health, disease, and health services through the mass media and the Internet (Green & Himelstein, 1998), and have even made it possible for patients and providers to consult in real time over long distances (Balas et al., 1997; Ritchie, 1998; Mitka, 1998; Wilson & Branigan, 1999). Nevertheless, the delivery of many health services still requires some form of direct contact between the provider of the service and the person who benefits from it. As outlined in the Introduction, direct personal contact can only be achieved if people's activities can be coordinated in time and space.

A *service delivery system* is "a cluster of diverse agencies within an organizational network that provides services to a common client population" (Alter, 1988, p. 91). The components of a health services delivery system include the client or patient population, the provider agencies, and the relationships that connect clients to providers. An early application of GIS technology (Achabal, Moellering, Osleb, & Swain, 1978) illustrates how interactive computer graphics can be used to display the locations of hospitals within a service area, the spatial distribution of the residential population, and the allocation of patients to service centers when patients are assigned to the hospitals so that no individual is required to travel more than a prespecified distance and no hospital is overutilized (Figure 10.1).

As this example shows, the components of a health service system are usually modeled in GIS as *objects* (see Chapter 2). At the community scale, health service facilities are represented as point features, populations served are represented as points or aggregated as count data for areas, and the assignments of service users to service providers are represented as lines. These points, lines, and areas form a *network* space for evaluating locational equity and efficiency in an existing or planned service delivery system.

Health service organizations must coordinate their activities in time and space as much as individuals do. Some organizations, like testing and counseling centers, operate at one or more fixed locations. These service centers represent nodes in the activity spaces of service providers and service users who travel to service sites. Other individuals or organizations that provide services to people move around or circulate (the visiting nurse or physician making a house call, the emergency medical response team, the home-delivered meals service). These services' activity patterns can be evaluated using time budget approaches like those described in the Introduction for analyzing individual travel and activity patterns. In addition to the location or set of locations where services are provided, there

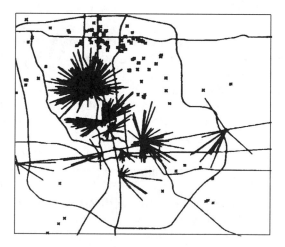

FIGURE 10.1. Allocation of residents to existing hospitals so that no individual must travel more than 6 kilometers and no hospital is overutilized. Reprinted from Achabal, Moellering, Osleeb, and Swain (1978), copyright 1978, with permission from Elsevier Science.

are other dimensions of community institutions (Alter, 1988) that have geographical implications.

Size can be interpreted as the number of service sites. In the case of the system modeled by Achabal et al. (1978), the hospital service system included nine major hospitals in the Columbus, Ohio, metropolitan area. The relationships between total size of a system (measured as the number of service sites) and *capacity*, or volume of service, are not always straightforward. Service centers located in communities of similar size can have different capacities and can provide varying volumes of service depending upon eligibility requirements and intake.

Threshold requirements, capacity constraints, and minimum standards are important characteristics of health services. A *threshold requirement* represents the minimum demand or volume of service needed to sustain service delivery. For example, the minimum number of deliveries in a community hospital obstetrics unit to make the provision of quality service viable is an example of a threshold. A *capacity constraint* is a maximum limit on the volume of service that can be provided. For example, the total number of hospital beds limits the number of patients who can be accommodated at any one time. An example of a *minimum standard for service delivery* would be that no person should live more than 10 minutes travel time from a first-response emergency service provider.

When there are threshold requirements, capacity constraints, and minimum standards for planned facilities, the optimal number, location, and capacities of service centers will be strongly influenced by the underlying geographical distribution of the population to be served. In fact, depending on the distribution of that population, it may be geographically infeasible to meet the threshold, capacity, and minimum service standards identified. This would happen if there were a small residential neighborhood that had too few people to meet the threshold requirement for a local facility and the neighborhood was located more than the desired travel distance or time from an existing provider. If provision of the service were necessary, one of the requirements would have to be broken. Either taxpayers would pay a subsidy to run a small health service center or patients would pay in excessive travel distance or time.

Centrality is another dimension of social service organizations. When the total volume of users flows through a single organization, that organization has a high degree of centrality. There is a strong relationship between differentiation of a service organization's functions and its degree of centrality.

The geographical relationships among service centers with varying degrees of centrality is the focus of central place theory (Christaller, 1933; King, 1984) and subsequent research on human settlement systems and public and private service systems (Foot, 1981; Ghosh & Rushton, 1987).

When a population is uniformly distributed, those service centers with smaller threshold requirements—for example, physicians' offices—will be more common in the landscape and spaced relatively close together. Those service centers with larger threshold requirements—for example, tertiary care centers—will be less common in the landscape and spaced relatively far apart. The service areas of small activity sites are commonly nested in the service areas of larger activity sites.

Integration refers to the relationships or forward and backward linkages among units within a system. In the case of health services systems in the United States, alternative pathways through the service hierarchy have generally been very common. Residents of a particular neighborhood are not generally "assigned" to a particular service center, although managed care systems may attempt to direct patients through the health service hierarchy of providers.

CLIENT POPULATION DISTRIBUTION

An important geographical pattern to investigate in planning and evaluating health services delivery systems is the distribution of the population who will be receiving care. The residential distribution of the population is usually considered the most relevant in health services planning, especially for home-delivered services, but also for services requiring the help seeker to travel to a fixed service delivery site. As noted in earlier chapters, the residential distribution of population is rarely uniform. GIS are effective tools for developing useful representations of population distribution.

This is particularly true for services designed to meet health problems affecting particular age or age/sex cohorts because these groups are probably not distributed equally across the distribution of the total residential population. Mammography, for example, is recommended for women aged 40 years and older on a regular basis. A map of the distribution of women aged 40 and older shows that the distribution of this age/sex group differs from the distribution of the total population (Figure 10.2).

Travel distance is an important consideration in locating health service centers. Time spent in travel—either by providers or by help seekers—increases the cost of providing care and decreases accessibility. For some types of care, like emergency medical service or home-delivered meals, there may be critical service response times after which the service is of little or no value. The importance of avoiding unnecessary travel means that opening service or dispatch sites at central locations within the distribution of the client population is a key objective of health services planning.

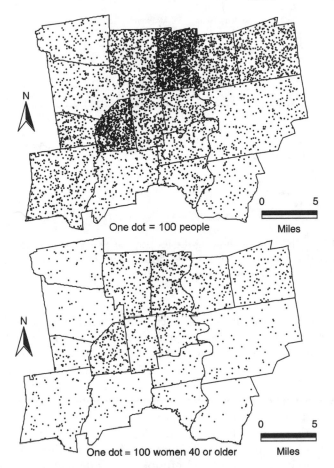

One dot = 100 people   Miles

One dot = 100 women 40 or older   Miles

FIGURE 10.2. Mapping the age/sex-specific need for mammography services. The map of women 40 years of age and older in the GIS study area shows that older women are somewhat more dispersed across the study area than the total population. The three most populous towns in the study area account for 46% of the study area's total population; the same three towns account for only 42% of the area's population of women 40 years and older.

THE MEANING OF "CENTRALITY" IN MODELS OF HEALTH SERVICE FACILITY LOCATION

The different operational meanings of a "central" location within a distribution of points can be explored through a simple example. In this hypothetical setting, the planning task is to open a single service center to meet the needs of nine people requiring care. The residential distribution of the population is shown in Figure 10.3. Again, to simplify, the population is

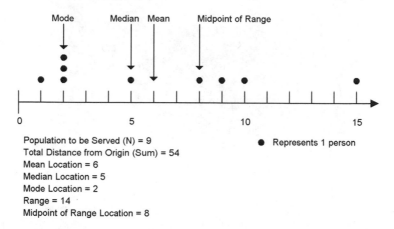

Population to be Served (N) = 9

Represents 1 person

Total Distance from Origin (Sum) = 54

Mean Location = 6

Median Location = 5

Mode Location = 2

Range = 14

Midpoint of Range Location = 8

FIGURE 10.3. An example showing the location of a single central facility to serve nine clients distributed along a single dimension. The location of the facility changes depending on how centrality is defined.

distributed in a one-dimensional space, along a hypothetical coastline or the foothills of a mountain range. In the example, location is measured in absolute terms from an arbitrary origin located outside the range of the data. Distance is calculated as difference between the starting and ending points along the number line.

Four measures of central tendency are available to define the "center" of this distribution of population: mean, median, mode, and midpoint of the range. To calculate the *mean* as the center of the distribution of residential locations, we would sum the distances of each residence to the origin and divide by the total number of residential locations. In this case, the mean is 6 and the "central facility" would be located at position 6, a place where no one actually resides. The mean—and therefore its associated location—has the special property of minimizing variance in travel distance. Position 6 is the location that ensures that the variation in distances people must travel to receive service is minimized; that is, the sum of the squared distances from each residence to position 6 is a minimum. Locating the facility at any other position would result in a greater sum of squared distances from the facility location.

To calculate the *median*, we can arrange the distances from the origin in order from lowest to highest and identify the distance value in the middle of the distribution. In this example, the median position is position 5. The median has the special property of minimizing total distance. That is, the sum of the absolute differences between position 5 and the other locations is a minimum. Locating the facility at any other position would result in a greater total distance traveled to the facility location.

To calculate the *mode*, we would identify the location that occurs most frequently in the residential distribution. This is position 2. The mode has the special property of maximizing access to the facility by locating it most conveniently for the greatest number of people. Position 2 is the location where the population to be served is concentrated.

Finally, to calculate the *midpoint* of the range, we would first calculate the range of the distribution. The range is a measure of dispersion and is the difference between the highest and lowest values in the ordered distribution. In this case, the range is 14. The midpoint of the range is calculated by dividing the range in half and adding that value to the lowest value in the distribution. When these calculations are performed for the hypothetical example, the midpoint of the range is 8. Locating the facility at position 8 minimizes the maximum distance that any single person would have to travel to obtain care—in this case, 7 units of distance. Locating the facility at any other position would increase the maximum travel distance for the most remotely located individual.

These measures can be also be computed in the bivariate space of the map (Figure 10.4) (Ebdon, 1985). As these hypothetical examples illustrate, there is more than one way to define a "central" location for a single facility depending on the particular travel distance function that the selected measure of centrality maximizes or minimizes. Facility locations based on measures of central tendency like the median or mode emphasize *locational efficiency* in the delivery of services because they minimize total travel effort or maximize accessibility (Morrill & Symons, 1977). Facility locations based on the mean or midpoint of the range emphasize *locational equity* in the delivery of services because they minimize variation in travel effort or reduce travel distances for those farthest from population centers.

NORMATIVE MODELS OF FACILITY LOCATION AND SERVICE DELIVERY

Normative Models and Mathematical Programming Methods

Normative models of facility location or service delivery do not seek to describe existing facility locations or flows. Instead, they are designed to identify the facility locations or flows that maximize or minimize a mathematical function that expresses the objective of the decision maker. *Allocation models* assume that facility locations are fixed—as they are in the short term—and identify the assignment of patients to facilities that maximizes or minimizes the objective function—for example, the assignment that minimizes total distance traveled to service sites. *Location models* seek the set of locations from among a set of candidate sites that maximize or minimize the objective function. *Location-allocation models* identify the optimal locations and assignments.

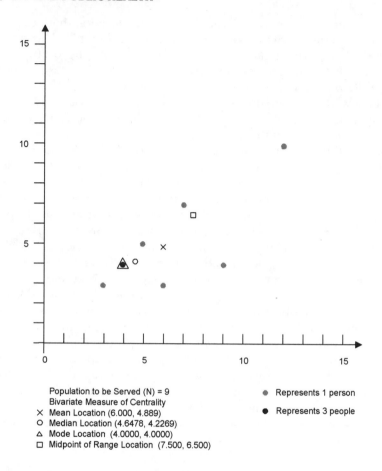

FIGURE 10.4. An example showing the location of a single central facility to serve nine clients distributed in a two-dimensional space. The location of the facility changes depending on how centrality is defined.

Location-allocation problems are solved through the application of mathematical programming techniques (Greenberg, 1978). *Mathematical programming* is a set of numerical methods for solving optimization problems. These methods are not based in multivariate inferential statistics. Most public health professionals have probably not received intensive training in these methods. Mathematical programming techniques, however, are applied in industrial and business planning to optimize various aspects of production, including facility location. Although other numerical methods, like calculus, can be used to solve an optimization problem (e.g., finding the minimum of an average cost function), mathematical programming methods are used when optimization problems involve quantities that cannot be negative. All location-allocation problems have these nonnegativity constraints. We cannot travel a negative number of miles to an outpatient facility or assign a negative number of patients to a hospital. Location-allocation models have been used within medical geography since the 1960s when the algorithms for solving them could be run on mainframe computers (Godlund, 1961; Gould & Leinbach, 1966; Rushton, 1975; Bennett, 1981; Mohan, 1983).

The Transportation Problem

A mathematical programming model is specified by an objective function and a set of constraints. One of the most commonly modeled problems is the transportation problem (Scott, 1970). It is an assignment or allocation problem because the geographical distributions of supply and demand are known and fixed. The objective of the transportation problem is to assign demand associated with a set of demand points to facilities that can supply the needed service (supply sites) so that the total cost of the assignment (total distance or travel time) is minimized (Table 10.1). This assignment is subject to the constraints that all demand must be served and the capacity of a supply site cannot be exceeded.

Mohan (1983) used the transportation problem to assess strategies for hospital location in the Durham Health District in England (Figure 10.5). The demand sites were represented by grid cells 1 kilometer square superimposed over the Durham Health District area; the volume of demand was total population per grid cell. In the initial analysis, the two existing supply sites (hospitals) were used and the minimum aggregate travel distance and the average travel distance for each hospital were calculated based on an optimal assignment of demand sites to service sites. Once the minimum aggregate travel achievable with optimal use of the existing hospital system was established as a benchmark, the impact of adding or modifying the existing hospital system could be evaluated. Two alternatives were examined. In the first, a third hospital facility was "added." In the second, one of the two existing hospitals was retained but the second existing hospital was "closed" and replaced with a facility at another location, Peterlee. Both of the alternative configurations resulted in substantial reductions in total travel time to obtain hospital service (Table 10.2). Locating a hospital at Peterlee instead of Chester-le-Street decreased aggregate travel distance by a third, from 1,570,021 to 1,054,316 kilometers.

As this research illustrates, total travel distance generally decreases as the number of service sites increases. But locating facilities in sparsely settled areas remote from large population centers may lead to facilities that are underutilized. The *bounded transportation problem* is a variant of the

TABLE 10.1. Mathematical Programming Formulation of the Transportation Problem

Objective function:	Minimize $Z = \sum_{i \in I} \sum_{j \in J} d_{ij} x_{ij}$

Subject to the constraints:

All demand at a demand site must be served $\quad \sum_{j \in J} x_{ij} \geq r_i$ for all i

The capacity at a supply site cannot be $\quad \sum_{i \in I} x_{ij} \leq q_j$ for all j
exceeded

The number of people assigned from a $\quad x_{ij}$ for all (i, j)
particular demand site to a particular facility
site cannot be negative

Where:

Z is the objective function

I is the set of demand areas, usually nodes on a network, and the subscript i is an index denoting a particular demand area

J is the set of candidate facility sites, usually nodes on a network, and the subscript j is an index denoting a particular facility site

d_{ij} is the distance or time (travel cost) separating place i from candidate facility site j

x_{ij} is the number of people from demand site i assigned to receive service at facility site j

r_i is the total number of people to be served at demand site i

q_j is the total capacity of facility site j to provide service

---

transportation problem that places a lower bound or service population threshold on each supply site as well as an upper bound on each site's capacity (Table 10.3). When a minimum level of service must be provided to ensure quality of care or economic viability, adding more service centers may actually increase the total travel cost of assigning patients to providers. This will happen if patients must be diverted to more distant service centers to ensure that threshold requirements are met there (Green, Cromley, & Semple, 1980).

Facility Location

Minimizing Travel Effort

One of the most commonly modeled location problems is the *p-median problem* (ReVelle & Swain, 1970; Church & Sorensen, 1996). The objective of the *p*-median problem is to locate a given number of facilities among a set of candidate facility sites so that the total travel distance or time to serve the population assigned to the facilities is minimized, using the median as the measure of central tendency. Unlike the transportation problem, in which the number and locations of supply sites are known in ad-

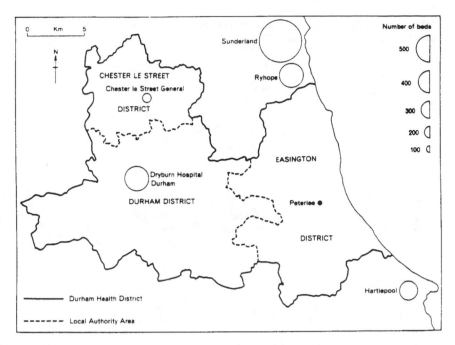

FIGURE 10.5. Hospital location in the Durham Health District showing the location of Peterlee New Town in relation to existing hospitals. Reprinted from *Social Science and Medicine*, *17*(8), Mohan, Location-allocation models, social science and health service planning: An example from North East England, pp. 493–499, Copyright 1983, with permission from Elsevier Science.

vance, the *p*-median problem specifies only the number of facilities, *p*, to be located from a larger set of possible facility sites.

The solution is subject to a set of constraints. Every place where users of the service originate (every demand site) must be assigned to one and only one facility, ensuring that all service needs will be met. Each potential facility site must either receive a facility or not receive a facility in the solution. The number of facilities located must equal the given number *p* exactly. These concepts can be written using mathematical programming notation (Table 10.4).

The following input is required to solve a *p*-median problem: the number of demand sites and the volume of demand at each site; the number of possible supply sites; the per-unit distance, time, or cost of travel from every demand site to every potential supply site; and *p*, the number of facilities to be opened.

The formulation of the problem reveals an important difference between the transportation problem and the *p*-median problem. All the vari-

TABLE 10.2. Aggregate and Average Travel Statistics for Various
Combinations of Hospital Locations

Hospital locations	Population served	Aggregate travel distance (km)	Average travel distance (km)
Two existing sites			
Dryburn	162,606	1,431,227	8.80
Chester-le-Street	49,442	138,794	2.80
Total	212,048	1,570,021	7.40
Two existing sites and one new site			
Dryburn	9,194	457,905	4.76
Chester-le-Street	49,439	138,745	2.80
Optimal site for third facility (Peterlee)	66,415	197,656	2.97
Total	212,048	794,306	3.74
One existing site and one new site			
Dryburn	144,485	845,021	8.85
Optimal site for second facility (Peterlee)	67,363	209,295	3.09
Total	212,048	1,053,316	4.97

Note. Adapted from *Social Science and Medicine, 17(8),* Mohan, Location-allocation models, social science and health service planning: An example from North East England, pp. 493–499, Copyright 1983, with permission from Elsevier Science.

ables in the transportation problem are continuous, but some of the variables in the p-median problem are discrete. The number of facilities to be located is an integer. It would not be possible to open half a facility. Similarly, a demand site is either assigned to a facility or it is not, so the decision variable to assign demand to a site is a zero–one integer variable. Integer programming problems are solved with different algorithms than those used to solve linear programming problems like the transportation problem.

In the research on evaluating hospital locations in Columbus mentioned earlier in this chapter, the optimal location for a new hospital among five candidate locations was identified by finding the location that minimized total travel distance for all user areas (Achabal et al., 1978). The candidate locations were concentrated in the north end of town after a model allocating population to the existing hospitals revealed that patients in that part of the city could not be allocated to existing hospitals.

For some facility location problems, however, the p-median problem may not be appropriate. The optimal solution minimizes total travel effort

TABLE 10.3. Mathematical Programming Formulation of the Bounded Transportation Problem

Objective function:	Minimize $Z = \sum_{i \in I} \sum_{j \in J} d_{ij} x_{ij}$

Subject to the constraints:

All demand at a demand site must be served	$\sum_{j \in J} x_{ij} = r_i$ for all i
The capacity at a supply site cannot be exceeded	$\sum_{i \in I} x_{ij} \leq q_j$ for all j
The minimum level of service provided at a facility site must exceed a threshold level	$\sum_{i \in I} x_{ij} \geq t_j$ for all j
The number of people assigned from a particular demand site to a particular facility site cannot be negative	$x_{ij} \geq 0$ for all (i, j)

Where:

Z is the objective function

I is the set of demand areas, usually nodes on a network, and the subscript i is an index denoting a particular demand area

J is the set of candidate facility sites, usually nodes on a network, and the subscript j is an index denoting a particular facility site

d_{ij} is the distance or time (travel cost) separating place i from candidate facility site j

x_{ij} is the number of people from demand site i assigned to receive service at facility site j

r_i is the total number of people to be served at demand site i

q_j is the total capacity of facility site j to provide service

t_j is the minimum amount of service (the threshold) that must be provided at facility site j

---

but it does not necessarily limit the travel effort of an individual service user. For many health services, critical travel or response time standards have been established. How can facilities be located to ensure that all users or as many users as possible will be served within the critical travel or response time?

One approach involves adding a constraint to the original p-median formulation to require each demand site to be served by a supply site within the critical distance or time. This formulation is known as the p-median with maximum distance constraints (Khumawala, 1973; Hillsman & Rushton, 1975). In the research on hospital locations in Columbus just mentioned, the researchers applied a maximum service distance of 6 kilometers in an urban area (Achabal et al., 1978). In the study of hospital location in rural Ohio, a maximum service distance of 40 miles was used (Green et al., 1980). Once these distance constraints were added, the question arose whether p facilities—the number specified at the outset of

TABLE 10.4. Mathematical Programming Formulation of the *p*-Median Problem

Objective function:	Minimize $Z = \sum_{i \in I} \sum_{j \in J} a_i d_{ij} x_{ij}$

Subject to the constraints:

An individual demand site must be assigned to a facility	$x_{ij} \leq x_{jj}$ for all (i, j)
Demand must be assigned to an open facility	$\sum_{j \in J} x_{ij} = 1$ for all i
Exactly *p* facilities must be located (the number of communities assigned to themselves equals the number of facilities to be located)	$\sum_{j \in J} x_{jj} = p$ for all j
All demand from an individual demand site is assigned to only one facility	$x_{ij} = (0, 1)$ for all (i, j)

Where:

Z is the objective function

I is the set of demand areas, usually nodes on a network, and the subscript i is an index denoting a particular demand area

J is the set of candidate facility sites, usually nodes on a network, and the subscript j is an index denoting a particular facility site

a_i is the number of people from demand site i

d_{ij} is the distance or time (travel cost) separating place i from candidate facility site j

x_{ij} is 1 if demand at place i is assigned to a facility opened at site j or 0 if demand at place i is not assigned to that site

p is the number of facilities to be located

---

analysis—would be sufficient to ensure that all users could be covered within the maximum service distance. If not, the problem would have an infeasible solution. The need to determine the minimum number of facilities that would be required to cover a set of demand sites gave rise to the location set covering problem (Church & Revelle, 1976).

Maximizing Coverage and Emergency Service Location

The *location set covering problem* (LSCP) identifies the minimal number and the locations of facilities required to "cover," or provide service to all users, within a prespecified critical travel distance or time (Toregas, Swain, ReVelle, & Bergman, 1971). The objective function of the LSCP is to minimize the total number of facilities to be "opened" from a set of potential facility locations (Table 10.5). This solution is subject to the constraint that every demand site must be within the critical distance or time of at least one open facility.

The mathematical formulation of the LSCP reveals that it, like the *p*-

TABLE 10.5. Mathematical Programming Formulation of the Location Set Covering Problem

Objective function: Minimize $Z = \sum_{j \in J} x_j$

Subject to the constraints:

An individual demand site must be within $\sum_{j \in Ni} x_j \geq 1$ for all i
the critical service distance or time of at least
one open facility site

A candidate facility site must be either $x_j = (0, 1)$ for all j
opened or closed

Where:

Z is the objective function

I is the set of demand areas, usually nodes on a network, and the subscript i is an index denoting a particular demand area

J is the set of candidate facility sites, usually nodes on a network, and the subscript j is an index denoting a particular facility site

x_j is 1 if a facility is opened at candidate site j or 0 if a facility is not opened at candidate site j

N_i is the set of facilities where the distance between demand site i and candidate facility site j is less than the critical distance or time, or $d_{ij} \leq s$

d_{ij} is the distance between a demand site i and a candidate facility site j

s is the critical service response distance or time

median problem, is an integer programming problem because the decision variable x_j is a zero–one integer variable: a candidate facility site will either be opened or it will not be opened in the solution. The following input is required to solve a LSCP: the number of demand sites, the number and location of possible supply sites, the critical service distance or time, and the distance or time from each demand site to each possible supply site. The latter makes it possible to identify the set of all possible supply sites that can serve an individual demand site within the critical service constraint.

An obvious limitation of the LSCP is that the number of facilities required to cover 100% of the population may be beyond the budget available for providing the service. To address this problem, analysts developed the *maximal covering problem*, incorporating elements of both the *p*-median problem and the LSCP (Church & ReVelle, 1974). The objective function of the maximal covering problem is to locate *p* facilities within a set of possible supply sites so that the number of users receiving service at a facility located within a critical service distance or time is as large as possible, or maximized. This is equivalent to minimizing the number of users beyond the critical distance (Table 10.6). The data required to solve a maximal covering problem are the same as for the LSCP, with the addi-

TABLE 10.6. Mathematical Programming Formulation of the Maximal Covering Problem

Objective function:	Minimize $Z = \sum_{i \in I} a_i y_i$

Subject to the constraints:

An individual demand site must be within the critical service distance or time of at least one open facility site or it is not covered	$\sum_{j \in N_i} x_j + y_i \geq 1$ for all i
Exactly p facilities must be located	$\sum_{j \in J} x_j = p$
A candidate facility site must be either opened or closed	$x_j = (0, 1)$ for all j
An individual demand site is either covered within the critical service distance of a facility or it is not	$y_i = (0, 1)$ for all i

Where:

Z is the objective function

I is the set of demand areas, usually nodes on a network, and the subscript i is an index denoting a particular demand area

J is the set of candidate facility sites, usually nodes on a network, and the subscript j is an index denoting a particular facility site

a_i is the number of people at demand site i

N_i is the set of facilities where the distance between demand site i and candidate facility site j is less than the critical distance or time, or $d_{ij} \leq s$

s is the critical service response distance or time

x_j is 1 if the facility is opened at site j or 0 if the facility at site j is not opened

y_i is 1 if the demand site i is not covered by an open facility within s and 0 if the demand site i is covered by an open facility within s

p is the number of facilities to be located

tion of the volume of demand at each demand site and the number of facilities to be opened.

Maximal covering problems are particularly appropriate for planning and evaluating the location of emergency service facilities. Emergency medical service (EMS) delivery is only effective if the response can be made within a critical time period. The maximal covering formulation was used as part of a study conducted in Austin, Texas, to determine what EMS services should be provided, by whom, using what numbers and types of equipment, and sited at which locations (Eaton, Daskin, Simmons, Bulloch, & Jansma, 1985). A software package to perform analyses of emergency call histories from various zones in the city, computer mapping programs, and a program to solve the maximal covering problem were used in the study.

Data from the call history analysis became inputs to both the computer mapping programs and the location model. Eight surrogates for EMS demand were modeled: total calls, critical calls, noncritical calls, total population, black population, Hispanic population, Anglo population, and elderly population. These were modeled with a range of vehicle fleet sizes and a variety of critical response times. Clear trade-offs in service became apparent. Locating 12 vehicles to maximize coverage of black residents allowed for 97% of the black population to be served within 5 minutes. The 12 vehicle sites that best covered the Anglo population would reach only 60% of the black population within 5 minutes. The final plan agreed upon after decision makers considered a variety of options deployed 12 vehicles in a two-tiered advanced and basic life-support system.

Maximizing Medical Outcomes

When the underlying distribution of demand for health services is not uniform, siting facilities to ensure coverage within the desired travel distance or time may lead to low utilization of facilities in less densely populated regions. Aside from the economic implications of this situation, there are also implications for health outcomes. The "*patient volume effect* . . . refers to the relationship between the number of patients treated in a facility and the rates of mortality and morbidity among those patients" (McLafferty & Broe, 1990, p. 298). Enhancing coverage by ensuring geographical accessibility and enhancing the level of care by centralizing services are two desirable objectives for the spatial organization of a health service system to improve patient outcomes. In some regions, however, satisfaction of both objectives may not be feasible.

In a study of coronary care services in upstate New York, the trade-offs between geographical accessibility and centralization of services were explored through the application of a location-allocation model designed to locate coronary care units to maximize patient survival (McLafferty & Broe, 1990). The objective function maximizes the difference between two terms. The first term shows the number of coronary care patients surviving after travel to the hospital, which is a function of distance to the hospital. The second term indicates the number of those patients who die in the coronary care unit (CCU), which is a function of the volume of care provided. The difference between the two terms is the total number of patients who survive, an important measure of health outcomes.

The results of the analysis suggested that the number of CCUs in the study region could be reduced and that a system with fewer but better located CCUs could provide better outcomes than the current system that has a greater number of dispersed units. Closing CCUs in small rural hospitals might, however, undermine the viability of those hospitals and result in an adverse effect on health if hospital closure led to a loss of other services.

Finding Optimal Routes for Service Delivery

As noted, health services delivery most commonly involves travel on the part of either the service provider or the patient. Most location models do not address the specific routes that patients might take in traveling for medical care.

Shortest Path Analysis

For services like EMS requiring service providers to travel to the person in need, the optimal route for the service provider to take from the dispatch site to the location where care will be delivered may also be an important issue. In general, this has been treated more as an operational issue than as a planning issue.

In location analysis, *shortest path algorithms* are used to find the shortest distance (or least cost) path from one point in a transportation network to another point. "The computation of shortest paths is an important task in many network and transportation related analyses" (Zhan & Noon, 1998, p. 65). Since the introduction of the problem in the late 1950s (Dijkstra, 1959), development, testing, and application of shortest path algorithms has been a research focus in geography, transportation, operations research, and management science (Gallo & Pallottino, 1988). Like most location-allocation models, shortest path algorithms assume a network consisting of a set of nodes or points connected by paths or arcs. Each arc begins at one node and ends at another node. Each arc also has associated with it a numerical value representing the distance or cost incurred when the arc is traversed. These kinds of networks are easily modeled in a vector GIS. As a consequence, shortest path algorithms, more than other types of normative models, have been incorporated into GIS software packages.

Routing Problems

For some types of service delivery, the design of effective systems is more complex than finding the shortest path between two points through a network. Home-delivered care, like the services provided by visiting nurses, requires the service provider to make a series of stops along a route. In rural areas, where travel times between stops are likely to be longer, less service can be delivered by a single provider because more time must be devoted to travel. In this case, the locations of the stops that have to be made are known, and the distances between each pair of stops can be readily determined. Finding the order in which the stops are made that minimizes the total distance traveled is an optimization problem known as the "Traveling Salesman Problem" (Lawler, Lenstra, Rinnooy Kan, & Shmoys, 1987).

This problem is one in an extended set of vehicle routing and scheduling problems that have been formulated for problems with multiple routes and dispatch sites. If there is a large number of homebound people requiring care, the home health agency likely has more than one nurse to schedule. This means that the agency will need to identify multiple routes, one for each provider, and assign each person needing care to a particular place on a particular route. Although the locations of the people needing care are fixed, at least in the short term, the agency needs to evaluate the best location for one or more dispatch sites. Variations in the length of time required to make each stop or visit can also be incorporated into these models.

INCORPORATING NORMATIVE MODELS OF FACILITY LOCATION AND SERVICE DELIVERY INTO GIS

Normative models of facility location and service delivery have been developed to address a wide range of health services delivery problems over the last several decades (Walsh, Page, & Gesler, 1997). Some software systems for the PC include algorithms to solve mathematical programming problems. With few exceptions, like shortest path, however, the computer algorithms for solving these problems have not, as yet, been fully integrated into GIS software systems. Several themes related to this integration have been identified (Church & Sorenson, 1996):

- Representing demand for services and the implications of demand aggregation.
- Identifying feasible sites for facility location.
- Modeling coverage areas based on the road network.
- Modeling service delivery routes.
- Finding solution methodologies that can be implemented in the GIS.

Approaches addressing these themes are evident in a variety of GIS applications.

Representing Demand for Services and Demand Aggregation

An emerging role for GIS in health services planning lies in defining and characterizing localities that represent demand areas for health planning purposes. In Delaware, a GIS application mapped counts and rates for census tracts for 10 factors related to community health needs: teen mothers, prenatal care, poverty, employment, public assistance, transportation, home ownership, education, language, and children in single-parent households (Berry & Jarrell, 1999). A composite score was calculated and then the scores were mapped to identify communities with the greatest need for a new service initiative integrating state departments, school districts, and nonprofit organizations in service delivery partnerships. Similar research is being conducted in the United Kingdom to define catchment areas for various health service providers; to generate demographic, social, and residential profiles for patients who use particular providers; and to examine patient travel patterns for other activities like work and school (Hirschfield, Brown, & Bundred, 1995; Bullen, Moon, & Jones, 1996).

In the development of service area or neighborhood profiles and the identification of demand sites for services, the people requiring services are usually grouped together by residence. Distances to care are usually not calculated from individual residential locations to service centers. Instead, demand or need is aggregated to a set of area centroids or other central points. For example, the number of children requiring immunization might be aggregated to census tract areas or the number of motor vehicle collisions requiring an emergency response might be aggregated to the nearest intersection. Demand aggregation reduces the complexity of location and routing problems but it has some important implications for location modeling (Current & Schilling, 1990).

When demand is aggregated, the true distance to accomplish health service delivery to an individual is replaced by the distance from the point of aggregation (Figure 10.6). In some cases, the true distance exceeds the modeled distance; in other cases, the true distance will fall short of the modeled distance. For models like the p-median problem, this will result in under- or overestimation of the true travel distance or cost, and the modeled optimal facility location pattern may not be optimal in fact. For covering problems, demand aggregation may result in an under- or overestimation of coverage. If the location of a person needing care is translated to an aggregate demand site that is closer to a proposed facility than the person's residence, the person's residence may lie outside the critical service distance or time even when the aggregate demand site can be served within the critical service distance or time.

Given the ability of GIS to manage large volumes of spatial data, one solution to this problem might be more disaggregate representations of demand. This would increase the number of demand sites and increase the computational effort required to solve most location-allocation problems. Alternatively, GIS can be used to assist health service analysts make intelligent choices in aggregating demand. Analysts who have studied the problems of demand aggregation suggest several strategies for reducing its effects (Daskin, Haghani, Khanal, & Malandraki, 1989; Current & Schilling, 1990). First, demand should only be aggregated to places where some demand is actually present (Figure 10.7). Second, demand should only be aggregated to a location if the demand would be covered by a fa-

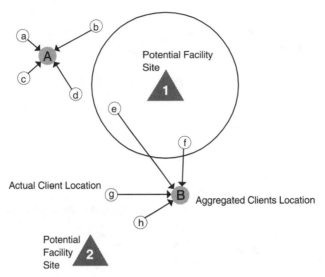

FIGURE 10.6. A schematic example of demand aggregation shows clients *e*, *f*, *g*, and *h* aggregated from their actual locations to location *B*. The true travel distance for client *h* to Potential Facility Site 1 would likely be underestimated as a result because location *B* is closer to Facility Site 1 than client *h* is. The true travel distance for client *e* would likely be overestimated as a result of this aggregation because location *B* is farther from Facility Site 1 than client *e* is. The true coverage would also be misrepresented by this aggregation. Clients *e* and *f* are actually within the critical distance from Facility Site 1, but this would not be apparent if they were aggregated to location *B*.

cility located at the aggregate site. Finally, analysts might wish to aggregate only those individuals covered by the same set of potential service sites.

Identifying Feasible Sites for Potential Facility Location

In addition to describing and analyzing the demand for health services, GIS analysis also has a role to play in identifying candidate facility locations. Most network models of facility location work with a set of potential facility sites from which the facilities to be opened are selected. In the traditional formulation of location-allocation models, candidate facility sites are usually nodes in the network space, included because they are also demand sites or because of their relative location to demand sites. Site characteristics affecting the feasibility of actually constructing a facility at the candidate supply site are generally ignored.

GIS, through its ability to integrate data layers spatially, provides an opportunity to take both location and site characteristics into account in

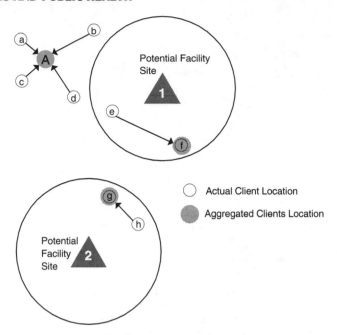

FIGURE 10.7. Error resulting from demand aggregation can be reduced by aggregating demand to locations where some clients are actually located and by aggregating demand only if the distance between the actual client location and the aggregated location is less than the critical distance specified in a covering problem.

identifying candidate facility locations. A team of planners from Maryland used a GIS to identify and rank sites for new primary medical care facilities (Marks, Thrall, & Arno, 1992). The GIS application included data layers describing parcel size, distance to facilities and demand centers, percent of local population older than 65 years, existing land use on the site, site availability, percent slope on the site, and availability of infrastructure like water and sewer systems.

Modeling Coverage Areas Based on Road Networks

Many early location-allocation models implemented outside a GIS environment required distances between demand and supply sites as direct data input. These distances might frequently be measured as straight-line Euclidean distances between sites. GIS provides an opportunity to improve measurement of coverage areas based on travel over actual street networks. Network analysis functions in the GIS make it possible to identify a node in the street network as a starting point and to identify the portions of street network segments within a specified travel distance from the starting point (Figure 10.8).

A standard of 30-minutes travel time to a primary care physician or a standard of 6 minutes for EMS response, for example, could be effectively modeled in a GIS using these techniques, leading to more accurate descriptions of underserved areas. Mapping coverage areas would indicate regions and populations in the larger study region that probably cannot be served at the minimum standard with the existing arrangement of resources. Utilization data showing longer actual travel or response times

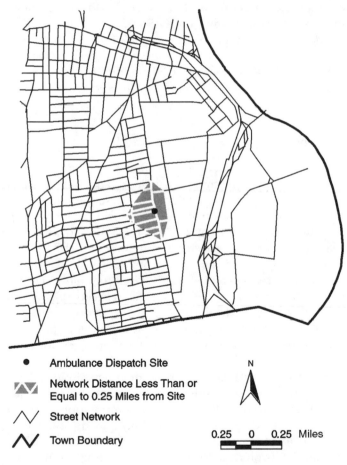

●   Ambulance Dispatch Site

   Network Distance Less Than or
   Equal to 0.25 Miles from Site

   Street Network

   Town Boundary

N

0.25   0   0.25   Miles

FIGURE 10.8. GIS network functions identify street network segments within a specified travel distance or travel time from a starting point.

than expected based on the modeled coverage area would indicate neighborhoods where barriers to service delivery exist.

Modeling Service Delivery Routes

GIS applications have also been useful for evaluating optimal routes for services delivered to those in need. GIS routing functions were used to evaluate the optimality of delivery routes in a meals-on-wheels program in southeastern Connecticut (Wong & Meyer, 1993). Five vans were used to deliver meals, with each van covering a particular route after it departed from the main kitchen. A single depot vehicle routing problem with time windows to account for meal delivery time was solved using the GIS. The application required a street network database. Residential locations of delivery stops were geocoded using the GIS and assigned to nodes on the street network. The routing procedure was used to allocate clients to five routes to minimize the time required to serve all clients, an important consideration in home-delivered meal service. Four of the five routes described in the results of the GIS analysis differed from the five actual routes.

Solution Methodologies

Exact solutions to optimization problems can be found through linear programming or integer programming algorithms. These algorithms guarantee an optimal solution if one can be found. These methods, however, are computationally intensive, especially for real-world problems like a p-median problem involving many demand and supply sites. If we want an exact solution, our analysis will be constrained by problem size. "Even though optimal solutions have been generated to problems where the numbers of demands and of sites reached 800–900, the resulting solution times are relatively large, and greater than what is considered acceptable by many to be of value in a good interactive decision-making environment" (Church & Sorenson, 1996). Integer programming solutions are more computationally complex than linear programming solutions even for problems of the same size.

The alternative to mathematical programming solutions is heuristics. A *heuristic* is an algorithm that finds an approximate solution to an optimization problem in a reasonable amount of computation time. The solution is not guaranteed to be optimal but may indeed be optimal. Benchmarking studies have evaluated the most commonly used heuristics for solving complex problems. Research investigating the most appropriate heuristics for integration into GIS is ongoing.

Although most GIS packages do not yet include functions to determine locations for new facilities or to select facilities for closure, data on distances between demand and supply sites can be exported from a GIS and imported into spreadsheets where simple calculations can be performed to compare the average travel distances of clients to services sites so that the facility patterns that minimize travel distances can be identified. Rushton (1999) illustrates this approach for closing some existing facilities and reopening them at other locations, for locating facilities in an unserved area, and for evaluating changing patterns of utilization associated with changes in the location and number of clinics.

The mathematical structure of shortest path problems makes solution by exact methods more practical. As a result, shortest path algorithms are commonly found in many GIS software packages. Many of these algorithms, however, were developed using hypothetical street networks. The development of GIS provides an opportunity to test them using real road networks. Real street networks differ from many of the hypothetical networks used in testing shortest path algorithms because road density is variable in real-world networks. Density is higher in urban centers that are in turn surrounded by suburban areas with distinct subnetworks, further surrounded by sparse rural roads. A test of 15 shortest path algorithms on two real road networks modeled in a GIS indicated that different algorithms would be preferred for different kinds of problems (Zhan & Noon, 1998).

Clearly, the effective integration of normative models of facility location and routing into a GIS would give the analyst the opportunity to select from a variety of problems and solutional techniques. Much of the literature emphasizes the value of altering estimates of demand, the set of candidate supply sites, critical service distances, and solutional techniques to evaluate alternatives (Birkin, Clarke, Clarke, & Wilson, 1996). Increasingly, GIS for health services delivery are being viewed as spatial decision support systems.

SPATIAL DECISION SUPPORT SYSTEMS

The concept of the spatial decision support system (SDSS) grew out of the decision support system (DSS) first championed by Geoffrion (1983). SDSS have the following in common with DSS: (1) an explicit approach to solving ill-defined problems, (2) easy-to-use interfaces, (3) flexibility in combining analytical models with data, (4) ability to evaluate alternatives, (5) models reflecting a variety of decision-making styles, and (6) support for interactive and recursive problem solving (Malczewski, 1999). Densham (1991) identified some distinguishing features of the SDSS. These include (1) support for spatial data input, (2) representation of spatial relations and structures, (3) availability of spatial analytic techniques, and (4) support for output in a variety of forms, including maps. The components of an SDSS include a geographic database, a set of models, a database management system (DBMS), and a user interface (Figure 10.9). The DBMS manages spatial and attribute data and provides the GIS with capabilities for data input, storage, retrieval, and manipulation. An SDSS called DOCLOC was designed to assist health practitioners make decisions about practice locations in Idaho (Jankowski & Ewart, 1996).

A DSS approach was used to identify routes for high-level radioactive waste shipments that could address the multiple facets of route choice and emergency response team siting comprising the waste shipment problem (List & Turnquist, 1998). Each of these facets had multiple objectives associated with it. For route choice, the objectives included finding the routes that would minimize population at risk, minimize probability of an accident, and minimize delays. For emergency response team siting, the objectives included minimizing distance to road links with the highest shipment volumes and minimizing the maximum distance a team would have to travel to reach any possible accident location. The siting of the response teams depends, in part, on the choice of routes. The system was tested using the anticipated shipments of waste from around the country to a Waste Isolation Pilot Project site in southeastern New Mexico.

CONCLUSION

GIS are reviving interest in the application of normative modeling techniques in services delivery planning, operation, and evaluation. These

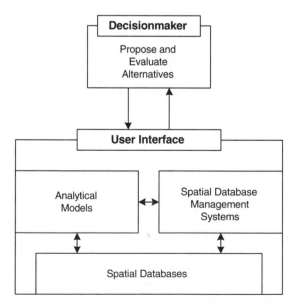

FIGURE 10.9. The components of a spatial decision support system.

techniques have sometimes been criticized because they do not attempt to describe observed patterns of behavior, but there are also drawbacks to relying solely on utilization data or manifest patterns of travel in planning health services. First, utilization patterns for existing services may be of little use in planning for new services because the new sites will alter the geographical set of opportunities for receiving care. If the service becomes more accessible through the addition or relocation of resources, then the true cost of the service will decrease and individuals will be able to utilize more of the service without increasing total out-of-pocket expenditures. Second, for some health services, like EMS, geographical areas must be covered whether there has been high utilization or not. Finally, given that utilization data are not always available, normative methods make it possible to study the pattern of health services that would result if particular objectives were desired. Even if conflicts in the multiple objectives that decision makers want to achieve make it difficult to implement optimal solutions in practice, the results of location-allocation models and the output from SDSS can establish quantitative benchmarks for what it is possible to achieve in designing a service delivery system.

In developing meaningful analyses of health services delivery systems, it is important to recognize that the location, hours of operation, and scale of service are not simply matters of convenience or economics. They truly impact the quality of care provided and the medical outcomes that result. In addition to the studies described in this chapter on the impact of distance on whether care can actually be provided, the research reviewed in Chapter 9 on the links between distance and utilization indicates that the geography of health services impacts health status. Numerous studies have shown that the volume of care provided is related to the quality of the care and the pattern of health outcomes.

More research is needed on the relationships between the timing of care and health outcomes. There is an increasing interest in the medical research literature on the relationships between biological clocks and human health (Hrushesky, 1985). Strokes and heart attacks are more likely to occur during the morning hours. What are the implications for EMS provision? The effectiveness of treatments like chemotherapy may be a function of when they are administered. Are health services designed so that therapy can be provided at the optimal time and place? GIS can support health services planning efforts to make sure that quality health services are available when and where we need them.

CHAPTER 11

GIS and Community Health

The themes, concepts, and applications discussed in this book demonstrate how to develop a geographical foundation for the study of health problems using GIS. The examples in the preceding chapters illustrate the different kinds of spatial data and spatial methods available for health-related GIS analyses. Many of the examples are drawn from the research of medical geographers, epidemiologists, and medical and public health professionals working in universities or federal and state agencies. These settings represent particular institutional contexts for GIS implementation. Some critiques of GIS emphasize the potentially harmful social consequences of the diffusion of GIS technology, including reinforcing the power of state agencies, facilitating surveillance, and promoting an—at best—naive, technocratic view of social problems (Goss, 1995; Sheppard, 1995; Campbell, 1996; Clark, 1998). At the same time, the development of GIS and the hardware, software, databases, and networking systems they rely on have also made it possible for the general public to have greater access to health and environmental information and to visualize and analyze that information in new and innovative ways.

This chapter explores the role of GIS in community-based efforts to improve health and well-being. We begin by examining the concepts that underpin the development of community-based or "public participation" GIS and how these GIS differ from the systems implemented in other institutional contexts. We then briefly review some of the grassroots efforts being made in the United States to broaden access to GIS data, to educate the general public to use GIS, and to provide access to the GIS that state and federal agencies use, so that residents can play more of a role in decision making. Though not necessarily limited to the public health field, these efforts suggest that individuals and organizations with local needs and concerns have entered into the GIS community. We then turn our attention to examples of community-based GIS for public health from around the country.

INSTITUTIONAL CONTEXTS AND PUBLIC PARTICIPATION GIS

A range of institutions and organizations have adopted GIS as an information technology. These organizations have different program responsibilities and information needs, and as a consequence different reasons for using GIS (Table 11.1). Equally important, the institutional context affects the kind and quality of geographic data available for GIS implementation. Federal and state agencies have developed important foundation databases for their own use and for public distribution, and they use databases that are spatially aggregated to larger units like states and counties. State agency data vary from place to place depending upon geographical conditions, state agency responsibilities, and state regulatory requirements. Local agencies and community groups often have access to detailed information about local conditions. The databases developed by private concerns may be very detailed but are less likely to be available for public distribution.

The expanding role of GIS in community-based health initiatives is

TABLE 11.1. Institutional Context and Interests in GIS Development

Institution	Data collection	Database management	Data analysis	Data distribution	Regulation	Scientific research	Education and training	Advocacy	Health service delivery	Software development
Federal agencies	×	×	×	×	×	×				
State agencies	×	×	×	×	×	×		×		
Local agencies	×	×	×	×				×		
Health care providers and insurers	×	×	×					×		
Universities and research institutes	×	×	×			×	×			×
Libraries and clearinghouses		×		×			×			
GIS vendors				×			×			×
Community groups	×	×	×	×				×	×	

connected to the broader movement to develop public participation GIS, linking the various institutions and organizations involved in GIS development. *Public participation GIS* (PPGIS) are systems that facilitate and enhance participation of individuals and groups in society around issues of local concern (Sheppard, Couclelis, Graham, Harrington, & Onsrud, 1999). The systems enable participants to explore local environmental and social issues, assess their significance, and communicate openly and effectively in attempting to address those issues.

One of the cornerstones of PPGIS is "to accommodate an equitable representation of diverse views" (Sheppard et al., 1999, p. 811). Historically, most GIS were developed for use by government agencies and private firms with relatively narrowly defined programmatic or commercial interests. Designed to facilitate spatial database management and to support decision making, the systems included powerful tools for managing the large spatial databases these organizations often rely on and for solving well-defined geographical problems, as described in earlier chapters of this book. In contrast, PPGIS are designed to accommodate a much more diverse set of participants and viewpoints. This implies enhancements to GIS design and functionality, as well as understanding of the sociopolitical contexts of community participation.

A key element of PPGIS is community involvement in the creation, evaluation, and analysis of spatial data. Local knowledge of environmental or health problems can be an important source of information for PPGIS, providing a more detailed, grounded summary of local conditions than can be gleaned from secondary data (Harris, Weiner, Warner, & Levin, 1995). Such local knowledge is often in the form of narratives, photos, sketch maps, or video images that may be linked to and integrated with foundation spatial data (Howard, 1999). Although these are not traditional GIS data formats, some GIS are now able to handle such diverse types of spatial information. In PPGIS, participant involvement also extends into analysis and interpretation of spatial data. This requires systems that permit multiple users and diverse forms of querying and that facilitate communication among users in the analysis process. Web-based GIS, mentioned in Chapters 1 and 4, hold great promise for the development of PPGIS.

PPGIS can be designed in different ways depending on the needs and goals of participants, along with technical and social constraints (Leitner, McMaster, Elwood, McMaster, & Sheppard, 1999). The structure of PPGIS within and across communities affects the degree and nature of public participation. Are community-based GIS networked together to facilitate sharing of information, strategies, and problems, or are they isolated, with each community operating its own independent system? How and where community participants are able to interact with GIS is also important. Often community interaction is limited to the use of predefined queries and mapping options. A more flexible approach allows participants to design their own queries, create new classifications, and even contribute data to the GIS; however, using these systems requires higher levels of skill and expertise on the part of community participants.

Finally, PPGIS differ in the involvement of key interest groups or stakeholders. Because maintaining and operating GIS requires technical expertise, most PPGIS involve partnerships between community groups and academic researchers, students, or trained public health professionals. Effective partnerships benefit all participants, providing teaching opportunities and grounded research applications for academic participants, technical assistance and training for community groups, and a direct connection to the community for governmental participants. Stakeholders also include individuals and institutions with a direct interest in the process and outcome of the GIS analysis—representatives of private industry, as well as representatives of the diverse groups and interests that exist in a particular community.

The very diversity of these interests, however, means that there are potential conflicts among the goals of the stakeholders involved in a partnership. The Community University Consortium for Regional Environmental Justice developed a partnership between community groups and Cornell University to document water and air quality conditions and potential hazards in neighborhoods (Larsen, 1999). The purpose of the partnership was to create a sustainable GIS website to provide demographic, commercial, and up-to-date environmental information. The maps and information produced by the GIS would assist community groups in their organizing and advocacy efforts. Because of the different institutional settings and priorities among program participants, one conclusion drawn from the project was that "the process and purpose of academic involvement in community organizations can be problematic" (Larsen, 1999, p. 147).

PPGIS are only beginning to emerge in communities across the United States, not just around health issues, but around a diverse array of social and environmental concerns. Clearly, the development of these systems depends on access to foundation spatial data, along with the hardware, software, and technical expertise needed to examine community concerns in a GIS environment.

GIS ACCESS AND EDUCATION FOR COMMUNITY GROUPS

One of the most important underpinnings of PPGIS in community settings is the availability of foundation spatial data. In the United States, GIS and the Internet are supporting public distribution of foundation data layers. A number of chapters in this book reference sites on the World Wide Web maintained by federal agencies from which spatial databases can be downloaded or ordered. The U.S. Bureau of the Census has made substantial efforts to improve positional accuracy, attribute accuracy, and completeness of the TIGER/Line database for the 2000 census for internal purposes. Because officials realized that the data are being widely used for purposes not necessarily related to the census, they are taking steps to ensure wide distribution of the updated TIGER/Line database.

The Bureau of the Census has also joined with the EPA, the U.S. Geological Survey, the Nuclear Regulatory Commission, the Department of Transportation, and the Federal Emergency Management Agency to develop LandView III (U.S. Bureau of the Census, 2000). LandView III is a mapping software system adapted by the EPA from software originally developed by the National Oceanic and Atmospheric Administration. The software displays a detailed network of roads and other linear features based on TIGER/Line 1995 data. Users can also display jurisdictional and statistical boundaries for states, congressional districts, metropolitan areas, minor civil divisions in the 20 states where they are governmental entities, and census blocks and block groups. Selected demographic and economic data from the 1990 census are included. LandView III can also be used to display EPA-regulated sites drawn from five EPA databases, including the Toxics Release Inventory. The software enables users to make thematic maps of census data, map street networks and EPA-regulated facilities, query the databases, and estimate the number of people with selected demographic characteristics within a radius from a user-selected point. Maps can be printed or saved directly as bitmap files. Tutorials are supplied with the software and data (Garson, 1999). Files for the entire country or regions within it can be ordered directly from the Bureau of the Census.

The Department of Housing and Urban Development (HUD) partnered with a GIS software vendor to produce Community 2020, a low-priced desktop GIS (U.S. Department of Housing and Urban Development, 1997). The objectives of this project were to enhance the ability of HUD grantees and the general public to access demographic and neighborhood information at a variety of spatial scales, present information about neighborhoods in map format, and foster collaboration between local government agencies and community groups to improve decision making about housing and economic development at the local level. In addition to providing GIS software at low cost, the program provided technical support and training. Databases of information on HUD block grant programs and tenant and site information for public housing programs were available with the software.

The distribution of government publications has shifted from paper and microform to digital media. In response, libraries around the country, including those that serve as federal depositories, have adapted their systems for acquiring, cataloguing, and making public information accessible to the community (Gorman, 1998).

Libraries and GIS

The shift from paper maps to GIS has required libraries to develop new methods for sharing spatial information with patrons. In the past, people interested in geographic information in the form of maps would access maps by traveling to a library and viewing the library's map collection. Many maps, especially old or rare maps, would not circulate. The development of computer-assisted mapping means that the range of documents users might wish to access has expanded. The services required to provide access have become more complicated too.

In addition to acquiring, cataloguing, and providing access to existing paper collections, librarians dealing with spatial data must consider five categories of documents and services (Cobb & Olivero, 1997): scanned map images, spatial database libraries and their catalogs, map generators, map browsers, and real-time maps and images. Many of these services are provided online; Cobb and Olivero provide selected URLs for sites of interest. The move to embrace GIS services began and is probably most advanced in academic libraries associated with schools of medicine and public health and in state library systems.

Many land-grant research universities, even those without geography or cartography programs, have added GIS as a specialized service within their reference sections (Suh & Lee, 1999). The Association of Research Libraries (ARL) initiated the ARL GIS Literacy Project, which has supported a range of GIS applications in research libraries (Association of Research Libraries, 1998). The New York State Library in Albany hosts the New York State GIS Clearinghouse. Hands-on GIS technology is available, again as an enhancement to reference services (Strasser, 1998). Within the reference framework, person-to-person interaction between reference librarians and patrons is emphasized.

In addition to providing access to digital geospatial data, libraries will fulfill a critical role in archiving and maintaining collections of digital geospatial data as the databases are replaced by updated versions. An important part of this task will be maintaining data in forms that will be accessible even when media and platforms change through time. The librarians' view of GIS as an essential reference tool and digital geospatial data as important databases for archival purposes reflects the fact that the need for spatial data is not tied to a single discipline or educational level.

GIS in the Schools

The diffusion of GIS technology into K–12 education has been slow (Bednarz & Audet, 1999), but it is occurring. Access to hardware and time constraints in the learning day have been identified as critical factors affecting the incorporation of GIS into the K–12 curriculum (Meyer, Butterick, Olkin, & Zack, 1999), although these are constraints that have to be addressed at any educational level. A GIS learning project introduced in a fifth-grade classroom was highly motivating for students but also frustrating (Keiper, 1999). Use of local data relevant to a real community issue and using a collaborative, mentoring approach were identified as means of introducing the technology successfully. Teacher training workshops and surveys designed to help educators assess GIS readiness are being used to encourage the diffusion of GIS technology into the public schools (Carlstrom & Quinlan, 1997; Audet & Paris, 1997). Some GIS software vendors have also recognized opportunities for GIS in K–12 education and developed programs for making software and data available to school systems.

Local Planning

Grassroots GIS efforts are also involving citizens more directly in managing their communities. Local government has used a GIS since 1987 in Pima County, Arizona (Barlas, 1998). In 1995, the county GIS manager began working with a Tucson neighborhood association to broaden the use of the county's spatial databases and GIS capability. The Midtown Neighborhood Association had already created the Virtual Neighborhood Association, a webpage advising other neighborhood groups on developing and publishing their own webpages. The transportation department provided the hardware and technical support and a vendor provided software. Several goals that emerged for the project were using the GIS to pick a site for a new library, testing the concept of involving neighborhood residents in data collection, and job training for local residents.

The availability of relatively high-quality foundation databases and software for viewing and querying the data, support services in libraries and community organizations, and technology education in the schools is creating an environment for broader community awareness of GIS and access to the technology. How have these developments affected community efforts to improve public health?

COMMUNITY-BASED PUBLIC HEALTH GIS

Community-based public health GIS applications are difficult to review because these efforts are not always well represented in the research literature. Nevertheless, a few general themes emerge from a review of these GIS activities. Community-based GIS applications usually deal with specific, localized communities, but they often seek to document a wide range of neighborhood conditions, reflecting a broad view of health. GIS technology is adopted by local groups as a tool to raise community awareness of neighborhood conditions and available services, to organize and mobilize local residents, and, ultimately, to effect change. Finally, community-based GIS applications frequently involve partnerships between community organizations, universities, and in some cases governmental agencies.

GIS Assessment of Neighborhood Conditions

A common use of GIS in community-based applications is developing information about available community resources and services to distribute to people in need. Social service agencies have been using information technology to promote data sharing, to understand individual pathways through diverse service systems, and to assess the best combination of health and social services to meet individual needs (Mayor, 1999).

A GIS developed in Wicomico County, Maryland, in collaboration with faculty at Salisbury State University displayed the residential patterns of recipients of temporary cash assistance and of abused and neglected children (Chen, Harris, Folkoff, Drudge, & Jackson, 1999). In addition to simply characterizing the community environments of these individuals within the county, the GIS was used to evaluate access to daycare services and to uncover the need for enhanced transportation services. An efficient route for transporting 23 clients to a potential employment site was modeled using the GIS.

In Akron, Ohio, the local health department developed a GIS to study patient-origin patterns at five community-based child health clinics where attendance had dropped dramatically over a several year period (Casey, Cazzolli, & Keck, 1999). The health department was considering consolidating services at two sites and improving full-time staffing at those sites. The GIS analysis and resulting maps were developed to help local government officials understand that each of the existing centers was already drawing children from all parts of the city, so that closing a center would not adversely impact a single neighborhood. The maps also displayed related service sites like childcare facilities and job centers.

GIS have also been used at the grassroots level to document neighborhood conditions and health problems. These efforts often take a broad view of health and the kinds of local land uses that are perceived to affect it negatively. Many community groups are concerned about the locations of bars and stores where alcohol can be purchased (Wieczorek & Hanson, 1997), outlets where guns can be purchased, vacant and abandoned properties, and the noise, odors, and truck traffic associated with centralized waste disposal facilities. As noted in earlier chapters, many public health investigations are initiated because local residents bring their concerns about environmental conditions or elevated levels of illness in their communities to the doorsteps of the local health department.

To foster understanding of the potential relationships between the environment and public health at the community and neighborhood level, an environmental exposure interview form was linked to a GIS as part of a project in Louisiana (Pine & Diaz, 2000). Software was developed to make it easy for health care providers to enter basic exposure records into a database. These records could then be geocoded by matching them to street addresses using LandView III, and then analyzed in the context of other data layers. This project, funded by the EPA and implemented by Louisiana State University and the Association of Occupational and Environmental Clinics, gives health service providers the opportunity to explore individual risk factors and environmental indicators that allow screening for local environmental exposures.

Although GIS hardware, software, and foundation databases are available to community groups—especially those that form partnerships with other organizations—data on health problems and morbidity may be more difficult to acquire without these kinds of screening tools or community surveys. In a number of projects, however, organizations have made effective use of state or local registry databases to implement public health interventions.

GIS and Community-Based Intervention

GIS analyses have been used by local health departments and local health care providers to support public health intervention activities. In Chautauqua County, New York, the health department identified an area of nitrate-contaminated groundwater in a rural community (Boria, Berke, Clark, & Reisenweber, 1999). Most of the drinking water in the community came from a single public water supply well, but public and private wells drew from the same unconfined aquifer. Exposure to nitrate-nitrogen in drinking water at concentrations of 10 milligrams per liter can lead to methemoglobinemia, a low blood oxygen condition; infants are particularly at risk. The health department routinely queries the New York State Electronic Birth Certificate database to identify families determined to be in the affected area and to notify them of the potential risk so that they can take measures to provide water from other sources to their infants. Regular reminders are sent to water users throughout the county.

The Connecticut Childhood Injury Prevention Center, based at the Connecticut Children's Medical Center, used a GIS to identify areas in greatest need to guide a community smoke detector campaign in Hartford (Lapidus, McGee, Cromley, & Banco, 1998). Digital fire incident data for all residential fires from 1992 through 1994 were obtained from the Hartford Fire Department. These records also go into a statewide fire reporting system. The locations of more than 900 house fires occurring in that time period in the city were geocoded. These fires had resulted in 41 civilian injuries and 9 civilian deaths, as well as 282 firefighter injuries. Census tracts in Hartford were grouped based on the frequency of house fires during the study period. The population, socieconomic, and housing data for each census tract were also considered in selecting neighborhoods for the smoke detector campaign. With the assistance of the fire department, local community members formed into a community fire safety coalition. The coalition installed more than 75 new smoke detectors and tested and replaced batteries in existing smoke detectors in one high-risk census tract.

These examples illustrate the wide range of GIS applications in community settings around health issues of local concern. In the diversity of issues and, in some cases, the active roles of community groups, we see the emergence of PPGIS, a trend that will likely accelerate as spatial data and GIS become more widely available and as communities learn more about their capabilities. As this process unfolds, the limitations of PPGIS for improving public health in localities will also become apparent.

CONSTRAINTS ON PPGIS

An important practical barrier to the implementation of PPGIS for community health is differences in community resources and capacity to adopt GIS technology (Leitner et al., 1999). Although the costs of hardware and software are falling and secondary data are becoming more widely available free of charge on the Internet, these trends are mitigated by increases in the size and complexity of spatial databases and the expertise required to manage and manipulate such databases. A GIS represents a significant investment of money, time, and staff, an investment that competes with other important needs for scarce community resources. Communities that lack resources and political clout are less likely to benefit from participatory health GIS.

Once a PPGIS is in place, local politics and power relations can create formidable barriers to effective and equitable participation. GIS exist in webs of social and political relations, and those relations shape GIS outcomes just as they affect other types of local decision making. Most communities are heterogeneous, consisting of diverse groups with differing needs, interests, and levels of political and economic clout. Little is known about the performance and outcomes of PPGIS in diverse communities and the varying capacities of diverse groups to ensure that their health interests and needs are addressed (Sheppard et al., 1999). These are very real concerns for marginalized groups, those disadvantaged on the basis of class, race, disability, or some other dimension of social exclusion.

Without full and democratic participation, PPGIS may become an additional force of marginalization for these groups rather than a progressive source of empowerment.

Finally, although PPGIS facilitate community participation in identifying and analyzing local health problems, they do not guarantee that those problems will be addressed. Many types of health problems have multiple, interrelated, and unknown causes for which there is no obvious public health solution. GIS analysis serves a useful purpose by identifying the health problem of interest and tracing its geographical distribution, but the analysis rings hollow when there are no prospects for improvement. As noted earlier, GIS maps can also lead to stigmatization or redlining, to the detriment of local residents. When health problems have solutions, the outcome of PPGIS will depend on whether the GIS analysis is tied to an effective public health response. The links of GIS to public health organizations and the ability of those organizations to work with community groups in responding to health problems are crucial for success. Here again, the "position" of PPGIS within wider networks of community groups and public health organizations is critically important.

CONCLUSION

This book has demonstrated the use of GIS in creating a geographic foundation for the study of human health problems. GIS in public health means more than just making maps. The design of a public health GIS raises a greater range of issues than conventional, nonspatial health data collection and analysis, and involves a greater number of actors. In order to develop meaningful GIS applications for public health, it is necessary for individuals interested in health problems to understand geographic data and methods.

Geographic data are complex. They are drawn from many sources relying on various data-collection techniques. Geographic data are compiled at many scales from the global to the local. The scale at which data are collected affects the level of detail. The management of geographic data involves decisions about how data will be aggregated and what kinds of data will be distributed. These factors work together to create a situation wherein the kind and quality of geographic data available vary from place to place.

Geographic entities are arranged in at least a two-dimensional space. Representing spatial arrangement requires information systems that are capable of storing and displaying these spatial relationships. Setting aside questions of scale, the same geographic entity can be represented with a wide range of symbols. A point feature can be represented by a dot, a graduated circle, or an icon, and these graphics can take on different colors and textures. GIS users are immediately confronted with many more decisions about data management and representation than analysts using spreadsheets and data in other tabular formats.

Geographic methods are also complex because they must measure or uncover the existence of particular spatial patterns. The examples in this book illustrate the challenges in identifying areas of high and low incidence and prevalence of disease and the associated factors that explain these patterns. The geographic methods for investigating the location of medical care resources to address health needs are equally challenging. Differences in the geographic patterns of population distribution and transportation networks from one region to another give rise to different location patterns for medical care facilities, even if the objectives for locating facilities are the same in both regions.

Institutional issues are important in shaping the diffusion and implementation of GIS in public health. The individuals, community groups, researchers, governmental and nonprofit organizations, and health care providers who want to use GIS differ not just in their access to GIS hardware, software, and technical training, but in their capabilities, resources, and political clout. Furthermore, these participants act in broader institutional settings that constrain how, when, and where GIS can and will be used. Data will continue to drive GIS implementation, as society debates the rapidly increasing availability of digital spatial data, including health data, from a wide variety of sources. Legal and ethical considerations will redefine public access to confidential health information.

GIS applications in public health require institutional settings that foster the conceptual understanding of geographic data and methods. The lack of this understanding is at least as important a barrier to the diffusion of GIS in public health as the technological issues raised by GIS implementation. Technological issues include differential access to hardware, software, and technical training.

The "technology gap" that limits access to computer-based communication has serious implications for GIS applications in public health. As it has in the past, technological change continues to drive the evolution of GIS, making it difficult to close this gap. Collaborative efforts between practitioners in public health agencies, researchers based in institutions of higher education, and community groups need to address both the conceptual and the technological issues in GIS implementation, despite the different primary interests of participants. Researchers and public health practitioners who are concerned about GIS as a surveillance technology, who see manipulation of service delivery systems by for-profit providers as decreasing access to care, and who decry the absence of interventions to address some of this country's most pressing health problems, can make a contribution by engaging with the forces that are shaping GIS applications in public health.

We hope that we have conveyed the amazing breadth of public health applications in GIS. While we have focused somewhat narrowly on the causes of ill health and the effective delivery of services to address health problems in most of the examples discussed in this book, the material in this concluding chapter suggests that GIS will continue to play an important and expanding role in our society into the 21st century. "Public health officials have the responsibility to continue to ensure that the promise of this wonderful new tool is realized" (Melnick & Fleming, 1999, p. x).

References

Aangeenbrug, R. T. (1997). Introduction. In R. T. Aangeenbrug, P. E. Leaverton, T. J. Mason, & G. A. Tobin (Eds.), *Proceedings of the International Symposium on Computer Mapping in Epidemiology and Environmental Health* (pp. iii–iv). Alexandria, VA: World Computer Graphics Foundation.

Abate, F. R. (Ed.). (1991). *OMNI gazetteer of the United States of America*. Detroit: Omnigraphics.

Achabal, D. D., Moellering, H., Osleeb, J. P., & Swain, R. W. (1978). Designing and evaluating a health care delivery system through the use of interactive computer graphics. *Social Science and Medicine, 12*(1D), 1–6.

Aday, L., & Anderson, R. (1981). Equity of access to medical care: A conceptual and empirical overview. *Medical Care, 19*(Suppl.), 4–27.

Alter, C. F. (1988). The changing structure of elderly service delivery systems. *Gerontologist, 28*(1), 91–98.

Amerasinghe, F. P., Breisch, N. L., Azad, A. F., Gimpel, W. F., Greco, M., Neidhardt, K., Pagac, B., Piesman, J., Sandt, J., Scott, T. W., & Sweeney, K. (1992). Distribution, density, and Lyme disease spirochete infection in *Ixodes dammini* (Acari: Ixodidae) on white-tailed deer in Maryland. *Journal of Medical Entomology, 29*(1), 54–61.

American Civil Liberties Union of Wisconsin. (1999). *In the balance: State government and medical records privacy*. [Online]. ACLU of Wisconsin. Available: http://www.aclu-wi.org/issues/data-privacy/reportx.html. [December 21, 1999].

American Geographical Society. (1944). A proposed atlas of diseases. *Geographical Review, 34*(4), 642–652.

American Hospital Association. (1999). *AHA guide to the health care field, 1999–2000 edition*. Chicago: Author.

American Medical Association. (1998). *About the AMA physician list and masterfile*. [Online]. American Medical Association. Available: http://mmslists.com/AMA_PHYSICIANS_LIST_BROCHURE.html. [February 10, 2000].

American Public Health Association. (1996). *Final program, American Public Health Association 124th annual meeting and exposition*. Washington, DC: Author.

Anderson, J. F., Andreadis, T. G., Vossbrinck, C. R., Tirrell, S., Wakem, E. M., French, R. A., Garmendia, A. E., & Van Kruiningen, H. J. (1999). Isolation of West Nile virus from mosquitoes, crows, and a Cooper's hawk in Connecticut. *Science, 286*(5448), 2331–2333.

Anscombe, F. J. (1973). Graphs in statistical analysis. *American Statistician, 27*(1), 17–21.

Anselin, L. (1995). Local indicators of spatial autocorrelation: LISA. *Geographical Analysis, 27*(2), 93–115.

Antenucci, J. C., Brown, K., Croswell, P. L., Kevany, M. J., & Archer, H. (1991). *Geographic information systems: A guide to the technology.* New York: Van Nostrand Reinhold.

Arlinghaus, S. L. (Ed.). (1994). *Practical handbook of digital mapping: Terms and concepts.* Boca Raton, FL: CRC Press.

Armstrong, C. J. (Ed.). (1995). *World databases in geography and geology.* London: Bowker Saur.

Armstrong, M. P., Rushton, G., & Zimmerman, D. L. (1999). Geographically masking health data to preserve confidentiality. *Statistics in Medicine, 18*(5), 497–525.

Ashact Ltd. & Dagh Watson, Spa. (1989). *INVENT: An industrial waste prediction model.* Washington, DC: United Nations.

Association of Research Libraries. (1998). ARL GIS Literacy Project FTP site. [Online]. Association of Research Libraries. Available: http://www.arl.org.info.gis.gislit.html. [March 23, 2000].

Audet, R. H., & Paris, J. (1997). GIS implementation model for schools: Assessing the critical concerns. *Journal of Geography, 96*(6), 293–300.

Aye, D. D., & Archambault, G. V. (1997). *Cancer incidence in Southington, CT 1968–91 in relation to emissions from solvents recovery services of New England,* ATSDR U50/ATU199044. Hartford, CT: Connecticut Department of Public Health.

Bailey, T. C. (1994). A review of statistical spatial analysis in geographical information systems. In S. Fotheringham & P. Rogerson (Eds.), *Spatial analysis and GIS* (pp. 13–44). Bristol, PA: Taylor & Francis.

Bailey, T. C., & Gatrell, A. C. (1995). *Interactive spatial data analysis.* Harlow, England: Longman Scientific & Technical.

Bakken, J. S., Dumler, J. S., Chen, S. M., Eckman, M. R., Van Etta, L. L., & Walker, D. H. (1994). Human granulocytic ehrlichiosis in the upper midwest United States: A new species emerging? *Journal of the American Medical Association, 272*(3), 212–218.

Balas, E. A., Jaffrey, F., Kuperman, G. J., Boren, S. A., Brown, G. D., Pinciroli, F., & Mitchell, J. A. (1997). Electronic communication with patients: Evaluation of distance medicine technology. *Journal of the American Medical Association, 278*(2), 152–159.

Barlas, S. (Ed.). (1998). GIS data gathering takes grassroots course. *American City and County, 113*(12), 12–14.

Barnard, N. D., & Kaufman, S. R. (1997). Animal research is wasteful and misleading. *Scientific American, 276*(2), 80–82.

Bashshur, R. L., Shannon, G. W., & Metzner, C. A. (1971). Some ecological differentials in the use of medical services. *Health Services Research, 6*(1), 61–75.

Beach, S. L. (1987). Ground water sampling strategies for a water resources geographic information system. In D. Brown & P. Gersmehl (Eds.), *File structure design and data specifications for water resources geographic information systems* (Special Report No. 10, pp. 14-1–14-22). St. Paul, MN: Water Resources Research Center, University of Minnesota.

Beck, L. R., Lobitz, B. M., & Wood, B. L. (2000). Remote sensing and human health: New sensors and new opportunities. *Emerging Infectious Diseases, 6*(3), 217–227.

Becker, K., Glass, G., Braithwaite, W., & Zenilman, J. (1998). Geographic epidemiology of gonorrhea in Baltimore, Maryland, using a geographic information system. *American Journal of Epidemiology, 147*(7), 709–716.

Becker, N. (1994). Cancer mapping: Why not use absolute scales? *European Journal of Cancer, 30A*(4), 699–706.

Bednarz, S. W., & Audet, R. H. (1999). The status of GIS in technology in teacher preparation programs. *Journal of Geography, 98*(2), 60–67.

Bennett, W. D. (1981). A location allocation approach to health care facility location: A study of the undoctored population in Lansing, Michigan. *Social Science and Medicine, 15D*(2), 305–312.

Berry, D., & Jarrell, T. W. (1999). Ranking priorities for a state family service integration initiative by census tract in northern New Castle County, Delaware, 1997. *Journal of Public Health Management Practice, 5*(2), 57–59.

Bertin, J. (1979). Visual perception and cartographic transcription. *World Cartography, 15*, 17–27.

Besag, J., & Newell, J. (1991). The detection of clusters in rare diseases. *Journal of the Royal Statistical Society, Series A, 154*(Part 1), 143–155.

Bicki, J. T., & Brown, R. B. (1991). On-site sewage disposal: The influence of system density on water quality. *Journal of Environmental Health, 53*(5), 39–42.

Bifani, P. J., Mathema, B., Liu, Z., Moghazeh, S. L., Shopsin, B., Tempalski, B., Driscol, J., Frothingham, R., Musser, J. M., Alcabes, P., & Kreiswirth, B. N. (1999). Identification of a W variant outbreak of Mycobacterium tuberculosis via population-based molecular epidemiology. *Journal of the American Medical Association, 282*(24), 2321–2327.

Billings, J., Zeitel, L., Lukomnik, J., Carey, T. S., Blank, A. E., & Newman, L. (1993). Impact of socio-economic status on hospital use in New York City. *Health Affairs, 12*(1), 162–173.

Birkin, M., Clarke, G., Clarke, M., & Wilson, A. (1996). *Intelligent GIS: Location decision and strategic planning.* Cambridge, England: Geoinformation International.

Bithell, J. F. (1995). The choice of test for detecting raised disease risk near a point source. *Statistics in Medicine, 14*(21–22), 2309–2322.

Blanchard, J., Moses, S., Greenaway, C., Orr, P., Hammond, G. W., & Brunham, R. C. (1998). The evolving epidemiology of chlamydial and gonococcal infections in response to control programs in Winnepeg, Canada. *American Journal of Public Health, 88*(10), 1496–1502.

Boone, J. D., McGwire, K. C., Otteson, E. W., DeBaca, R. S., Kuhn, E. A., Villard, P., Brussard, P. F., & St. Jeor, S. C. (2000). Remote sensing and geographic information systems: Charting Sin Nombre virus infections in deer mice. *Emerging Infectious Diseases, 6*(3), 248–258.

Boria, W., Berke, R., Clark, M., & Reisenweber, G. M. (1999). Public notification to families with newborns at risk of methemoglobinemia from drinking water exposure, Clymer, New York, 1996–1998. *Journal of Public Health Management Practice, 5*(2), 37–38.

Bosley, M. (1997, November 21). Laboratory-based surveillance for rotavirus— United States, July 1996–June 1997. *Morbidity and Mortality Weekly Report, 46*(46), 1092–1094.

Botting, J. H., & Morrison, A. R. (1997). Animal research is vital to medicine. *Scientific American, 276*(2), 83–85.

Bowman, J. D. (2000). GIS model of power lines used to study EMF and childhood leukemia. *Public Health GIS News and Information, 32,* 7–10.

Bowman, J. D., Thomas, D. C., Jiang, L., Jiang, F., & Peters, J. M. (1999). Residential magnetic fields predicted from wiring configurations: I. Exposure model. *Bioelectromagnetics, 20*(7), 399–413.

Bracken, I., Higgs, G., Martin, D., & Webster, C. (1989). *A classification of geographical information systems literature and applications,* CATMOG 52. Norwich, England: Environmental Publications, University of East Anglia.

Brassel, K., Bucher, F., Stephan, E., & Vckovski, A. (1995). Completeness. In S. C. Guptill & J. L. Morrion (Eds.), *Elements of spatial data quality* (pp. 81–108). Oxford, England: Elsevier Science.

Bretsky, P. M. (1995). *Rabies epizootic in Connecticut: Analysis and human risk reduction strategies.* Unpublished master's thesis, Yale University, New Haven, CT.

Brewer, C., MacEachren, A., Pickle, L., & Herrman, D. (1997). Mapping mortality: Evaluating color schemes for choropleth maps. *Annals of the Association of American Geographers, 87*(3), 411–438.

Brown, R. N., & Lane, R. S. (1992). Lyme disease in California: A novel enzootic transmission cycle of Borrelia burgdorferi. *Science, 26*(5062), 1439–1442.

Brugge, D., Leong, A., & Lai, Z. (1999). Can a community inject public health values into transportation issues? *Public Health Reports, 114*(1), 40–47.

Brutsaert, W. (1982). *Evaporation into the atmosphere: Theory, history, and applications.* Boston: Reidel.

Bullen, N., Moon, G., & Jones, K. (1996). Defining localities for health planning: a GIS approach. *Social Science & Medicine, 42*(6), 801–816.

Burke, L. M. (1993). *Environmental equity in Los Angeles (Technical Report 93–6).* Santa Barbara, CA: National Center for Geographic Information and Analysis.

Buttenfield, B. P., & Mackaness, W. A. (1991). Visualization. In D. J. Maguire, M. F. Goodchild, & D. W. Rhind (Eds.), *Geographical information systems: Principles and applications: Vol. 1. Principles* (pp. 427–443). Harlow, England: Longman Scientific & Technical.

Callahan, G. M., & Broome, F. R. (1984). The joint development of a national 1:100,000 scale digital cartographic database. In *Technical papers of the annual meeting of the American Congress on Surveying and Mapping* (pp. 246–253). Falls Church, VA: American Congress on Surveying and Mapping.

Campbell, H. (1996). A social interactionist perspective on computer implementation. *Journal of the American Planning Association, 62*(1), 99–107.

Campbell, J. (1991). *Map use and analysis.* Dubuque, IA: Brown.

Carlstrom, D., & Quinlan, L. A. (1997). Students investigate local communities with geographic information systems (GIS). *Tech Trends, 42*(3), 4–6.

Casey, N. M., Cazzolli, J., & Keck, C. W. (1999). Active patients attending the North Hill Child Health Clinic, Akron, Ohio, 1997. *Journal of Public Health Management Practice, 5*(2), 51–52.

Centers for Disease Control and Prevention. (1993a). 1993 revised classification systems for HIV infection and expanded surveillance case definition for AIDS among adolescents and adults. *Journal of the American Medical Association, 269*(6), 729–730.

Centers for Disease Control and Prevention. (1993b). Impact of the expanded AIDS surveillance case definition on AIDS case reporting—United States, first quarter, 1993. *Journal of the American Medical Association, 269*(19), 2492.

Centers for Disease Control and Prevention. (1993c). Update: Impact of the expanded AIDS surveillance case definition for adolescents and adults on case reporting—United States, 1993. *Journal of the American Medical Association, 271*(13), 976–978.

Centers for Disease Control and Prevention. (1997a). Case definitions for infectious conditions under public health surveillance. *Morbidity and Mortality Weekly Report, 46*(RR-10), 1–55.

Centers for Disease Control and Prevention. (1997b). Summary of notifiable diseases, United States, 1996. *Morbidity and Mortality Weekly Report, 45*(53), 1–87.

Centers for Disease Control and Prevention. (1998). Human rabies—Texas and New Jersey, 1997. *Morbidity and Mortality Weekly Report, 47*(1), 1–5.

Centers for Disease Control and Prevention. (1999a). CDC guidelines for national human immunodeficiency virus case surveillance, including monitoring for human immunodeficiency virus infection and acquired immune deficiency syndrome. *Morbidity and Mortality Weekly Report, 48*(RR-13), 1–28.

Centers for Disease Control and Prevention. (1999b). *AIDS cases dot map summary.* [Online]. Division of HIV/AIDS Prevention, CDC. Available: http://www.cdc.gov/nchstp/hiv_aids/graphics/dotmapa.htm. [January 20, 2000].

Centers for Disease Control and Prevention. (2000). Guidelines for surveillance, prevention, and control of West Nile virus infection—United States. *Morbidity and Mortality Weekly Report, 49*(2), 25–28.

Chakraborty, J., & Armstrong, M. P. (1995). Using geographic plume analysis to assess community vulnerability to hazardous accidents. *Computers, Environment, and Urban Systems, 19*(5–6), 1–17.

Chang, S. W., Katz, M. H., & Hernandez, S. R. (1992). The new AIDS case definition: Implications for San Francisco. *Journal of the American Medical Association, 267*(7), 973–975.

Chen, F. M., Breiman, R. F., Farley, M., Plikaytis, B., Deaver, K., & Cetron, M. S. (1998). Geocoding and linking data from population-based surveillance and the U.S. Census to evaluate the impact of median household income on the epidemiology of invasive Streptococcus pneumonia infections. *American Journal of Epidemiology, 148*(12), 1212–1218.

Chen, M., Harris, D., Folkoff, M., Drudge, R., & Jackson, C. (1999). Developing a collaborative GIS project in social services. *Geo Info Systems, 9*(7), 44–47, 52.

Chernin, P. R. (1995). Demonstrating watershed protection using GIS. *Journal of the New England Water Works Association, 109*(2), 132–139.

Childs, J. E., McLafferty, S. L., Sadek, R., Miller, G. L., Khan, A. S., DuPree, E. R., Advani, R., Mills, J. N., & Glass, G. E. (1998). Epidemiology of rodent bites and prediction of rat infestation in New York City. *American Journal of Epidemiology, 148*(1), 78–87.

Choynowski, M. (1959). Maps based on probabilities. *Journal of the American Statistical Association, 54*(286), 385–388.

Chrisman, N. (1997). *Exploring geographic information systems.* New York: Wiley.

Christaller, W. (1933). *Central places in southern Germany* (C. W. Baskin, Trans.). Englewood Cliffs, NJ: Prentice-Hall.

Church, R. L., & ReVelle, C. S. (1974). The maximal covering location problem. *Papers of the Regional Science Association, 32,* 101–118.

Church, R. L., & ReVelle, C. S. (1976). Theoretical and computational links between the *p*-median, location set-covering, and the maximal covering location problem. *Geographical Analysis, 8*(4), 406–415.

Church, R. L., & Sorenson, P. (1996). Integrating normative location models into GIS: Problems and prospects with the *p*-median model. In P. Longley & M. Batty (Eds.), *Spatial analysis: Modelling in a GIS environment* (pp. 167–184). Cambridge, England: GeoInformation International.

Clark, M. J. (1998). GIS: Democracy or delusion? *Environment and Planning A, 30*(2), 303–316.

Clarke, K. C. (1986). Advances in geographic information systems. *Computers, Environment, and Urban Systems, 10*(3–4), 175–184.

Clayton, D., & Kaldor, J. (1987). Empirical Bayes estimates of age-standardized relative risks for use in disease mapping. *Biometrics, 43*(3), 671–681.

Cliff, A., & Haggett, P. (1988). *Atlas of disease distributions: Analytical approaches to epidemiological data.* Oxford, England: Blackwell.

Cliff, A., & Haggett, P. (1996). The impact of GIS on epidemiological mapping and modeling. In P. Longley & M. Batty (Eds.), *Spatial analysis: Modeling in a GIS environment* (pp. 321–343). Cambridge: GeoInformation International.

Cobb, D. A., & Olivero, A. (1997). Online GIS service. *Journal of Academic Librarianship, 23*(6), 484–497.

Colten, C. E. (1991). A historical perspective on industrial wastes and groundwater contamination. *Geographical Review, 81*(2), 215–228.

Colwell, R. R. (1996). Global climate and infectious disease: The cholera paradigm. *Science, 274*(5295), 2025–2031.

Congalton, R. G. (1991). A review of assessing the accuracy of classifications of remotely sensed data. *Remote Sensing of Environment, 37*(1), 35–46.

Cook, R., Royce, R., Thomas, J., & Hanusa, B. (1999). What's driving an epidemic? The spread of syphilis along an interstate highway in rural North Carolina. *American Journal of Public Health, 89*(3), 369–373.

Coppock, J. T., & Rhind, D. W. (1991). The history of GIS. In D. J. Maguire, M. F. Goodchild, & D. W. Rhind (Eds.), *Geographical information systems: Principles and applications: Vol. 1, Principles* (pp. 21–43). Harlow, England: Longman Scientific & Technical.

Council of State and Territorial Epidemiologists. (1999). *Reporting requirements for health care providers and laboratories diseases and conditions under national surveillance.* [Online]. CSTE. Available: http://www.cste.org/ndtable1a.html. [January 15, 2000].

Cowen, D. J. (1988). GIS versus CAD versus DBMS: What are the differences? *Photogrammetric Engineering and Remote Sensing, 54*(11), 1551–1555.

Craig, W. (1995). Why we can't share geographic information. In H. Onsrud & G. Rushton (Eds.), *Sharing geographic information* (pp. 107–118). New Brunswick, NJ: Center for Urban Policy Research.

Cressie, N. (1992). Smoothing regional maps using empirical Bayes predictors. *Geographical Analysis, 24*(1), 75–95.

Cresswell, M. P., Morse, A. P., Thomson, M. C., & Connor, S. J. (1999). Estimating surface air temperatures, from Meteosate land surface temperatures, using an empirical solar zenith angle model. *Internal Journal of Remote Sensing, 20*(6), 1125–1132.

Cromley, E. K. (2001). Case study of the use of GIS to inventory and understand the pattern of traffic accidents in Connecticut. In K. C. Clarke, *Getting started with geographical information systems* (3rd ed., pp. 257–261). Upper Saddle River, NJ: Prentice-Hall.

Cromley, E. K., Archambault, G., Aye, D., & McGee, S. (1997). *Accuracy of residential address locations geocoded by geographic information system address-matching procedures.* Unpublished manuscript, Department of Geography, University of Connecticut, Storrs, CT.

Cromley, E. K., Cartter, M. L., Mrozinski, R. D., & Ertel, S. -H. (1998). Residential setting as a risk factor for Lyme disease in a hyperendemic region. *American Journal of Epidemiology, 147*(5), 472–477.

Cromley, E. K., & Cromley, R. G. (1996). An analysis of alternative classification schemes for medical atlas mapping. *European Journal of Cancer, 32A*(9), 1551–1559.

Cromley, E. K., & Joy, K. P. (1995). Estimating childhood exposure to electromagnetic field associated with electric power transmission lines. In S. D. Majumdar, E. W. Miller, & F. J. Brenner (Eds.), *Environmental contaminants, ecosystems, and human health* (pp. 328–340). Easton, PA: Pennsylvania Academy of Science.

Cromley, E. K., & Shannon, G. W. (1986). Locating ambulatory medical care facilities for the elderly. *Health Services Research, 21*(4), 499–514.

Cromley, R. G. (1996). A comparison of optimal classification strategies for choroplethic displays of spatially aggregated data. *International Journal of Geographic Information Systems, 10*(4), 405–424.

Cromley, R. G., & Mrozinski, R. D. (1999). The classification of ordinal data for choropleth mapping. *Cartographic Journal, 36*(2), 101–109.

Croner, C., Pickle, L., Wolf, D., & White, A. (1992). A GIS approach to hypothesis generation in epidemiology. In A. W. Voss (Ed.), *ASPRS/ACSM technical papers, Vol. 3. GIS and cartography* (pp. 275–283). Washington, DC: ASPRS/ACSM.

Current, J. R., & Schilling, D. A. (1990). Analysis of errors due to demand data aggregation in the set covering and maximal covering location problems. *Geographical Analysis, 22*(2), 116–126.

Curry, M. (1998). *Digital places: Living with geographic technologies.* New York: Routledge.

Curry, M. (1999). *In plain and open view: Geographic information systems and the problem of privacy.* [Online]. Department of Geography, University of California, Los Angeles. Available: http://www.spatial.maine.edu/tempe/curry.html. [January 20, 2000].

Curtis, S., & Taket, A. (1989). The development of geographical information systems for locality planning in health care. *Area, 21*(4), 391–399.

Curtis, S., & Woods, K. (1984). Health care in London: Planning issues and the contribution of local morbidity surveys. In M. Clarke (Ed.), *Planning and analysis in health care systems* (pp. 57–77). London: Pion.

Cutter, S. (1993). *Living with risk: The geography of technological hazards.* London: Arnold.

Cuzick, J., & Edwards, R. (1990). Spatial clustering for inhomogeneous populations. *Journal of the Royal Statistical Society, Series B, 52*(1), 73–104.

Dale, P. F. (1991). Land information systems. In D. J. Maguire, M. F. Goodchild, & D. W. Rhind (Eds.), *Geographical information systems: Principles and applications: Vol. 2. Applications* (pp. 85–99). Harlow, England: Longman Scientific & Technical.

Dale, P. F., & McLaren, R. A. (1999). GIS in land administration. In P. A. Longley, M. F. Goodchild, D. J. Maguire, & D. W. Rhind (Eds.), *Geographical information systems: Volume 2. Management issues and applications* (2nd ed., pp. 859–875). New York: Wiley.

Dangermond, J. (1984). A classification of software components commonly used in geographical information systems. In D. Marble, H. Calkins, & D. Peuquet (Eds.), *Basic readings in geographic information systems* (pp. 1-23–1-57). Amherst, NY: SPAD Systems.

Dangermond, J., & Morehouse, S. (1987). Trends in hardware for geographic information systems. In N. R. Chrisman (Ed.), *AUTO-CARTO 8 proceedings* (pp. 380–385). Falls Church, VA: American Society for Photogrammetry and Remote Sensing and American Congress on Surveying and Mapping.

Daskin, M. S., Haghani, A. E., Khanal, M., & Malandraki, C. (1989). Aggregation effects in maximal covering models. *Annals of Operations Research, 18*, 115–40.

Davis, K., & Stapleton, J. (1991). Migration to rural areas by HIV patients: Impact on HIV-related healthcare use. *Infection Control and Hospital Epidemiology, 12*(9), 540–543.

Davis, R. M., & Flores, P. I. (1992). Identifying potential pollutant point sources in an area of high ground water consumption. *Ground Water Monitoring Review, 12*(2), 116–119.

de Lepper, M. J. C., Scholten, H. J., & Stern, R. M. (Eds.). (1995). *The added value of geographical information systems in public and environmental health.* Dordrecht, The Netherlands: Kluwer Academic .

DeMers, M. N. (2000). *Fundamentals of geographic information systems* (2nd ed.). New York: Wiley.

Dennis, D. T. (1991). Lyme disease: Tracking an epidemic. *Journal of the American Medical Association, 266*(9), 1269–1270.

Densham, P. J. (1991). Spatial decision support systems. In D. J. Maguire, M. F. Goodchild, & D. W. Rhind, (Eds.), *Geographical information systems: Principles and applications: Vol. 1. Principles* (pp. 403–412). Harlow, England: Longman Scientific & Technical.

Devasundaram, J., Rohn, D., Dwyer, D., & Israel, E. (1998). A geographic information systems application for disease surveillance. *American Journal of Public Health, 88*(9), 1406–1407.

Devine, O., & Lewis, T. (1994). A constrained empirical Bayes estimator for incidence rates in areas with small populations. *Statistics in Medicine, 13*(11), 1119–1133.

DiBiasi, D., MacEachren, A., Krygier, J., & Reeves, C. (1992). Animation and the role of map design in scientific visualization. *Cartography and Geographic Information Systems, 19*(4), 215–227.

Diehr, P. (1984). Small area statistics, large statistical problems. *American Journal of Public Health, 74*(4), 313–314.

Dijkstra, E. W. (1959). A note on two problems in connection with graphs. *Numeriche mathematik, 1,* 269–271.

Doa, M. J. (1992). The Toxics Release Inventory. *Hazardous Waste and Hazardous Materials, 9*(1), 61–72.

Drummond, J. (1995). Positional accuracy. In S. C. Guptill & J. L. Morrison (Eds.), *Elements of spatial data quality* (pp. 31–58). Oxford, England: Elsevier Science.

Drummond, W. J. (1995). Address matching: GIS technology for mapping human activity patterns. *Journal of American Planning Association, 61*(2), 240–251.

Dyck, I. (1990). Context, culture and client: Geography and the health for all strategy. *Canadian Geographer, 34*(4), 338–341.

Eaton, D. J., Daskin, M. S., Simmons, D., Bulloch, B., & Jansma, G. (1985). Determining emergency medical service vehicle deployment in Austin, Texas. *Interfaces, 15*(1), 96–108.

Ebdon, D. (1985). *Statistics in geography* (2nd ed.). New York: Basil Blackwell.

Elliott, P., Cuzick, J., English, D., & Stern, R. (Eds.). (1992). *Geographical and environmental epidemiology: Methods for small area studies.* New York: Oxford University Press.

Environmental Protection Agency. (1995). *1997–1993 Toxics Release Inventory* (EPA 749/C-95-004). Washington, DC: U.S. Government Printing Office.

Environmental Protection Agency. (2000). Toxics Release Inventory: Community right to know. [Online]. U. S. Environmental Protection Agency. Available: http://www.epa.gov/opptintr/tri. [January 18, 2000].

Ewald, P. W. (1994). *The evolution of infectious diseases.* Oxford, England: Oxford University Press.

Ewald, P. W., & Cochran, G. (1999). Catching on to what's catching. *Natural History, 108*(1), 34–37.

Eylenbosch, W. J., & Noah, N. D. (Eds.). (1988). *Surveillance in health and disease.* Oxford, England: Oxford University Press.

Federal Geographic Data Committee. (1998). Content standard for digital geospatial metadata. CSDGM-Version 2–FGDC-STD-001–1998. [Online]. Federal Geographic Data Committee. Available: http://www.fgdc.gov/metadata/constan.html. [January 15, 2000].

Federal Geographic Data Committee. (2000). FGDC Geospatial Data Clearinghouse. [Online]. Federal Geographic Data Committee. Available: http://www.fgdc.gov/clearinghouse/clearinghouse.html. [January 15, 2000].

Finkel, A. M., & Golding, D. (Eds.). (1994). *Worst things first? The debate over risk-based national environmental priorities.* Washington, DC: Resources for the Future.

Fleiss, J. L. (1981). *Statistical methods for rates and proportions* (2nd ed.). New York: Wiley.

Flowerdew, R., & Green, M. (1989). Statistical methods for inference between incompatible zoning systems. In M. F. Goodchild & S. Gopal (Eds.), *Accuracy of spatial databases* (pp. 239–248). London: Taylor & Francis.

Flowerdew, R., & Green, M. (1994). Areal interpolation and types of data. In S. Fotheringham & P. Rogerson (Eds.), *Spatial analysis and GIS* (pp. 121–145). Bristol, PA: Taylor & Francis.

Folland, S. (1983). Predicting hospital market shares. *Inquiry, 20*(1), 34–44.

Foot, D. (1981). *Operational urban models: An introduction.* New York: Methuen.

Foresman, T. W. (Ed.). (1998). *The history of geographic information systems: Perspectives from the pioneers.* Upper Saddle River, NJ: Prentice-Hall.

Fotheringham, S., & Rogerson, P. (1994). *Spatial analysis and GIS.* Bristol, PA: Taylor & Francis.

Fotheringham, S., & Zhan, B. (1996). A comparison of three exploratory methods for cluster detection in spatial point patterns. *Geographical Analysis, 28*(3), 200–218.

Frank, A. L. (1992). *Taking an exposure history (Case studies in environmental medicine no. 26).* Atlanta, GA: Agency for Toxic Substances and Disease Registry, U.S. Department of Health and Human Services.

Friede, A., & O'Carroll, P. (1996). CDC and ATSDR electronic information resources for health officers. *Environmental Health, 59*(4), 13–22.

Friis, R., & Sellers, T. (1996). *Epidemiology for public health practice.* Gaithersburg, MD: Aspen Publications.

Fry, C. M. (1988). Maps for the physically disabled. *Cartographic Journal, 25*(11), 20–28.

Gallo, G., & Pallottino, S. (1988). Shortest paths algorithms. *Annals of Operations Research, 13*, 3–79.

Garbe, E., & Blount, S. (1992). Chronic disease surveillance. In W. Halperin & E. Baker (Eds.), *Public health surveillance* (pp. 130–139). New York: Van Nostrand Reinhold.

Garson, G. D. (1999). Analyzing hazardous waste facility location by racial composition of census tract with Land View III: A brief tutorial. *Social Science Computer Review, 17*(1), 64–68.

Gatrell, A. C., & Bailey, T. C. (1996). Interactive spatial data analysis in medical geography. *Social Science and Medicine, 42*(6), 843–855.

Gatrell, A. C., Bailey, T. C., Diggle, P. J., & Rowlingson, B. S. (1996). Spatial point pattern analysis and its application in medical geography. *Transactions of the Institute of British Geographers, NS, 21*(1), 256–274.

Gatrell, A. C., & Löytönen, M. (Eds.). (1998). *GIS and health.* London: Taylor & Francis.

Geertman, S., & Ritsema Van Eck, J. (1995). GIS and models of accessibility potential: An application in planning. *International Journal of Geographical Information Systems, 9*(1), 67–80.

General Accounting Office. (1995). *Health care shortage areas: Designations not a useful tool for directing resources to the underserved* (GAO/HEHS-95-200). Washington, DC: U.S. General Accounting Office.

Geoffrion, A. M. (1983). Can OR/MS evolve fast enough? *Interfaces, 13*(1), 10–25.

Geography and Map Division, Library of Congress. (1991). *Fire insurance maps in the Library of Congress.* Washington, DC: Library of Congress.

Gesler, W. M., & Meade, M. S. (1988). Locational and population factors in health care-seeking behavior in Savannah, Georgia. *Health Services Research, 23*(3), 443–462.

Getis, A., & Ord, J. (1992). The analysis of spatial association by the use of distance statistics. *Geographical Analysis, 24*(3), 189–206.

Ghosh, A., & Rushton, G. (Eds.). (1987). *Spatial analysis and location-allocation models*. New York: Van Nostrand Reinhold.

Gilbert, E. W. (1958). Pioneer maps of health and disease in England. *Geographical Journal, 124*(2), 172–183.

Ginsberg, H. S. (1993). Geographic spread of *Ixodes dammini* and *Borrelia burgdorferi*. In H. S. Ginsberg (Ed.), *Ecology and environmental management of lyme disease* (pp. 63–81). New Brunswick, NJ: Rutgers University Press.

Ginsberg, H. S. (1994). Lyme disease and conservation. *Conservation Biology, 8*(2), 343–353.

Glass, G. E., Amerasinghe, F. P., Morgan, J. M., III, & Scott, T. W. (1994). Predicting *Ixodes scapularis* abundance on white-tailed deer using geographic information systems. *American Journal of Tropical Medicine and Hygiene, 51*(5), 538–544.

Glass, G. E., Cheek, J. E., Patz, J. A., Shields, T. M., Doyle, T. J., Thoroughman, D. A., Hunt, D. K., Enscore, R. E., Gage, K. L., Irland, C., Peters, C. J., & Bryan, R. (2000). Using remotely sensed data to identify areas at risk for hantavirus pulmonary syndrome. *Emerging Infectious Diseases, 6*(3), 238–247.

Glass, G. E., Morgan, J. M., III, Johnson, D. T., Noy, P. M., Israel, E., & Schwartz, B. S. (1992). Infectious disease epidemiology and GIS: A case study of Lyme disease. *Geo Info Systems, 3*(3), 65–69.

Glass, G. E., Schwartz, B. S., Morgan, J. M., Johnson, D. T., Noy, P. M., & Israel, E. (1995). Environmental risk factors for Lyme disease identified with GIS. *American Journal of Public Health, 85*(7), 944–948.

Godlund, S. (1961). *Population, regional hospitals, transportation facilities, and regions: Planning the location of regional hospitals in Sweden* (Lund studies in geography series B: Human geography No. 21). Lund, Sweden: Department of Geography, Royal University of Lund.

Gold, M. (1999). The changing U.S. health care system: Challenges for responsible public policy. *Milbank Quarterly, 77*(1), 3–37.

Golledge, R. G., & Stimson, R. J. (1997). *Spatial behavior: A geographic perspective*. New York: Guilford Press.

Goodchild, M. F. (1984). Geocoding and geosampling. In G. L. Gaile & C. Willmott (Eds.), *Spatial statistics and models* (pp. 33–53). Dordrecht, The Netherlands: Reidel.

Goodchild, M. F. (1992). Geographic data modeling. *Computers and Geosciences, 18*(4), 311–319.

Goodchild, M. F. (1995a). Attribute accuracy. In S. C. Guptill & J. L. Morrison (Eds.), *Elements of spatial data quality* (pp. 59–80). Oxford, England: Elsevier Science.

Goodchild, M. F. (1995b). GIS and geographic research. In J. Pickles (Ed.), *Ground truth: The social implications of geographic information systems* (pp. 31–50). New York: Guilford Press.

Goodchild, M. F., Haining, R., Wise, S., Arbia, G., Anselin, L., Bossard, E., Brunsdon, C., Diggle, P., Flowerdew, R., Green, M., Griffith, D., Hepple, L.,

Krug, T., Martin, R., & Openshaw, S. (1992). Integrating GIS and spatial data analysis: Problems and possibilities. *International Journal of Geographical Information Systems, 6*(5), 407–423.

Goodchild, M. F., & Lam, N. (1980). Areal interpolation: A variant of the traditional spatial problem. *Geo-Processing, 1,* 297–312.

Goodman, D., Fisher, E., Stukel, T., & Chang, C. (1997). The distance to community medical care and the likelihood of hospitalization: Is closer always better? *American Journal of Public Health, 87*(7), 1144–1150.

Goodman, D., & Wennberg, J. (1999). Maps and health: The challenges of interpretation. *Journal of Public Health Management and Practice, 5*(4), xiii–xvii.

Gorman, P. C. (1998). Learn as you go: Creating an electronic publishing capability. *Library Hi Tech, 16*(3–4), 73–79.

Goss, J. (1995). "We know who you are and we know where you live": The instrumental rationality of geodemographic systems. *Economic Geography, 71*(2), 171–198.

Gould, P. R. (1995). *The coming plague.* New York: Blackwell.

Gould, P. R., & Leinbach, T. R. (1966). An approach to the geographic assignment of hospital services. *Tijdschrift voor economische in social geografie, 57*(5), 203–206.

Green, H., & Himelstein, L. (1998). A cyber revolt in health care. *Business Week, 3600,* 154–156.

Green, M. B., Cromley, R. G., & Semple, R. K. (1980). The bounded transportation problem. *Economic Geography, 56*(1), 30–44.

Greenberg, M. R. (1978). *Applied linear programming.* New York: Academic Press.

Greenberg, M. R., & Schneider, D. (1992). Region of birth and mortality of blacks in the United States. *International Journal of Epidemiology, 21*(2), 324–328.

Greenberg, M. R., & Wartenberg, D. (1991). Communicating to an alarmed community about cancer clusters: A fifty state survey. *Journal of Community Health, 16*(2), 71–82.

Griffith, D. A., Doyle, P. G., Wheeler, D. C., & Johnson, D. L. (1998). A tale of two swaths: Urban childhood blood-lead levels across Syracuse, New York. *Annals of the Association of American Geographers, 88*(4), 640–665.

Grimson, R. (1999). Community breast cancer maps. [Online]. Manuscript, Department of Preventive Medicine, State University of New York at Stony Brook. Available: http://www/esri.com/conservation/scgis/ScgNews2/ctspsection/ct99huntington.html [February 27, 2000].

Guptill, S. C. (1995). Temporal information. In S. C. Guptill & J. L. Morrison (Eds.), *Elements of spatial data quality* (pp. 153–165). Oxford, England: Elsevier Science.

Guthe, W. G., Tucker, R. K., & Murphy, E. A. (1992). Reassessment of lead exposure in New Jersey using GIS technology. *Environmental Research, 59*(2), 318–325.

Habicht, F. H. II. (1994). EPA's vision for setting national environmental priorities. In A. M. Finkel & D. Golding (Eds.), *Worst things first? The debate over risk-based national environmental priorities* (pp. 33–46). Washington, DC: Resources for the Future.

Hales, S., Weinstein, P., Souares, Y., & Woodward, A. (1999). El Niño and the dynamics of vectorborne disease transmission. *Environmental Health Perspectives, 107*(2), 99–102.

Hales, S., Weinstein, P., & Woodward, A. (1997). Public health impacts of global climate change. *Reviews on Environmental Health, 12*(3), 191–199.

Hallenbeck, W. H. (1993). *Quantitative risk assessment for environmental and occupational health* (2nd ed.). Boca Raton, FL: Lewis.

Halperin, W., & Baker, E. (Eds.). (1992). *Public health surveillance*. New York: Van Nostrand Reinhold.

Hammen, J. L., & Gerla, P. J. (1994). A geographic information systems approach to wellhead protection. *Water Resources Bulletin, 30*(5), 833–839.

Han, L. L., Popovici, F., Alexander, J. P., Jr., Laurentia, V., Tengelsen, L. A., Cernescu, C., Gary, H. E., Jr., Ion Nedelcu, N., Campbell, G. L., & Tsai, T. F. (1999). Risk factors for West Nile virus infection and meningoencephalitis, Romania, 1996. *Journal of Infectious Diseases, 179*(1), 230–233.

Hanchette, C. (1998). GIS implementation of 1997 CDC guidelines for childhood lead screening in North Carolina. In *GIS in Public Health, 3rd national conference abstracts*. San Diego, CA. [Online]. Agency for Toxic Substances Disease Registry. Available: http://www.atsdr.cdc.gov/gis/conference98/index.html. [July 28, 2000].

Handy, S. L., & Niemeier, D. A. (1997). Measuring accessibility: An exploration of issues and alternatives. *Environment and Planning A, 29*(7), 1175–1194.

Harris, T., Weiner, D., Warner, T., & Levin, R. (1995). Pursuing social goals through participatory geographic information systems: Redressing South Africa's historical political ecology. In J. Pickles (Ed.), *Ground truth: The social implications of geographic information systems* (pp. 196–222). New York: Guilford Press.

Hattis, D. (1996). Drawing the line: Quantitative criteria for risk management. *Environment, 38*(6), 10–15, 35–39.

Hay, S. I., & Lennon, J. J. (1999). Deriving meteorological variables across Africa for the study and control of vector-borne disease: A comparison of remote sensing and spatial interpolation of climate. *Tropical Medicine and International Health, 4*(1), 58–71.

Haynes, K., & Fotheringham, S. (1984). *Gravity and spatial interaction Models*. Beverly Hills, CA: Sage.

Haynes, R. M., & Bentham, C. G. (1982). The effects of accessibility on general practitioner consultations, out-patient attendances, and in-patient admissions in Norfolk, England. *Social Science and Medicine, 16*(5), 561–569.

Haynes, R. M., Bentham, G., Lovett, A., & Gale, S. (1999). Effects of distances to hospital and GP surgery on hospital inpatient episodes, controlling for needs and provision. *Social Science and Medicine, 49*(3), 425–433.

Healy, R. G. (1991). Database management systems. In D. J. Maguire, M. F. Goodchild, & D. W. Rhind (Eds.), *Geographical information systems: Principles and applications: Vol. 1. Principles* (pp. 427–443). Harlow, England: Longman Scientific & Technical.

Hearne, S. A. (1996). Tracking toxics: Chemical use and the public's "right-to-know." *Environment, 38*(6), 4–9, 28–34.

Hearnshaw, H. M., & Unwin, D. J. (Eds.). (1994). *Visualization in geographical information systems*. Chichester, England: Wiley.

Hillsman, E., & Rushton, G. (1975). The *p*-median problem with maximum distance constraints. *Geographical Analysis, 7*(1), 85–89.

Hirschfield, A., Brown, P. J. B., & Bundred, P. (1995). The spatial analysis of community health services on Wirral using geographic information systems. *Journal of the Operational Research Society, 46*(2), 147–159.

Howard, D. (1999). Geographic technologies and community planning: Spatial empowerment and public participation. [Online]. National Center for Geographic Information and Analysis. Available: http://www.ncgia.ucsb.edu/varenius/ppgis/papers/howard.html. [March 30, 2000].

Hrushesky, W. J. (1985). Circadian timing of cancer chemotherapy. *Science, 228*(4965), 73–75.

Hsueh, Y., & Rajagopal, R. (1988). Modeling ground water quality sampling decisions. *Ground Water Monitoring Review, 8*(4), 121–134.

Hunter, J. M. (1974). The challenge of medical geography. In J. M. Hunter (Ed.), *The geography of health and disease* (Studies in Geography No. 6, pp. 1–31). Chapel Hill, NC: University of North Carolina, Chapel Hill.

Huxhold, W., & Levinsohn, A. (1995). *Managing GIS projects*. New York: Oxford University Press.

Ihrig, M. M., Shalat, S. L., & Baynes, C. (1998). A hospital-based case-control study of stillbirths and environmental exposure to arsenic using an atmospheric dispersion model and a geographical information system. *Epidemiology, 9*(3), 290–294.

Isaaks, E., & Srivastava, R. (1989). *An introduction to applied geostatistics*. Oxford, England: Oxford University Press.

Istre, G. (1992). Disease surveillance at the state and local levels. In W. Halperin & E. Baker (Eds.), *Public health surveillance* (pp. 42–55). New York: Van Nostrand Reinhold.

Jacquez, G. M. (1996). Disease cluster statistics for imprecise space–time locations. *Statistics in Medicine, 15*(7–9), 873–885.

Jankowski, P., & Ewart, G. (1996). Spatial decision support system for health practitioners: Selecting a location for rural health practice. *Geographical Systems, 3*(2), 279–299.

Jenks, G. F. (1977). *Optimal data classification for choropleth maps* (Occasional Paper No. 2). Lawrence, KS: Department of Geography, University of Kansas.

Jenks, G. F., & Caspall, F. C. (1971). Error on choroplethic maps: Definition, measurement, reduction. *Annals of the Association of American Geographers, 61*(2), 217–244.

Jensen, J. R. (1996). *Introductory digital image processing: A remote sensing perspective* (2nd ed.). Upper Saddle River, NJ: Prentice-Hall.

Jensen, J. R. (2000). *Remote sensing of the environment: An earth resource perspective*. Upper Saddle River, NJ: Prentice-Hall.

Jia, X. Y., Briese, T., Jordan, I., Rambaut, A., Chi, H. C., Mackenzie, J. S., Hall, R. A., Scherret, J., & Lipkin, W. I. (1999). Genetic analysis of West Nile New York 1999 encephalitis virus. *Lancet, 354*(9194), 1971–1972.

Jones, C. G., Ostfeld, R. S., Richard, M. P, Schauber, E. M., & Wolff, J. O. (1998). Chain reactions linking acorns to gypsy moth outbreaks and Lyme disease risk. *Science, 279*(13), 1023–1026.

Jones, N., Bloomfield, A., Rainger, W., & Taylor, P. (1998). Epidemiology and control of the 1997 measles epidemic in Auckland. *New Zealand Public Health Report, 5*(8), 57–60.

Joseph, A., & Phillips, D. (1984). *Accessibility and utilization: Geograhical perspectives on health care delivery*. New York: Harper & Row.

Joy, K. P. (1994). *Estimating child exposure to electromagnetic fields associated with transmission lines in Hartford County, Connecticut*. Unpublished master's thesis, Department of Geography, University of Connecticut, Storrs, CT.

Kafadar, K. (1996). Smoothing geographical data, particularly rates of disease. *Statistics in Medicine, 15*(23), 2539–2560.

Kainz, W. (1995). Logical consistency. In S. C. Guptill & J. L. Morrion (Eds.), *Elements of spatial data quality* (pp. 109–135). Oxford, England: Elsevier Science.

Kearns, R. A. (1993). Place and health: Towards a reformed medical geography. *Professional Geographer, 45*(2), 139–147.

Keating, J. (1993). *The geopositioning selection guide for resource management*. Cheyenne, WY: Bureau of Land Management.

Keiper, T. A. (1999). GIS for elementary students: An inquiry into a new approach to learning geography. *Journal of Geography, 98*(2), 47–59.

Keister, K. (1993). Charts of change. *Historic Preservation, 45*(3), 42–48, 91–92.

Kelsey, J. L., Whittemore, A. S., Evans, A. S., & Thompson, W. D. (1996). *Methods in Observational Epidemiology* (2nd ed.). New York: Oxford University Press.

Kennedy, H. (1999). Mapping health care networks. *ArcUser, 2*(2), 30–31.

Kessler, B. L. (1992). Glossary of GIS terms. *Journal of Forestry, 90*(11), 37–45.

Khumawala, B. M. (1973). An efficient algorithm for the p-medical problem with maximum distance constraints. *Geographical Analysis, 5*(4), 309–321.

King, L. J. (1984). *Central place theory* (Scientific Geography Series, Vol. 1). Beverly Hills and Newbury Park, CA: Sage.

King, R. (1999). State plane coordinate system—Designations. [Online]. Available: http://www.pipeline.com/~rking/csmeta.htm. [January 30, 2000].

Kingham, S., Gatrell, A., & Rowlingson, B. (1995). Testing for clustering of health events within a geographical information systems framework. *Environment and Planning A, 27*(5), 809–821.

Kirby, R. (1996). Toward congruence between theory and practice in small area analysis and local public health data. *Statistics in Medicine, 15*(17–18), 1859–1866.

Kitagawa, E. M. (1966). Theoretical considerations in the selection of a mortality index, and some empirical comparisons. *Human Biology, 38*(3), 293–308.

Kitron, U., Jones, C. J., Bouseman, J. K., Nelson, J. A., & Baumgartner, D. L. (1992). Spatial analysis of the distribution of *Ixodes dammini* (Acari: Ixodidae) on white-tailed deer in Ogle County, Illinois. *Journal of Medical Entomology, 29*(2), 259–266.

Knapp, M., Archambault, G., & Aye, D. (1998). Methodology to simulate control populations for the spatial analysis of surveillance data. In *GIS in public health: Third national conference abstracts*. San Diego, CA. [Online]. Agency for Toxic Substances and Disease Registry. Available: http://www.atsdr.cdc.gov/gis/conference98/index.html. [July 28, 2000].

Knox, P. (1978). The intraurban ecology of primary care: Patterns of accessibility and their policy implications. *Environment and Planning A, 10*(4), 415–435.

Kohli, S., Sahlen, K., Lofman, O., Sivertun, A., Foldevi, M., Trell, E., & Wigertz, O. (1997). Individuals living in areas with high background radon: A GIS method to identify populations at risk. *Computer Methods and Programs in Biomedicine, 53*(2), 105–112.

Kovner, A. R. (Ed.). (1990). *Health care delivery in the United States* (4th ed.). New York: Springer.

Kraak, M.-J. (1999). Visualising spatial distribution. In P. A. Longley, M. F. Goodchild, D. J. Maguire, & D. W. Rhind (Eds.), *Geographical information systems: Vol. 1. Principles and technical issues* (2nd ed., pp. 157–173). New York: Wiley.

Kraak, M.-J., & Brown, A. (Eds.). (2000). *Web cartography: Development and prospects.* London: Taylor & Francis.

Krebs, J. R., Anderson, R. M., Clutton-Brock, T., Donnelly, C. A., Frost, S., Morrison, W. I., Woodroffe, R., & Young, D. (1998). Badgers and bovine TB: Conflicts between conservation and health. *Science, 279*(5352), 817–818.

Krebs, J. W., Strine, T. W., & Childs, J. E. (1993). Rabies surveillance in the United States during 1992. *Journal of the American Veterinary Association, 203*(12), 1718–1726.

Krebs, J. W., Wilson, M. L., & Childs, J. E. (1995). Rabies: Epidemiology, prevention, and future research. *Journal of Mammalogy, 76*(3), 681–694.

Kronick, R., Goodman, D. C., Wennberg, J., & Wagner, E. (1993). The demographic limitations of managed competition. *New England Journal of Medicine, 328*(2), 148–152.

Kulldorff, M. (1997). A spatial scan statistic. *Communications in Statistics: Theory and Methods, 25*(6), 1481–1496.

Kulldorff, M. (1998). Statistical methods for spatial epidemiology. In A. Gatrell & M. Loytonen (Eds.), *GIS and health* (pp. 49–62). London: Taylor & Francis.

Kulldorff, M., Feuer, E., Miller, B., & Freedman, L. (1997). Breast cancer clusters in the northeast United States: A geographic analysis. *American Journal of Epidemiology, 146*(2), 161–170.

Kulldorff, M., Rand, K., Gherman, G., Williams, G., & DiFrancesco, D. (1998). SaTScan: Software for calculating the space, time, and space–time scan statistics. [Online]. Division of Cancer Prevention, National Cancer Institute. Available: http://dcp.nci.nih.gov/bb/satscan.html. [December 28, 2000].

Kwan, M. P. (1999). Gender and individual access to urban opportunities: A study using space–time measures. *Professional Geographer, 51*(2), 210–227.

Lam, N. S.-N. (1983). Spatial interpolation methods: A review. *American Cartographer, 10*(2), 129–149.

Lanciotti, R. S., Roehrig, J. T., Deubel, V., Smith, J., Parker, M., Steele, K., Crise, B., Volpe, K. E., Crabtree, M. B., Scherret, J. H., Hall, R. A., MacKenzie, J. S., Cropp, C. B., Panigrahy, B., Ostlund, E., Schmitt, B., Malkinson, M., Banet, C., Weissman, J., Komar, N., Savage, H. M., Stone, W., McNamara, T., & Gubler, D. J. (1999). Origin of the West Nile virus responsible for an outbreak of encephalitis in the northeastern United States. *Science, 286*(5448), 2333–2337.

Langford, I. (1994). Using empirical Bayes estimates in the geographical analysis of disease risk. *Area, 26*(2), 142–149.

Langran, G. (1992). *Time in geographic information systems.* London: Taylor & Francis.

Lapidus, G., McGee, S., Cromley, E., & Banco, L. (1998). Using a geographic information system to guide a community based smoke detector campaign. In *GIS in public health: Third national conference abstracts.* San Diego, CA. [Online]. Agency for Toxic Substances and Disease Registry. Available: http://www.atsdr.cdc.gov/gis/conference98/index.html. [July 28, 2000].

Larsen, S. (1999). Community–university partnerships using Internet based GIS to communicate air and water quality conditions. In E. Kendy (Ed.), *Science into policy: Water in the public realm* (Technical Publication Series TPS-99-3, pp. 147–152). Herndon, VA: American Water Resources Association.

Laurini, R., & Thompson, D. (1992). *Fundamentals of spatial information systems.* San Diego, CA: Academic Press.

Laveissiere, C., & Meda, A. H. (1999). Incidence of sleeping sickness and settlement density in the forests of Cote d'Ivoire: Predicting high risk areas for the establishment of an efficient surveillance network. *Tropical Medicine and International Health, 4*(3), 199–206.

Lawler, E. L., Lenstra, J. K., Rinnooy Kan, A. H. G., & Shmoys, D. B. (Eds.). (1987). *The traveling salesman problem: A guided tour of combinatorial optimization.* Chichester, England: Wiley.

Lawson, A. B., & Waller, L. A. (1996). A review of point pattern methods for spatial modeling of events around sources of pollution. *Environmetrics, 7*(5), 471–487.

Lawson, J., & Floyd, J. (1996). The future of epidemiology: A humanist response. *American Journal of Public Health, 86*(7), 1029.

Leitner, H., McMaster, R., Elwood, S., McMaster, S., & Sheppard, E. (1999). Models for making GIS available to community organizations: Dimensions of difference and appropriateness. [Online]. National Center for Geographic Information and Analysis. Available: http://www.ncgia.ucsb.edu/varenius/ppgis/papers/index.html. [March 30, 2000].

Lepofsky, M., Abkowitz, M., & Cheng, P. (1993). Transportation hazard analysis in integrated GIS environment. *Journal of Transportation Engineering, 119*(2), 239–254.

Lewis-Michl, E. L., Melius, J. M., Kallenbach, L. R., Ju, C. L., Talbot, T. O., Orr, M. F., & Lauridsen, P. E. (1996). Breast cancer risk and residence near industry or traffic in Nassau and Suffolk Counties, Long Island, New York. *Archives of Environmental Health, 51*(4), 255–265.

List, G. F., & Turnquist, M. A. (1998). Routing and emergency-response team siting for high-level radioactive waste shipments. *IEEE Transactions on Engineering Management, 45*(2), 141–152.

Loaiciga, H. A. (1989). An optimization approach for groundwater quality monitoring network design. *Water Resources Research, 25*(8), 1771–1782.

Lobitz, B., Beck, L., Huq, A., Wood, B., Fuchs, G., Faruque, A. S., & Colwell, R. (2000). Climate and infectious disease: Use of remote sensing for detection of *Vibrio cholerae* by indirect measurement. *Proceedings of the National Academy of Sciences of the United States, 97*(4), 1438–1443.

Love, D., & Lindquist, P. (1995). Geographical accessibility of hospitals to the aged: A geographic information systems analysis within Illinois. *Health Services Research, 29*(6), 629–651.

Lowe, J., & Sen, A. (1996). Gravity model applications in health planning: Analysis of an urban hospital market. *Journal of Regional Science, 36*(3), 437–461.

Lowry, J. H. Jr., Miller, H. J., & Hepner, G. F. (1995). A GIS-based sensitivity analysis of community vulnerability to hazardous contaminants on the Mexico/

U.S. border. *Photogrammetric Engineering and Remote Sensing, 61*(11), 1347–1359.

Lundstrom, J. O. (1999). Mosquito-borne viruses in western Europe: A review. *Journal of Vector Ecology, 24*(1), 1–39.

Luzzader-Beach, S. (1995). Evaluating the effects of spatial monitoring policy on groundwater quality portrayal. *Environmental Management, 19*(3), 383–392.

MacEachern, A. M. (1994). *Some truth with maps: A primer on symbolization and design.* Washington, DC: Association of American Geographers.

MacEachren, A. M. (1995). *How maps work: Representation, visualization, and design.* New York: Guilford Press.

MacEachren, A. M., Buttenfield, B., Campbell, J., DiBiase, D., & Monmonier, M. (1992). Visualization. In R. Abler, M. Marcus, & J. Olson (Eds.), *Geography's inner worlds: Pervasive themes in contemporary American geography* (pp. 99–137). New Brunswick, NJ: Rutgers University Press.

Mahoney, R. P. (1991). GIS and utilities. In D. J. Maguire, M. F. Goodchild, & D. W. Rhind (Eds.), *Geographical information systems: Principles and applications: Vol. 2. Applications* (pp. 101–114). Harlow, England: Longman Scientific & Technical.

Malczewski, J. (1999). *GIS and multicriteria decision analysis.* New York: Wiley.

Maling, D. H. (1992). *Coordinate systems and map projections* (2nd ed.). Oxford, England: Pergamon Press.

Marks, A. P., Thrall, G. I., & Arno, M. (1992). Siting hospitals to provide cost-effective health care. *Geo Info Systems, 2*(8), 58–66.

Marshall, R. J. (1991). A review of methods for the statistical analysis of spatial patterns of disease. *Journal of the Royal Statistical Society, Series A, 154*(Part 3), 421–441.

Martens, P. (2000). Malaria and global warming in perspective? *Emerging Infectious Diseases, 6*(3), 313–314.

Marx, R. W. (1986). The TIGER system: Automating the geographic structure of the United States Census. *Government Publications Review, 13*(2), 181–201.

Mather, T. N., Nicholson, M. C., Donnelly, E. F., & Matyas, B. T. (1996). Entomologic index for human risk of Lyme disease. *American Journal of Epidemiology, 144*(11), 1066–1069.

Mattos, N. M., Meyer-Wegener, K., & Mitschang, B. (1993). Grand tour of concepts for object-orientation from a database point of view. *Data and Knowledge Engineering, 9*(3), 321–352.

Maxcy, K. F. (1926). An epidemiological study of endemic typhus (Brill's disease) in the southeastern United States with special reference to its mode of transmission. *Public Health Reports, 41*(52), 2967–2995.

Mayhew, L. D., Gibbard, R. W., & Hall, H. (1986). Predicting patient flows and hospital case-mix. *Environment and Planning A, 18*(5), 619–638.

Mayor, T. (1999). Pathways connects Atlanta's homeless, poor to services. *civic. com, 3*(12), 18–19.

McCormac, J. C. (1995). *Surveying* (3rd ed.). Englewood Cliffs, NJ: Prentice-Hall.

McCormack, E. (1999). Using a GIS to enhance the value of travel diaries. *ITE Journal, 69*(1), 38–43.

McCormick, B. H., DeFanti, T. A., & Brown, M. D. (Eds.). (1987). Visualization in scientific computing. *ACM SIGGRAPH Computer Graphics, 21*(6) (Special Issue).

McDonnell, W. F., Kehrl, H. R., Abdul Salaam, S., Ives, P. J., Folinsbee, L. J., Devlin, R. B., O'Neil, J. J., & Horstman, D. H. (1991). Respiratory response of humans exposed to low levels of ozone for 6.6 hours. *Archives of Environmental Health, 46*(3), 145–150.

McFadden, F. R., & Hoffer, J. A. (1994). *Modern database management* (4th ed.). Redwood City, CA: Benjamin/Cummings.

McGuirk, M. A., & Porell, F. W. (1984). Spatial patterns of hospital utilization: The impact of time and distance. *Inquiry, 21*(1), 84–95.

McLafferty, S. (1988). Predicting the effect of hospital closure on hospital utilization patterns. *Social Science and Medicine, 27*(3), 255–262.

McLafferty, S., & Broe, D. (1990). Patient outcomes and regional planning of coronary care services: A location-allocation approach. *Social Science and Medicine, 30*(3), 297–304.

McManus, J. (1993). Mapping helps Met track its health care networks. *National Underwriter, 97*(23), 38.

McSorley, K. (1999). *A geography of dental health needs in NJ: Prioritizing at-risk communities using GIS.* Unpublished master's thesis, Department of Geography, Hunter College, New York.

Melnick, A. L., & Fleming, D. W. (1999). Modern geographic information systems: Promise and pitfalls. *Journal of Public Health Management and Practice, 5*(2), viii–x.

Meyer, J. W., Butterick, J., Olkin, M., & Zack, G. (1999). GIS in the K–12 curriculum: A cautionary note. *Professional Geographer, 51*(4), 571–578.

Meyers, J. (1999). GIS in the utilities. In P. A. Longley, M. F. Goodchild, D. J. Maguire, & D. W. Rhind (Eds.), *Geographical information systems: Vol. 2. Management issues and applications* (2nd ed., pp. 801–818). New York: Wiley.

Mitka, M. (1998). Developing countries find telemedicine forges links to more care and research. *Journal of the American Medical Association, 280*(15), 1295–1296.

Moellering, H. (Ed.). (1987). *A draft proposed standard for digital cartographic data* (American Congress on Surveying and Mapping Report #8). Bethesda, MD: National Committee for Digital Cartographic Standards, American Congress on Surveying and Mapping.

Moellering, H. (Ed.). (1991). *Spatial database transfer standards: Current international status.* Oxford, England: Elsevier Science.

Mohan, J. (1983). Location-allocation models, social science, and health service planning: An example from north east England. *Social Science and Medicine, 17*(8), 493–499.

Monmonier, M. (1996). *How to lie with maps* (2nd ed.). Chicago: University of Chicago Press.

Moochhala, S. M., Shahi, G. S., & Cote, I. L. (1997). The role of epidemiology, controlled clinical studies, and toxicology in defining environmental risks. In G. S. Shahi, B. S. Levy, A. Binger, T. Kjellstrom, & R. Lawrence (Eds.), *International perspectives on environment, development, and health: Toward a sustainable world* (pp. 341–352). New York: Springer.

Moon, G., & Gillespie, R. (Eds.). (1995). *Society and health: An introduction to social science for health professionals.* London: Routledge.

Moore, J. E., Sandquist, G. M., & Slaughter, D. M. (1994). A route-specific system for risk assessment of radioactive materials transportation accidents. *Nuclear Technology, 112*(1), 63–78.

Morrill, R. L., & Earickson, R. (1968). Hospital variation and patient travel distances. *Inquiry, 5*(4), 26–34.

Morrill, R. L., & Symons, J. (1977). Efficiency and equity aspects of optimum location. *Geographical Analysis, 9*(3), 215–225.

Morrison, D., Alexander, D., Fisk, J., & McGuire, J. (1999). Improving delivery of health and community services to welfare recipients, Columbia, SC, 1997. *Journal of Public Health Management and Practice, 5*(2), 49–50.

Morrison, J. L. (1995). Spatial data quality. In S. C. Guptill & J. L. Morrison (Eds.), *Elements of spatial data quality* (pp. 1–12). Oxford, England: Elsevier Science.

Muehrcke, P., & Muehrcke, J. (1992). *Map use: Reading, analysis, and interpretation* (3rd ed.). Madison, WI: JP Publications.

Myers, G., MacInnes, K., & Myers, L. (1993). Phylogenetic moments in the AIDS epidemic. In S. Morse (Ed.), *Emerging viruses* (pp. 120–137). New York: Oxford University Press.

Nasca, P. C. (1997). Current problems that are likely to affect the future of epidemiology. *American Journal of Epidemiology, 146*(11), 907–911.

National Academy of Sciences, Mapping Science Committee. (1993). *Toward a coordinated spatial data infrastructure for the nation.* Washington, DC: National Academy Press.

National Academy of Sciences, Mapping Science Committee. (1995). *A data foundation for the National Spatial Data Infrastructure.* Washington, DC: National Academy Press.

National Cancer Institute. (1999). The Long Island Breast Cancer Study Project. [Online]. National Cancer Institute. Available: http://www-dccps.ims.nci.nih.gov/LIBCSP. [August 11, 2000].

National Cancer Institute. (2000). GIS-H Long Island. [Online]. National Cancer Institute. Available: http://www.healthgis-li.com. [November 16, 2000].

National Center for Health Statistics. (1979). *Proceedings of the 1976 Workshop on Automated Cartography and Epidemiology* (DHEW Publication No. [PHS] 79–1254). Hyattsville, MD: Department of Health, Education, and Welfare.

National Center for Health Statistics. (1995). *Proceedings, 25th Public Health Conference on Records and Statistics and the National Committee on Vital and Health Statistics 45th Anniversary Symposium* (DHHS Publication No. [PHS] 96–1214). Hyattsville, MD: Department of Health and Human Services.

National Center for Health Statistics. (2000). GIS and public health. [Online]. Centers for Disease Control and Prevention, Hyattsville, Maryland. Available: http://www.cdc.gov/nchs/about/otheract/gis/gis_home.htm. [November 15, 2000].

National Institute of Standards and Technology. (1994a). *Codes for named populated places, primary county divisions, and other locational entities of the United State, Puerto Rico, and the outlying areas* (FIPS-55–DC3). [Online]. National Institute of Standards and Technology. Available: http://www.itl.nist.gov/fipspubs/fip55-3.htm [January 16, 2000].

National Institute of Standards and Technology. (1994b). *Federal information processing standard publication 173 (Spatial data transfer standard part 1, version 1.1)*. Gaithersburg, MD: Author.

National Science and Technology Council, Office of Science and Technology Policy, Office of the President of the United States. (1995). *Infectious disease: A global health threat*. Washington, DC: U.S. Government Printing Office.

Neibert, D., & Reichardt, M. (2000, January 25 and February 15). *Managing confidentiality: Building blocks for the protection of and access to health data* (CDC/ATSDR GIS Lecture Series). Hyattsville, MD: National Center for Health Statistics.

Nelson, J. D., & Ward, R. C. (1981). Statistical considerations and sampling techniques for ground-water quality monitoring. *Ground Water, 19*(6), 617–625.

Neutra, R., Swan, S., & Mack, T. (1992). Clusters galore: Insights about environmental clusters from probability theory. *Science of the Total Environment, 127*(1-2), 187–200.

Nicholson, M. C., & Mather, T. N. (1996). Methods for evaluating Lyme disease risks using geographic information systems and geospatial analysis. *Journal of Medical Entomology, 33*(5), 711–720.

Nizeyimana, E., Petersen, G. W., Anderson, M. C., Evans, B. M., Hamlett, J. M., & Baumer, G. M. (1996). Statewide GIS/census data assessment of nitrogen loadings form septic systems in Pennsylvania. *Journal of Environmental Quality, 25*(2), 346–354.

Nolen, R. S. (2000). Multistate surveillance system in place for West Nile virus. *Journal of the American Veterinary Medical Association, 216*(1), 11.

Obermeyer, N. (1995). Reducing inter-organizational conflict to facilitate sharing geographic information. In H. Onsrud & G. Rushton (Eds.), *Sharing geographic information* (pp. 138–148). New Brunswick, NJ: Center for Urban Policy Research.

O'Brien, M. (1994). A proposal to address, rather than rank, environmental problems. In A. M. Finkel & D. Golding (Eds.), *Worst things first?: The debate over risk-based national environmental priorities* (pp. 87–106). Washington, DC: Resources for the Future.

Olea, R. A. (1984). Sampling design optimization for spatial functions. *Mathematical Geology, 16*(4), 365–391.

Onsrud, H., & Rushton, G. (1995). *Sharing geographic information*. New Brunswick, NJ: Center for Urban Policy Research.

Openshaw, S. (1984). *The modifiable areal unit problem (Concepts and Techniques in Modern Geography, No. 38)*. Norwich, England: Geo Books.

Openshaw, S., Charlton, M., & Craft, A. (1988). Searching for leukemia clusters using a geographical analysis machine. *Papers of the Regional Science Association, 64*, 95–106.

Osleeb, J., & Kahn, S. (1999). Integration of geographic information. In V. Dale & M. English (Eds.), *Tools to aid environmental decision making* (pp. 161–189). New York: Springer Verlag.

Pappas, G., Hadden, W., Kozak, L., & Fisher, G. (1997). Potentially avoidable hospitalization: Inequalities in rates between U.S. socioeconomic groups. *American Journal of Public Health, 87*(5), 811–816.

Parker, E., & Campbell, J. (1998). Measuring access to primary medical care: Some examples of the use of geographical information systems. *Health and Place,* *4*(2), 183–193.

Parrott, R., & Stutz, F. P. (1991). Urban GIS applications. In D. J. Maguire, M. F. Goodchild, & D. W. Rhind (Eds.), *Geographical information systems: Principles and applications: Vol. 2. Applications* (pp. 247–260). Harlow, England: Longman Scientific & Technical.

Patz, J. A., Strzepek, K., Lele, S., Hedden, M., Greene, S., Noden, B. Hay, S. I., Kalkstein, L., & Beier, J. C. (1998). Predicting key malaria transmission factors, biting, and entomological inoculation rates, using modelled soil moisture in Kenya. *Tropical Medicine and International Health, 3*(10), 818–827.

Patz, J. A., Epstein, P. R., Burke, T. A., & Balbus, J. M. (1996). Global climate change and emerging infectious diseases. *Journal of the American Medical Association, 275*(3), 217–223.

Pearce, N. (1996). Traditional epidemiology, modern epidemiology, and public health. *American Journal of Public Health, 86*(5), 678–683.

Pearson, F. II. (1990). *Map projections: Theory and applications.* Boca Raton, FL: CRC Press.

Penchansky, R., & Thomas, J. W. (1981). The concept of access: Definition and relationships to consumer satisfaction. *Medical Care, 19*(2), 127–140.

Peterson, M. P. (1997). Cartography and the Internet: Introduction and research agenda. *Cartographic Perspectives, 26,* 3–12.

Peuquet, D. J. (1984). A conceptual framework and comparison of spatial data models. *Cartographica, 21*(4), 66–113.

Phair, M. (Ed.). (1997). Standards open GIS data access. *ENR, 239*(9), 15.

Phibbs, C., & Luft, H. (1995). Correlation of travel time on roads versus straight line distances. *Medical Care Research and Review, 52*(4), 532–542.

Pickles, J. (1995). Representations in an electronic age: Geography, GIS, and democracy. In J. Pickles (Ed.), *Ground truth: The social implications of geographic information systems* (pp. 1–30). New York: The Guilford Press.

Pine, J. C., & Diaz, J. H. (2000). Environmental health screening with GIS: Creating a community environmental health profile. *Journal of Environmental Health, 62*(8), 9–15.

Plewe, B. (1997). *GIS online: Information retrieval, mapping, and the Internet.* Sante Fe, NM: OnWord Press.

Poiker, T. K. (1985). Geographic information systems in the geographic curriculum. *Operational Geographer, 3*(8), 38–41.

Puckett, L. J. (1994). Nonpoint and point sources of nitrogen in major watersheds of the United States (Water Resources Investigations Report 94-001). Reston, VA: U.S. Geological Survey.

Pyle, G. (1979). *Applied medical geography.* Washington, DC: Winston.

Reed, K. D., Mitchell, P. D., Persing, D. H., Kolbert, C. P., & Cameron, V. (1995). Transmission of human granulocytic ehrlichiosis. *Journal of the American Medical Association, 273*(1), 23.

ReVelle, C. S., & Swain, R. W. (1970). Central facilities location. *Geographical Analysis, 2*(1), 30–42.

Richards, T. B., Croner, C. M., Rushton, G., Brown, C. K., & Fowler, L. (1999). Geographic information systems and public health: Mapping the future. *Public Health Reports, 114*(4), 359–373.

Rifai, H. S., Hendricks, L. A., Kilborn, K., & Bedient, P. B. (1993). A geographic information system (GIS) user interface for delineating wellhead protection areas. *Ground Water, 31*(3), 480–488.

Ritchie, C. (1998). British Army establishes telemedicine unit in Bosnia. *Lancet* (North American ed.), *352*(9121), 46.

Rockland County Planning Department GIS. (2000). *Rockland County, New York, Number of dead wildlife per square mile.* Rockland County, NY: Author.

Rodkay, G. K. (Ed.). (1995). *GIS world sourcebook 1996.* Fort Collins, CO: GIS World.

Roper, F., & Boorkman, J. (1994). *Introduction to reference sources in the health sciences* (3rd ed.). Chicago: Medical Library Association.

Rothenberg, R. (1983). The geography of gonorrhea transmission: Empirical demonstration of core group transmission. *American Journal of Epidemiology, 117*(6), 688–694.

Rouhani, S. (1985). Variance reduction analysis. *Water Resources Research, 21*(6), 837–846.

Roush, S., Birkhead, G., Koo, D., Cobb, A., & Fleming, D. (1999). Mandatory reporting of disease and conditions by health care professionals and laboratories. *Journal of the American Medical Association, 282*(2), 164–170.

Rowan, A. N. (1997). The benefits and ethics of animal research. *Scientific American, 276*(2), 79.

Ruckleshaus, W. D. (1983). Science, risk, and public policy. *Science, 221*(4615), 1026–1028.

Rupprecht, C. E., Smith, J. S., Fekadu, M., & Childs, J. E. (1995). The ascension of wildlife rabies: A cause for public health concern or intervention? *Emerging Infectious Diseases, 1*(4), 107–114.

Rushton, G. (1975). *Planning primary health services for rural Iowa: An interim report* (Technical Report No. 39). Iowa City: Center for Locational Analysis, Institute of Urban and Regional Research, University of Iowa.

Rushton, G. (1997). Improving public health through geographical information systems: An instructional guide to major concepts and their implementation. [CD ROM and Online]. Department of Geography, University of Iowa, Iowa City. Available: http://www.uiowa.edu/~geog. [November 12, 2000].

Rushton, G. (1998). Improving the geographic basis of health surveillance using GIS. In A. Gatrell & M. Löytönen (Eds.), *GIS and health* (pp. 63–79). London: Taylor & Francis.

Rushton, G. (1999). Methods to evaluate geographic access to health services. *Journal of Public Health Management Practice, 5*(2), 93–100.

Rushton, G., & Armstrong, M. (1997). Mapping: Choropleth advisor, improving public health through geographical information systems, GIS lab section. [Online]. Available: http://www.uiowa.edu/~geog/health/mapping/choro. html. [January 16, 2000].

Rushton, G., Krishnamurthy, R., Krishnamurti, D., Lolonis, P., & Song, H. (1996). The spatial relationship between infant mortality and birth defect rates in a U.S. city. *Statistics in Medicine, 15*(17–18), 1907–1019.

Rushton, G., & Lolonis, P. (1996). Exploratory spatial analysis of birth defect rates in an urban population. *Statistics in Medicine, 15*(7–9), 717–726.

Scott, A. J. (1970). Location-allocation systems: A review. *Geographical Analysis,* 2(2), 95–119.

Selvin, S. (1991). *Statistical analysis of epidemiologic data.* New York: Oxford University Press.

Shannon, G. W. (1980). The utility of medical geography research. *Social Science and Medicine, 14D*(1), 1–2.

Shannon, G. W. (1981). Disease mapping and early theories of yellow fever. *Professional Geographer, 33*(2), 221–227.

Shannon, G. W., Bashshur, R. L., & Metzner, C. A. (1969). The concept of distance as a factor in accessibility and utilization of health care. *Medical Care Review, 26*(2), 143–161.

Sheppard, E. (1995). Sleeping with the enemy, or keeping the conversation going? *Environment and Planning A, 27*(7), 1026–1028.

Sheppard, E., Couclelis, H., Graham, S., Harrington, J. W., & Onsrud, H. (1999). Geographies of the information society. *International Journal of Geographical Information Science, 13*(8), 797–823.

Siegel, C., Davidson, A., Kafadar, K., Norris, J. M., Todd, J., & Steiner, J. (1997). Geographic analysis of pertussis infection in an urban area: A tool for health services planning. *American Journal of Public Health, 87*(12), 2022–2025.

Slocum, T. A. (1999). *Thematic cartography and visualization.* Upper Saddle River, NJ: Prentice-Hall.

Smith, N. (1992). Real wars, theory wars. *Progress in Human Geography, 16*(2), 257–271.

Snyder, J. P. (1987). *Map projections: A working manual* (U.S. Geological Survey Professional Paper 1395). Washington, DC: U.S. Government Printing Office.

Sol, V. M., Lammers, P. E. M., Aiking, H., De Boer, J., & Feenstra, J. F. (1995). Integrated environmental index for application in land-use zoning. *Environmental Management, 19*(3), 456–467.

Sperling, J. (1995). Development of the TIGER database: Experiences in spatial data sharing at the U.S. Bureau of Census. In H. Onsrud & G. Rushton (Eds.), *Sharing geographic information* (pp. 377–396). New Brunswick, NJ: Center for Urban Policy Research.

Stallones, L., Nuckols, J. R., & Berry, J. K. (1992). Surveillance around hazardous waste sites: Geographic information systems and reproductive outcomes. *Environmental Research, 59*(2), 81–92.

Steere, A. C., Broderick, T. F., & Malawista, S. E. (1978). Erythema chronicum migrans and Lyme arthritis: Epidemiological evidence for a tick vector. *American Journal of Epidemiology, 108*(4), 312–321.

Stern, J. E. (1989). *State Plane Coordinate System of 1983* (NOAA Manual NOS NGS 5). Rockville, MD: National Geodetic Information Center, NOAA.

Stockwell, J. R., Sorensen, J. W., Eckert, J. W. Jr., & Carreras, E. M. (1993). The U.S. EPA geographic information system for mapping environmental releases of Toxic Chemical Release Inventory (TRI) chemicals. *Risk Analysis, 13*(2), 155–164.

Strasser, T. C. (1998). Geographic information systems and the New York State Library: Mapping new pathways for library service. *Library Hi Tech, 16*(3–4), 43–50, 56.

Stroup, N. E., Zack, M. M., & Wharton, M. (1994). Sources of routinely collected data for surveillance. In S. M. Teutsch & R. E. Churchill (Eds.), *Principles and practice of public health surveillance* (pp. 31–85). New York: Oxford University Press.

Suh, H.-S. (J.), & Lee, A. (1999). Embracing GIS services in libraries: The Washington State University experience. *Reference Librarian, 64*, 125–137.

Susser, M., & Susser, E. (1996a). Choosing a future for epidemiology: 1. Eras and paradigms. *American Journal of Public Health, 86*(5), 668–673.

Susser, M., & Susser, E. (1996b). Choosing a future for epidemiology: 2. From black box to Chinese boxes and eco-epidemiology. *American Journal of Public Health, 86*(5), 674–677.

Swanson, J. M. (1997). Mouseover mapping. [Online]. Available: http://maps.unomaha.edu/NACIS/cp26/Techniques/imagine.html. [October 19, 2000].

Talen, E. (1998). Visualizing fairness: Equity maps for planners. *Journal of the American Planning Association, 64*(1), 22–38.

Thacker, S. B., Redmond, S., Rothenberg, R. B., Spitz, S. B., Choi, K., & White, M. C. (1986). A controlled trial of disease surveillance strategies. *American Journal of Preventive Medicine, 2*(6), 345–350.

Thacker, S. B., Stroup, D. F., Parrish, R. G., & Anderson, H. A. (1996). Surveillance in environmental public health: Issues, systems, and sources. *American Journal of Public Health, 86*(5), 633–641.

Thomas, D. C., Bowman, J. D., Jiang, L., Jiang, F., & Peters, J. M. (1999). Residential magnetic fields predicted from wiring configurations: II. Relationships to childhood leukemia. *Bioelectromagnetics, 20*(7), 414–422.

Thomas, J., & Tucker, M. (1996). The development and use of the concept of a sexually transmitted disease core. *Journal of Infectious Diseases, 174*(Suppl. 2), S134–S143.

Thomas, R. (1992). *Geomedical systems: Intervention and control.* New York: Routledge.

Tim, U. S. (1995). The application of GIS in environmental health sciences: Opportunities and limitations. *Environmental Research, 71*(2), 75–88.

Timander, L., & McLafferty, S. (1998). Breast cancer in West Islip, NY: A spatial clustering analysis with covariates. *Social Science and Medicine, 46*(12), 1623–1635.

Timyan, J., Griffey Brechin, S., Measham, D., & Ogunleye, B. (1993). Access to care: More than a problem of distance. In M. Koblinsky, J. Timyan, & J. Gay (Eds.), *The health of women: A global perspective* (pp. 217–234). Boulder, CO: Westview Press.

Tobler, W. R. (1959). Automation and cartography. *Geographical Review, 5*(4), 426–534.

Tobler, W. R. (1973). Choropleth maps without classes intervals? *Geographical Analysis, 5*(3), 262–265.

Tomlin, C. D. (1990). *Geographic information systems and cartographic modeling.* Englewood Cliffs, NJ: Prentice-Hall.

Tomlinson, R. F. (1987). Current and potential uses of geographical information systems: The North American experience. *International Journal of Geographical Information Systems, 1*(3), 203–218.

Tomlinson, R. F., & Boyle, A. R. (1981). The state of development of systems for handling national resources inventory data. *Cartographica, 18*(4), 65–95.

Toregas, C., Swain, R., ReVelle, C., & Bergman, L. (1971). The location of emergency service facilities. *Operations Research, 19*(5), 1363–1373.

Torok, T. J., Kilgore, P. E., Clarke, M. J., Holman, R. C., Bresee, J. S., & Glass, R. I. (1997). Visualizing geographic and temporal trends in rotavirus activity in the United States, 1991–1996. *Pediatric Infectious Disease Journal, 16*(10), 941–946.

Tsai, T. F., Popovici, F., Cernescu, C., Campbell, G. L., & Nedelcu, N. I. (1998). West Nile encephalitis epidemic in southeastern Romania. *Lancet, 352*(9130), 767–771.

Tufte, E. R. (1983). *The visual display of quantitative information.* Cheshire, CT: Graphics Press.

Tukey, J. W. (1977). *Exploratory data analysis.* Reading, MA: Addison-Wesley.

U.S. Bureau of the Census. (1992). *TIGER/Line (TM) Files, 1992.* Chapter 5: Data quality. [Online]. U. S. Department of Commerce. Available: http://www.census.gov/geo/www/tiger/chapter5.asc. [February 10, 2000].

U.S. Bureau of the Census. (1993). *A guide to state and local Census geography* (CPH-I-18). Washington, DC: U.S. Department of Commerce.

U.S. Bureau of the Census. (2000). LandView III specialized computer mapping application. [Online]. U.S. Census Bureau, Department of Commerce. Available: http://www.census.gov/geo/www/tiger/landview.html. [March 23, 2000].

U.S. Department of Housing and Urban Development. (1997). Community 2020 HUD Community Planning Software fact sheet. [Online]. U. S. Department of Housing and Urban Development. Available: http://www.hud.gov/adm/c2020fct.html. [December 15, 2000].

U.S. Geological Survey. (1997). *The evolution of topographic mapping in the USGS's national mapping program.* [Online]. Available: http://mapping.usgs.gov/misc/evolution.html. [February 10, 2000].

U.S. Geological Survey. (1998). *Digital line graphs (DLGs).* [Online]. U.S. Geological Survey. Available: http://edcwww.cr.usgs.gov/nsdi/gendlg.htm. [January 15, 2000].

U.S. Geological Survey. (2000). *EarthExplorer.* [Online]. U.S. Geological Survey. Available: http://edcsns17.cr.usgs.gov/EarthExplorer. [September 29, 2000].

Van Sickle, J. (1996). *GPS for land surveyors.* Chelsea, MI: Ann Arbor Press.

Veregin, H., & Hargitai, P. (1995). An evaluation matrix for geographical data quality. In S. C. Guptill & J. L. Morrison (Eds.), *Elements of spatial data quality* (pp. 167–188). Oxford, England: Elsevier Science.

Villalon, M. (1999). GIS and the Internet: Tools that add value to your health plan. *Health Management Technology, 20*(9), 16–18.

Vogt, R. L. (1992). National survey of state epidemiologists to determine the status of Lyme disease surveillance. *Public Health Reports, 107*(6), 644–646.

Vogt, R. L., LaRue, D., Klaucke, D. N., & Jillson, D. A. (1983). Comparison of an active and passive surveillance system of primary care providers for hepatitis, measles, rubella, and salmonellosis in Vermont. *American Journal of Public Health, 73*(7), 795–797.

Wagenet, R. J., & Hutson, J. L. (1996). Scale-dependency of solute transport modeling/GIS applications. *Journal of Environmental Quality, 25*(3), 499–510.

Wakeford, R. (1990). Some problems in the interpretation of childhood leukemia clusters. In R. Thomas (Ed.), *Spatial epidemiology* (pp. 79–89). London: Pion.

Walker, D. H., Barbour, A. G., Oliver, J. H., Lane, R. S., Dumler, J. S., Dennis, D.

T., Persing, D. H., Azad, A. F., & McSweegan, E. (1996). Emerging bacterial zoonotic and vector-borne diseases: Ecological and epidemiological factors. *Journal of the American Medical Association, 275*(6), 463–469.

Wallace, D., & Wallace, R. (1998). *A plague on your houses: The war on the urban poor*. London: Verso.

Walsh, S. J., Page, P. H., & Gesler, W. M. (1997). Normative models and healthcare planning: Network-based simulations within a geographic information system environment. *Health Services Research, 32*(2), 243–260.

Warnecke, L., Johnson, J. M., Marshall, K., & Brown, R. S. (1992). *State geographical information activities compendium*. Lexington, KY: Council of State Government.

Weise, F. (Ed). (1997). *Health statistics: An annotated bibliographic guide to information resources*. Lanham, MD: Medical Library Association and the Scarecrow Press.

Weisner, C. G. (1994). *Pediatric asthma and outdoor air pollution in Brooklyn and Queens: A geographical analysis*. Unpublished master's thesis, Department of Geography, Hunter College, City University of New York, New York, NY.

Wennberg, J. (Ed.). (1998). *The Dartmouth atlas of health care*. Chicago: American Hospital.

Wennberg, J., & Gittelsohn, A. (1982). Variations in medical care among small areas. *Scientific American, 246*(4), 120–134.

Wieczorek, W. F., & Hanson, C. E. (1997). New modeling methods: geographic information systems and spatial analysis. *Alcohol Health and Research World, 21*(4), 331–339.

Wilson, J. D. (1998). GIS goes mobile. *GeoWorld, 11*(12), 54–57.

Wilson, J. L., & Branigan, A. (1999). Location of East Carolina University School of Medicine telemedicine sites in relation to primary care health professional shortage areas for North Carolina's Health Service Area VI, 1997. *Journal of Public Health Management and Practice, 5*(2), 45–46.

Wilson, M. L., Bretsky, P. M., Cooper, G. H., Egbertson, S. H., Van Kruiningen, H. J., & Cartter, M. L. (1997). Emergence of raccoon rabies in Connecticut, 1991–1994: Spatial and temporal characteristics of animal infection and human contact. *American Journal of Tropical Medicine and Hygiene, 57*(4), 457–463.

Winch, P. (1998). Social and cultural responses to emerging vector-borne diseases. *Journal of Vector Ecology, 23*(1), 47–53.

Wolch, J. (1996). Community-based human service delivery. *Housing Policy Debate, 7*(4), 649–670.

Wong, D. W. S., & Meyer, J. W. (1993). A spatial decision support system approach to evaluate the efficiency of a meals-on-wheels program. *Professional Geographer, 45*(3), 332–341.

Wood, M. (1994). The traditional map as a visualization technique. In H. M. Hearnshaw, & D. J. Unwin (Eds.), *Visualization in geographical information systems* (pp. 9–17). Chichester, England: Wiley.

Woodward, M. (1999). *Epidemiology: Study design and data analysis*. Boca Raton, FL: Chapman & Hall/CRC.

Worboys, M. F. (1995). *GIS: A computing perspective*. Bristol, PA: Taylor & Francis.

Worboys, M. F. (1999). Relational databases and beyond. In P. A. Longley, M. F.

Goodchild, D. J. Maguire, & D. W. Rhind (Eds.), *Geographical information systems: Vol. 1. Principles and technical issues* (2nd ed., pp. 373–384). New York: Wiley.

Working Group on Emerging and Re-emerging Infectious Diseases. (1995). *Infectious disease: A global threat.* Washington, DC: Committee on International Science, Engineering, and Technology, National Science and Technology Council.

Yearsley, C., Worboys, M., Story, P., Jayawardena, P., & Bofakos, P. (1994). Computational support for spatial information systems: Models and algorithms. In M. Worboys (Ed.), *Innovations in GIS 1* (pp. 75–88). Bristol, PA: Taylor & Francis.

Yeh, A. G. -O. (1999). Urban planning and GIS. In P. A. Longley, M. F. Goodchild, D. J. Maguire, & D. W. Rhind (Eds.), *Geographical information systems: Vol. 2. Management issues and applications* (2nd ed., pp. 877–888). New York: Wiley.

Yorke, J., Hethcote, H., & Nold, A. (1978). Dynamics and control of the transmission of gonorrhea. *Sexually Transmitted Diseases, 5*(2), 51–56.

Young, R. (1999). Prioritising family health needs: A time–space analysis of women's health-related behaviours. *Social Science and Medicine, 48*(6), 797–813.

Zenilman, J., Ellish, N., Fresia, A., & Glass, G. (1999). The geography of sexual partnerships in Baltimore: Applications of core theory dynamics using a geographic information system. *Sexually Transmitted Diseases, 26*(2), 75–81.

Zhan, F. B., & Noon, C. E. (1998). Shortest path algorithms: An evaluation using real road networks. *Transportation Science, 32*(1), 65–73.

Index

About the Authors

Ellen K. Cromley, PhD, is Professor of Geography at the University of Connecticut, Storrs, Connecticut, and is affiliated with the Department of Community Medicine and Health Care, University of Connecticut Health Center, Farmington, Connecticut. Her research is primarily concerned with geographical patterns of health and disease, health facility location, and GIS design to support public health surveillance and intervention programs. She has published in geography, epidemiology, public health, and health services journals.

Sara L. McLafferty, PhD, is Professor of Geography at the University of Illinois at Urbana–Champaign, Urbana, Illinois. In her research she explores the use of spatial analysis methods and GIS for health and social issues in cities, as well as gender and racial disparities in geographical access to services and employment opportunities. She has published in geography, epidemiology, and urban studies journals and serves on the editorial boards of *Economic Geography* and *Health and Place*.